Stoma Care

Edited by Jennie Burch

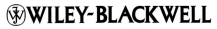
WILEY-BLACKWELL

A John Wiley & Sons, Ltd., Publication

This edition first published 2008
© 2008 John Wiley & Sons Ltd

Wiley-Blackwell is an imprint of John Wiley and Sons, formed by the merger of Wiley's global Scientific, Technical and Medical business with Blackwell Publishing.

Registered office
John Wiley & Sons Ltd, The Atrium, Southern Gate, Chichester, West Sussex, PO19 8SQ, United Kingdom

Editorial office
John Wiley & Sons Ltd, The Atrium, Southern Gate, Chichester, West Sussex, PO19 8SQ, United Kingdom

For details of our global editorial offices, for customer services and for information about how to apply for permission to reuse the copyright material in this book please see our website at www.wiley.com/wiley-blackwell.

The right of the author to be identified as the author of this work has been asserted in accordance with the Copyright, Designs and Patents Act 1988.

Wiley also publishes its books in a variety of electronic formats. Some content that appears in print may not be available in electronic books.

Designations used by companies to distinguish their products are often claimed as trademarks. All brand names and product names used in this book are trade names, service marks, trademarks or registered trademarks of their respective owners. The publisher is not associated with any product or vendor mentioned in this book. This publication is designed to provide accurate and authoritative information in regard to the subject matter covered. It is sold on the understanding that the publisher is not engaged in rendering professional services. If professional advice or other expert assistance is required, the services of a competent professional should be sought.

Library of Congress Cataloging-in-Publication Data

Stoma care / edited by Jennie Burch.
p. ; cm.
Includes bibliographical references and index.
ISBN 978-0-470-03177-3 (pbk. : alk. paper)   1. Enterostomy – Nursing.
2. Urinary diversion – Nursing.   I. Burch, Jennie.
[DNLM: 1. Enterostomy – nursing.   2. Surgical Stomas.   3. Enterostomy – rehabilitation.
4. Perioperative Nursing – methods.   5. Rehabilitation Nursing – methods.
WY 161 S8753 2008]
RD540.S835 2008
617.5'540231 – dc22
2008007539

A catalogue record for this book is available from the British Library.

Set in 10 on 11.5 pt Palatino by SNP Best-set Typesetter Ltd., Hong Kong

Printed in Singapore by Markono Print Media Ptd Ltd

1   2008

Books are to be returned on or before
the last date below.

S

Dedication

I would like to dedicate this to my friends and family all of whom I love very much. It has been hard work and thank you for all your support.

Contents

List of Contributors

Jennie Burch RN (Adult), BSc (Hons), ENB 980, ENB 998, Preparation in stoma care and inflammatory bowel disease modules at BSc level (editor)
Jennie currently works with people with bowel diseases, including inflammatory bowel disease, as the lead physiology research nurse at St Mark's Hospital, part of the North West London Hospitals NHS Trust. Previously she was a clinical nurse specialist – stoma care at St Mark's Hospital for seven years, working with ostomates, patients with enterocutaneous fistulae, intestinal pouches and intestinal failure.

Gemma Conn MBChb, MRCS, MSc
Gemma currently works as a general surgical registrar on the North East Thames rotation.

Julie Duncan MSc RGN, ENB 216
Julie is currently a PhD student at King's College London, working jointly at the Royal Marsden Hospital NHS Foundation Trust researching effective management of radiation induced bowel injury and at the Burdett Institute of GI Nursing as a research fellow/lecturer. Julie's clinical background has been mainly based at St Mark's Hospital where she was the lead clinical nurse specialist for bowel control.

Sharon Fillingham RN, BSc (Hons), MSc, Dip.Counselling, ENB 978, 980, 870, 998 and 216
Sharon is Clinical Nurse Specialist Urinary Diversion/Psychosexual and Gender Therapist at the University College London Hospitals. She currently works as a CNS Urinary Diversion with individuals undergoing reconstructive bladder surgery. Sharon qualified as a Stoma Care Nurse in 1986 and has worked as a urology stoma nurse since then.

Kay Neale MSc, RGN
Kay is a Nurse Specialist in the Polyposis Syndromes. She is currently the Manager of the St Mark's Hospital Polyposis Registry, having worked there since 1984.

Christine Norton PhD, MA, RN
Christine is Burdett Professor of Gastrointestinal Nursing, Associate Dean (Research), King's College London, and Nurse Consultant – Bowel Control, St Mark's Hospital. She has worked in continence nursing since 1979, both urinary and bowel. She was the Chair of the NICE guidelines on faecal incontinence (2007) and Chairs the RCN Gastroenterology and Stoma Care Forum.

Morag Pearson BSc(Hons), RD
Morag is Advanced Specialist Dietitian in Gastroenterology, St Mark's Hospital, specialising in intestinal failure, the management of intestinal stomas, pouches and enterocutaneous fistulae, inflammatory bowel disease and functional bowel disorders.

Zarah Perry-Woodford RN (Adult) Diploma in Nursing 1999, ENB 998, NVQ Assessor (D33/34), Foundations in stoma care, inflammatory bowel disease and Stoma care nursing modules at BSc level
Post registration, Zarah served in the Royal Air Force for three years as a military nurse on a general ward. She has worked as the Clinical Nurse Specialist in Pouch Care at St Mark's since 2005, developing the service and the nurse-led clinic. Previously she was employed as a clinical nurse specialist in stoma care at St Mark's working with ostomates, patients with enterocutaneous fistulae and intestinal failure.

Jo Sica RN (Adult) ENB 216
Jo currently works as Global Clinical Manager, Ostomy, Hollister Inc. Previously she worked as clinical specialist, Stoma Care in various hospitals including St George's University Hospital, London. She is Honorary Officer, WCET UK 2006 to present date.

Deep Tolia-Shah BSc, RN
Deep is currently Colorectal Clinical Nurse Specialist, Broomfield Hospital, Chelmsford, Essex. Previously she worked for ten years with people with colorectal disorders as a Macmillan colorectal cancer nurse specialist at St Mark's Hospital and more recently as a colorectal clinical nurse specialist.

Alistair C.J. Windsor MD FRCS FRCS(Ed)
Alistair is Consultant Colorectal Surgeon at University College Hospital in London and Honorary Senior Lecturer at the University College London. His clinical and research interests remain in sepsis and nutrition and since moving from St Mark's he has retained a busy tertiary referral practice focused mainly on the management of surgical catastrophe which includes, to a large extent, the management of enterocutaneous fistulae and complex Crohn's disease.

Jacquie Wright BSc RN DN, ENB 998, ENB 860
Jacquie worked as a Nurse Practitioner at St Mark's Hospital and specialised in caring for patients with the various Polyposis Syndromes for several years before a recent change of career.

Steve Wright RN (Adult), ENB 998, ENB 980, ENB R36, Preparation in stoma care level III
Steve is currently practising as a Perioperative Specialist Practitioner with colorectal surgical inpatients at St Mark's Hospital, caring for patients with a variety of complex bowel disorders. His previous roles include working as a stoma care nurse and senior charge nurse.

Acknowledgements

I would like to say thank you to all the people who have helped me by answering my never-ending questions when writing this book and in general. I have not named you all but a *big thank you!*

In particular, thanks to all those who contributed to the chapters and those who advised me on them – Chris Burch, Terry Burch, Brigitte Collins, Natalie Crawley, Julie Duncan, Ailsa Hart, Adam Haycock, David Lloyd, Yas Maeda, Jo Malone, Marian O'Connor, Zarah Perry-Woodford, Anna Swatton and Jo Sica.

Preface

Stoma care is a field of great interest, although not a glamorous subject, for nurses and allied health care professionals. This book aims to give the reader detailed information on stoma care and related topics to help develop the care of ostomates (people with stomas) and to improve their quality of life.

Working as a specialist nurse within a specialist hospital has given me knowledge and experience that I would like to share with others. I have also worked with many exceptional people; some have contributed to this book either directly or indirectly.

This book is written for readers with an interest in stoma care and related issues. It is also written so that it may be dipped into for information or read fully. The aim is to discuss comprehensively the subject which has been written about in many books and journals, pulling together many of the numerous issues related to stoma care.

Bodily function is not a glamorous subject and when something goes wrong with these systems, patients need knowledge-based help from their health care professionals. The objective of this book is to provide a comprehensive resource to assist in this process. This book will be a valuable aid for all health care professionals involved in the care of patients with gastrointestinal problems.

Jennie Burch

Introduction

This book is written to assist health care professionals when caring for ostomates; before, immediately after stoma forming surgery and in the long term. Many specialist nurses, doctors and dietitians wrote the book. The book is divided into chapters to make reading easier and to enable the reader to gain quick access to the topic of interest.

The contents of each chapter are subdivided into related information. Practical information is provided for use in the clinical area. This advice aims to assist the health care professional in caring for and giving guidance to the ostomate.

Many related subjects such as bowel diseases and continence will be discussed. This will assist the reader in understanding some of the complications and processes that the person with a stoma has encountered prior to their surgery. However, other stoma types such as tracheostomies will not be discussed in this book.

Illustrations and pictures are included to assist the reader. Tables and bullet points are used to simplify issues, making reading more simple.

Chapter 1

Stomas: The Past, Present and Future

Jennie Burch

Introduction

A stoma is a Greek word meaning mouth or opening (McCahon 1999) and they have been written about for over 2000 years. This chapter provides a history of stoma care through to the present day and offers thoughts for the future. The types of stomas that are generally formed to pass faeces or urine from the body under involuntary control by the patient are discussed. The other types of stoma such as the tracheostomy and gastrostomy will not be explored.

The history of stomas

The history of stoma care gives perspective and is examined from the 1700s to date. In Aristotle's time (384–322 BC) surgery for intestinal obstruction was reported; the results, however, are not discussed (MacKeigan 1997). In Celsus' time (55 BC–AD 7) there were poor survival outcomes from an abdominal injury to the colon, but a repair was worth attempting, as no intervention would result in certain death (Lewis 1999). However, during these times it was not thought worth attempting surgery for ileal damage.

In the 1700s there were several successful surgically exteriorised bowels. Stomas were formed as a consequence of faecal fistulae resulting from war, trauma or a strangulated hernia. The earliest recorded success in stoma care was a battle wound. George Deppe was injured in 1706. His abdominal wounds discharged faeces and he lived for 14 years with a prolapsed colostomy (Cromar 1968). During the eighteenth century to collect the faeces a tin or some cloth was used over the stoma and although this was problematic at least the person lived. Mr William Cheselden in 1756 operated on Margaret White when she was 73 years old. She had a prolapsed umbilical hernia that became gangrenous. After the surgeon formed a transverse colostomy, she lived for many years (Black 2000). An obstructing carcinoma led Pillore in 1776 to perform a cecostomy but the patient died 28 days later when the carcinoma perforated (MacKeigan 1997). Infant surgery was also successfully described. In 1798 a French surgeon, Duret, created a colostomy on a four-day-old baby with an anorectal defect. The patient lived for over 40 years (Webster 1985). In 1795 following a farming injury a French surgeon Daguesceau created a colostomy that the farmer lived with using a small, leather drawstring bag to collect the faeces (Cromar 1968).

During the 1800s mortality was high due to peritonitis as a result of faecal contamination (Black 2000). Mr Simon described urinary diversion surgery after operating on a child with a bladder abnormality in 1851. A channel was created between the ureters and the rectum. Despite the surgical technique being successful the child died several months later. Martini in 1879 performed a procedure similar to a Hartmann's (MacKeigan 1997). In 1887 William Allingham described formation of a loop colostomy with a glass rod (Lewis 1999). Using a rod with a loop stoma is often still undertaken, although the rod is now made from plastic.

Moving on to the twentieth century bowel resections and closures were undertaken successfully, but mortality remained high. Von Mikulicz in 1903 formed a double-barrel colostomy and this was closed using a crushing enterotome (Black 2000). In 1911 Coffey diverted urine by implanting the ureters into the sigmoid colon (Coffey 1911). The output was wet faeces, which was malodorous and caused peri-anal skin excoriation and infection. Mortality was very high at approximately 50%, predominantly due to infection. Hartmann in 1923 is attributed with the procedure that currently bears his name (Black 2000). Hartmann described an elective resection of a recto-sigmoid cancer and formation of an end colostomy. Miller in Canada performed in 1949 the first panproctocolectomy with formation of a permanent ileostomy, with 24 procedures performed without mortality (Miller *et al.* 1949). Bricker in 1950 formed the ileal conduit. Bryan Brooke from the UK addressed the difficulty with ileostomy management in 1952 by devising the spouted ileostomy (Brooke 1952). A spouted ileostomy reduces the risk of peri-stomal skin excoriation and was later revised to the '554 ileostomy' (Hall *et al.* 1995). In the 1950s the abdominoperineal resection of the rectum (AP, APR or APER) was introduced, resulting in the formation of a permanent colostomy (Black 2000).

A number of pouches were devised in the late twentieth century. In an attempt to improve the patients' quality of life, in 1969 a Swedish surgeon named Kock created an internal pouch to act as a faecal reservoir (Kock 1969). The Kock pouch was made continent by a valve and emptied regularly using a catheter passed through the abdominal stoma. This is rarely performed now since Parks further improved this in 1978, when he formed an ileoanal pouch that was attached to the anus and thus retained faecal continence (Parks *et al.* 1980). In Germany in the 1970s a magnetic colostomy system was developed to provide a continent stoma (Taylor-Mahood 1982). Although this was successful it is no longer used in the UK. Mitrofanoff in the 1980s devised the urinary pouch that required emptying with a catheter via a small opening in the abdomen. The Mitrofanoff pouch has proved effective after a 15-year follow up (Liard *et al.* 2001); for more information see Chapter 11 on urological pouches.

More recent changes include the increasing use of laparoscopic surgery. There has also been a reduction in the length of hospital stays, which reduces the time available for stoma training (MacKeigan 1997).

Stomas

A stoma is a surgically formed opening from the inside of an organ to the outside (Hyland 2002). In general the beginning of the name explains where the opening originates. The bowel that is attached to the abdomen is referred to as a stoma or an ostomy. There are three main types of stoma that are formed using the bowel: the colostomy, ileostomy and urostomy. There are other variations such as the rare jejunostomy.

There are a reported 100 000 ostomates (people with stomas) in the UK (Williams & Ebanks 2003). This figure remains largely unchanged over recent times (Lee 2001). The number of newly formed stomas in the UK appears to have remained fairly constant for the last ten years. In 2006 there were 21 351 stomas formed, in 2001 figures were 19 911 and in 1996 they stood at 19 806 (IMS 2007). To assist those with less experience of stomas the various terms for stomas are explained more fully.

End stomas

An end stoma is formed when one end of the bowel is brought through the surface of the abdomen. The edges of the bowel are turned back and stitched to the abdominal skin with dissolvable sutures. The other end of the bowel might be removed, as in an abdominoperineal resection of the rectum, or over-sewn such as in a Hartmann's procedure. An end stoma can be temporary or permanent but generally is permanent.

Loop stomas

Loop stomas are formed when the distal bowel is defunctioned, for example to protect an anastomosis. A loop of bowel is brought through the surface of the abdomen. A rod or bridge may be used under the bowel to reduce the risk of retraction, but this is not always required. The bowel loop is partially opened and the bowel edges are folded back and sutured to the skin with dissolvable sutures (Davenport & Sica 2003) resulting in two openings. Through the proximal (afferent) loop will pass faeces. Through the distal (efferent) loop will pass either nothing or a little mucus (Hyland 2002). As two loops of bowel are brought to the skin, loop stomas tend to be larger than end stomas. Loop stomas are generally temporary stomas, formed to make easy access to the distal bowel limb for rejoining at a later stage.

Split/divided stomas (Devine operation)

Split stomas are formed when both ends of the bowel are brought to the skin surface, but at different incision sites (Williams & Ebanks 2003). This may be following a subtotal colectomy when the ileum is formed into an ileostomy and the rectum into a colostomy (mucous fistula). A split stoma is usually temporary.

Double-barrelled stomas (Bloch-Paul-Miculicz)

A double-barrelled stoma may be used following resection of diseased bowel. The proximal stoma will pass faeces and the distal bowel will be non-functioning but both ends are exteriorised. This can appear like a loop stoma, but no rod is required. Closure of the temporary stoma will require further surgery.

Defunctioning stoma

A defunctioning stoma is intended only to be present for about three to six months and is used to defunction an anastomosis, for example. This can be as a loop stoma or an end stoma with closure of the distal limb. A loop stoma will not fully defunction the distal bowel, as it is possible for faeces to pass from the proximal to the distal bowel and not into the appliance. However a loop stoma does well enough in most cases (Nicholls 1996) to prevent complications.

Trephine stoma

A trephine stoma is created laparoscopically through an incision on the abdomen prior to the abdomen being opened. This means that the stoma is formed on secure muscles (Nicholls 1996). Often a midline abdominal incision is not required for a trephine colostomy, such as one formed for faecal incontinence.

Temporary stomas

In 2006 the number of temporary stomas formed was 10 301 which was a rise from 9067 in 2001 and an increase from 7925 in 1996 (IMS 2007). It should be noted that the number of temporary ileostomies has more than doubled in a ten-year period to 5749 in 2006 and the number of temporary transverse colostomies has more than halved to 760 in the same time period (IMS 2007). There are a variety of situations that may require the formation of a temporary stoma, in the emergency situation where there is sepsis, for example, and thus a risk to an anastomosis (Kirkwood 2005). A temporary stoma may be formed to protect an anastomosis until healing has occurred. Generally a temporary stoma is reversed or closed three or more months after the initial surgery in a smaller operation.

Permanent stomas

The number of permanent stomas has remained stable at about 11 000 newly formed each year (IMS 2007). Permanent stomas are generally formed if anal sphincters will be compromised during surgery. This could be in situations where incontinence may follow resection of a low rectal tumour, for example. A permanent stoma is also formed when the distal portion of the bowel or urinary tract is removed, for example in an abdominoperineal resection of the rectum.

Colostomy

In 2006 there were 6673 permanent colostomies formed and 4552 temporary colostomies (IMS 2007). A colostomy is a surgical procedure in which the colon is diverted to the abdomen to pass faeces from the body. This is currently the most common type of stoma. Colostomies may be temporary, after a trauma for example, or permanent for an anal cancer. A colostomy is usually situated in the left iliac fossa and is red, warm, moist and flush or minimally raised (Stephenson *et al.* 1995). The size and shape may vary, but an average is 30–35 mm in diameter.

A colostomy can be formed as an end or a loop stoma. It is important to note that when caring for an ostomate with a loop colostomy any medication or irrigation needs to be given via the correct route (Hyland 2002). A temporary end colostomy is formed when the colon is divided, in a Hartmann's procedure, for example.

The output from a colostomy is flatus and usually formed or soft faeces. The more distal the stoma, the more formed the faeces will be; this means that a transverse colostomy will have a more loose faecal output than a sigmoid colostomy, for example. A colostomy may be formed from the sigmoid colon, descending colon, transverse colon or the caecum (Hess 2003).

The appliance generally used by a colostomate is a closed bag. The appliance will need replacing when approximately a third to a half full. Colostomy appliances are therefore replaced once or twice daily, but this will vary depending on the colostomate's bowel function, which is generally every few days to three times daily. Most two-piece appliances can be used for up to seven days (Shollenberger *et al.* 2000), but not generally more than four days. Colostomy irrigation is also a method of management and the appliance used in this situation would be a stoma cap (see Chapter 17 on bowel irrigation).

Ileostomy

An ileostomy is the diversion of the ileum to the abdominal surface to pass faeces. Generally the terminal ileum is used to form an ileostomy. In 2006 there were 5749 temporary ileostomies and 2894 permanent ileostomies formed (IMS 2007). An ileostomy may also be temporary, permanent, an end or a loop stoma. The output from an ileostomy is loose faeces, often porridge-like in consistency. However, the faeces will vary throughout the day depending on what is consumed by the ileostomate. The average daily faecal output passed from an ileostomy is 600 to 800 ml (Black 2000), thus the appliance used is a drainable bag. An ileostomy appliance is generally emptied four to five times daily, when a third to half full (Shollenberger *et al.* 2000). The appliance is generally replaced on alternate days, but this can vary from daily to up to four days' wear.

An ileostomy is usually situated within the right iliac fossa and is warm, red and moist with a small spout. The spout is ideally 2.5 cm in length

(McCahon 1999) and the average diameter is smaller than a colostomy at about 30 mm.

Urostomy

A urostomy is the least common of the three main types of stoma. In 1996 there were 2218 new urostomies formed, reducing to 1962 in 2001 and further dropping in 2006 to 1483 (IMS 2007). A urostomy is formed to pass urine from the body via the abdomen. A small segment of bowel is used as a passage (conduit), often the ileum, giving the name ileal conduit. The bowel is isolated and one end is over sewn and the ureters are attached. Generally immediately after surgery there are stents in situ to prevent the anastomosis between the ureter and bowel from stenosing. Ileal conduits are an improvement on the ureterostomy, where the ureters were brought to the surface of the skin (Harvey 1997) often resulting in problems such as stenosis of the ureters. A urostomy is nearly always a permanent, end stoma. The appropriate appliance to use is a drainable bag with a tap or bung. As part of the bowel is used to form the urostomy the urine will also contain small amounts of mucus. The appliance is usually emptied four to six times daily, as the appliances have a maximum capacity of about 400 ml (Fillingham 1997). This is about the same frequency as a bladder requires emptying. The appliance is generally replaced on alternate days, but may be more or less frequent. The volume passed will vary depending on the volumes consumed, but can be about 1.5 litres daily (Burch & Sica 2004).

A urostomy is usually situated in the right iliac fossa and is similar in appearance to an ileostomy. The urostomy is warm, red and moist with a 2.5 cm spout and is about 30 mm in diameter.

Mucous fistula

When a person has a mucous fistula formed they will have two stomas. One is formed to pass faeces and the other to release mucus from the body. A mucous fistula is fairly uncommon, but might be formed when there is a low rectal cancer or in the case of emergency surgery for ulcerative colitis. A mucous fistula allows the disconnected portion of the intestine to pass any mucus from the body that cannot pass out of the anus, for example past a tumour (Hyland 2002). Usually the amount of mucus is minimal and may be intermittent and jellylike, collected using a stoma cap or dressing. The mucus can be quite malodorous and patients should be advised of this fact. Ostomates who have had a subtotal colectomy with a mucous fistula formed from their retained rectal stump may pass liquid mucus. To contain the mucus a small drainable appliance may be appropriate.

Jejunostomy

A rarely formed stoma is the jejunostomy. A jejunostomy will be formed in situations such as a bowel infarct or following an extensive resection of small bowel. A jejunostomy is formed from the jejunum and will have a high faecal output, usually over one litre daily. Thus the frequency of emptying the loose or liquid faeces is high (Erwin-Toth & Doughty 1992). Some ostomates will attach further drainage facilities to overcome this issue. Ideally the jejunostomy will look like an ileostomy, with a spout, but as the stoma is often formed in an emergency situation this is not always possible and stoma management may be difficult.

The appliance used for a jejunostomy can be an ileostomy appliance but there are also a limited number of specially designed appliances on the market. The high output appliances are slightly larger than the general ileostomy appliance and have a connector on the bottom that can be attached to a drainage bag. The appliance is generally changed on alternate days, but this may vary.

If there is under 100 cm of small bowel before the jejunostomy then parenteral nutrition will be required (see Chapter 16 on fistulae and intestinal failure). Any type of jejunostomy will generally require the ostomate to reduce oral hypotonic fluids and to take rehydration solution. Medications are also generally used to slow the gut and to reduce secretions, in addition, to try and reduce the faecal output (Nightingale 2003).

A feeding jejunostomy should not be confused with a faecal jejunostomy and is not discussed.

Stoma care nursing

The first mention of stoma care was in the 1930s when Plumley described how a patient worked out the care of his own ileostomy as there was no one to advise him (Black 2000). At this time the only help available was from other patients or to use one's own ingenuity (Elcoat 2003).

The issue of support for ostomates was first addressed in 1958 by an ileostomate Norma Gill (Broadwell & Jackson 1982). Ms Gill was not a health care professional but assisted Dr Turnbull in Cleveland, USA as an ostomy technician (Anderson 1982). Ms Gill helped to organise the United Ostomy Association and form the World Council of Enterostomal Therapists (Elcoat 2003). Dr Turnbull and Ms Gill started the first training programme for professionals in 1961, designed to assist ostomates to adjust to their stoma.

In 1969 a UK ward sister, Barbara Saunders at St Bartholomew's Hospital, London, set up a stoma clinic with her surgeon Ian Todd. Ms Saunders became the first stoma specialist nurse in the UK in 1971 (Black 2000).

In 1977 the Royal College of Nursing formed the Stoma Care Forum. Nurses with an interest in stoma care could, and still can, belong to this forum (Black 2000). This has now been expanded to include any nurse working in gastrointestinal nursing (Elcoat 2003). A year later the Department of Health and Social Services brought out 'The Provision of Stoma Care', a paper detailing to health authorities how to appoint a trained stoma specialist nurse. It was considered important to care for the small number of ostomates, as it was felt that this group faced significant problems coming to terms with their stoma.

Stoma care nursing is both acute and long-term, therefore patients are never discharged from the service. Patients can range from neonates to the elderly and the primary aim of the stoma specialist nurse is to promote independent living if possible. The advent of specialist nurses to improve the care for ostomates (Comb 2003) has resulted in over 400 stoma specialist nurses in the UK (Wallace 2002).

The WCET (World Council of Enterostomal Therapy) is a worldwide stoma care forum to support stoma specialist nurses. Every few years the council meets in different countries to exchange stoma care experience and knowledge. There is also the ECET (European Council of Enterostomal Therapy) in Europe and the WCET UK with meetings across Europe and the UK respectively.

Roles of the stoma specialist nurse

There are various perceptions on the role and qualities of the specialist nurse, with many centring on good communication and respect for the patients with an extensive knowledge of conditions and treatments (Rush & Cook 2006). The role of a specialist nurse includes:

- educator
- researcher
- expert
- clinician
- consultant
- resource
- administrator.
     (Black 2000)

Benner (1984) suggested that when becoming a specialist the nurse went through various stages from novice, advanced beginner, competence, proficiency, to becoming an expert. Specialisation has led to increasing independence for the practising nurse and thus greater accountability, for quality care, cost effectiveness, patient satisfaction and patient education (Jackson & Broadwell 1982). There is a perceived risk that the specialist nurse will simply take over medical roles that have been delegated to them. However, the nursing elements are still prevalent and important (Castledine 2002).

Training

The first UK stoma care course for trained nurses was in 1972 at St Bartholomew's Hospital (Black 2000). Training became popular and in 1980 the stoma care course had an 18-month waiting list (Yeo 1995). Later more training schools established stoma care courses. Currently, stoma care nursing courses have been given academic awards at diploma, degree and masters level. These modules can be used as 'stand alone' modules or as part of a programme to obtain a qualification. There are courses designed to assist registered nurses working with ostomates and others to prepare registered nurses to function as an expert in stoma care. These courses disseminate knowledge and expertise in stoma care (Elcoat 2003).

Link nurses

Link nurses are nurses with an interest in a specific area of nursing, such as stoma care. The aim for the link nurse is to enhance practice and therefore improve patient care. The link nurse can be seen as a two-way communicator between the specialist nurse and the ward nurses (Perry-Woodford 2005). The disadvantages are the time needed by the specialist nurse and the ward nurses to disseminate the information. This can be assisted by a computer-based training tool developed to be interactive and to underpin basic principles and practices in stoma care (Williams *et al.* 2007).

Deskilling

The role of specialist nurses is seen as many different things, ranging from providing expert care to deskilling other nurses to providing continuity of care. Elcoat (2003) suggests that the specialist nurse role should complement rather than detract from the skills of other health care professionals involved in the patient's care. To prevent nurses from losing their stoma care skills and competencies it is suggested that a referral is made to the stoma specialist nurse for advice rather than to take over the care (Dimond 2006). Following a survey undertaken by a community stoma specialist nurse her recommendations were, among other suggestions, that good communication was necessary between specialist nurses and others involved in the care of ostomates. Education by specialist nurses should be provided to prevent deskilling other nurses (Skingley 2006). Thus link nurses are ideal to assist the specialist nurse in the prevention of deskilling ward or community-based nurses. It is also essential for student nurses to gain a comprehensive knowledge of stoma care (Finlay 1990).

Present day stoma care

Stoma care, along with nursing in general and the National Health Service (NHS), are rapidly altering. Money and its effective use are more important than ever before. However, patients' expectations are also increasing and standards need to be maintained and improved. There are many generic nursing issues that affect stoma care, but specific areas include sponsorship of stoma nurse posts and the regulation of this.

The *Essence of Care* document (Department of Health 2001) discussed benchmarking to help improve the quality of care given to patients. Over the years those working in stoma care have attempted to achieve this by setting guidelines within their work remit. *Principle* was developed and published in conjunction with the Royal College of Nursing (RCN) and was designed as a framework for nurses to meet the needs of ostomates (Garnett *et al.* 1987). Wallace (2002) provided a more up-to-date set of competencies and nursing role with a booklet entitled *Competencies in Nursing: Caring for People with Colorectal Problems*.

Support groups

The first ostomy support groups were set up in America. Currently in the UK, professionals and ostomates run both national and local support groups for people with stomas. The practical advice and help that these groups provide to the ostomates is invaluable. The ones mentioned below are some of the support groups and the list is not exhaustive.

National support groups for colostomates

The Colostomy Welfare Group was formed in 1966 (McCahon 1999). This later became the British Colostomy Association (BCA), which folded 31 December 2005, partially due to funding problems (Gould 2006). A new organisation named the Colostomy Association was launched in November 2005, the website is www.colostomyassociation.org.uk. The association aims to support people with, or about to have, a colostomy and their families and carers (Hulme & Brierley 2007).

National support groups for ileostomates

The ileostomy association of Great Britain and Ireland *(ia)* was formed in 1956 (McCahon 1999). This association changed its name and function slightly to incorporate small bowel pouches such as the ileoanal pouch. The name is currently the Ileostomy and Internal Pouch Support Group; the website is www.the-ia.org.uk. The association aims to support people who require surgery to remove their colon and have an ileostomy or ileoanal pouch formed.

National support groups for urostomates

The Urostomy Association aims to support people who are to undergo, or have undergone, surgery to divert urine. The association was formed in 1971 as the Urinary Conduit Association. In 1984 the name changed to the Urostomy Association (UA). The website is www.uagbi.org.

National support groups for pouch patients

The Red Lion Group is a UK charity for people who have, or who are considering having, a pouch operation. The website is www.redliongroup.org.

The future of stoma care

The government regularly updates and alters its policies related to health care provision. There have been, on various occasions, proposals to revise the way that the NHS supplies and delivers stoma appliances. In many cases provision of personal assistance to patients may be lost for ostomates under the proposals that took effect in Scotland in 2005. More analysis of the situation is being undertaken before final decisions are made in the UK.

The NHS spends more than £630 million each year in England on products such as stoma appliances, incontinence pads and dressings. The reimbursements system for over 200 suppliers requires review. However, some people are concerned that company-sponsored nurses will only promote their own companies' products which compromises patient choice (Gould 2006). However, it can be argued that in the current climate sponsorship of nurse posts actually saves the Trusts' money (Black 2006). Additionally most specialist nurses consider that choice is important. In a survey of stoma specialist nurses, it was demonstrated that there were strong feelings from the nurses about the quality of products available to stoma patients. The research also showed that many of the newer products are far superior to the older products, and comparisons on a cost basis alone were short-sighted and jeopardise product availability and the current high standards of stoma care (Berry *et al.* 2007).

Patient empowerment is desirable if not essential (Christensen & Hewitt-Taylor 2006). Nurses are in the ideal position to facilitate patient empowerment. Appropriately informed autonomous patients can therefore be responsible for their own health decisions.

What is the future for nurses? Currently nurses are discovering it difficult to find new jobs, with potential budgets cuts and posts not being replaced (Foss 2006). Nurses need to remain flexible and adapt to change as they have for many years (Porrett 1996). There are, however, fears about the ability of nursing to continue to evolve in a situation where many hospital jobs including specialist nurse posts have been cut (Mallender 2006), downgraded or are under threat (Norton & Porrett 2006). The RCN magazine stated that the Health Service could not afford to lose specialist nursing posts (Thomas 2007) but many nursing jobs are still at risk.

To conclude, it is a huge change in an ostomate's life to have stoma forming surgery. However with appropriate support and advice the ostomate can enjoy a good quality of life.

References

Anderson FJ (1982) History of enterostomal therapy. In: Broadwell DC & Jackson BS (eds) *Principles of Ostomy Care*. London: The CV Mosby Co.

Benner P (1984) *From Novice to Expert*. California: Addison-Wesley.

Berry J, Black P, Smith R & Stuchfield B (2007) Assessing the value of silicone and hydrocolloid products in stoma care. *British Journal of Nursing*. **16(13)**: 778–88.

Black P (2000) *Holistic Stoma Care*. London: Baillière Tindall.

Black P (2006) Patients need specialist, sponsored nursing posts. *British Journal of Nursing*. **15(22)**: 1209.

Broadwell DC & Jackson BS (1982) A primer: definitions and surgical techniques. In: Broadwell DC & Jackson BS (eds) *Principles of Ostomy Care*. London: The CV Mosby Co.

Brooke BN (1952) The management of an ileostomy including its complications. *The Lancet*. **2(3)**: 102–4.

Burch J & Sica J (2004) Urostomy products: an update of recent developments. *British Journal of Nursing*. **9(11)**: 482–6.

Castledine G (2002) The important aspects of nurse specialist roles. *British Journal of Nursing.* **11(5)**: 350.

Christensen M & Hewitt-Taylor J (2006) Empowerment in nursing: paternalism or maternalism. *British Journal of Nursing.* **15(13)**: 695–9.

Coffey RC (1911) Physiologic implantation of the severed ureter or common bile-duct into the intestine. *Journal of American Medical Association.* **56(6)**: 397–403.

Comb J (2003) Role of the stoma care nurse: patient with cancer and colostomy. *British Journal of Nursing.* **12(14)**: 852–6.

Cromar CDL (1968) The evolution of colostomy. *Diseases of the colon and rectum.* **11(4, 5, 6)**: 256–80, 367–90, 423–46.

Davenport R & Sica J (2003) A new modern drainable appliance for people with ileostomies. *British Journal of Nursing.* **12(9)**: 571–5.

Department of Health (2001) *The Essence of Care: Patient-focused benchmarking for health care practitioners.* London: Department of Health.

Dimond B (2006) Generalist and specialist nurses: caring for a patient with a stoma. *British Journal of Nursing.* **15(14)**: 769–70.

Elcoat C (2003) Introduction. In: Elcoat C (ed) *Stoma Care Nursing.* London: Hollister.

Erwin-Toth P & Doughty DB (1992) Principles and procedures of stomal management. In: Hampton BG & Bryant RA (eds) *Ostomies and Continent Diversions Nursing Management.* London: Mosby Year Book.

Fillingham S (1997) Urological stomas. In: Fillingham S & Douglas J (eds) *Urological Nursing.* 2nd edn. London: Baillière Tindall.

Finlay TMD (1990) From text book to reality – student nurse training needs in stoma care. *Professional Nurse.* **5(12)**: 617–22.

Foss TD (2006) Editorial – the law of supply and demand: a different take. *British Journal of Nursing.* **15(13)**: 691.

Garnett EM, Russell E & Evans Y (1987) *Principle.* London: Royal College of Nursing.

Gould M (2006) A market in unmentionables in need of 'modernisation'. *Health Service Journal.* **116(5988)**: 14–15.

Hall C, Myers C & Phillips RKS (1995) The 554 ileostomy. *British Journal of Surgery.* **82**: 1385.

Harvey H (1997) Urological stomas. In: Fillingham S & Douglas J (eds) *Urological Nursing.* London: Baillière Tindall.

Hess CT (2003) Ostomy pearls. *Advances in Skin and Wound Care.* **16(3)**: 146–52.

Hulme E & Brierley R (2007) Life with a colostomy. *Gastrointestinal Nursing.* **5(2)**: 22–4.

Hyland J (2002) The basics of ostomies. *Gastroenterology Nursing.* **25(6)**: 241–4.

IMS (2007) referenced as © 2007 IMS Health Incorporated or its affiliates. All rights reserved. *New Stoma Patient Audit GB* – August 2007.

Jackson BS & Broadwell DC (1982) Role of the enterostomal therapy practitioner. In: Broadwell DC & Jackson BS (eds) *Principles of Ostomy Care.* London: The CV Mosby Co.

Kirkwood L (2005) An introduction to stomas. *Journal of Community Nursing.* **19(7)**: 20–5.

Kock NG (1969) Intra-abdominal 'reservoir' in patients with permanent ileostomy. *Archives of Surgery.* **99**: 223–31.

Lee J (2001) Common stoma problems: a brief guide for community nurses. *British Journal of Community Nursing.* **6(8)**: 407–13.

Lewis L (1999) History and evolution of stomas and appliances. In: Taylor P (ed) *Stoma Care in the Community.* London: Nursing Times Books.

Liard A, Séguier-Lipszyc E, Mathiot A & Mitrofanoff P (2001) The Mitrofanoff procedure: 20 years later. *The Journal of Urology.* **165(6, part 2 of 2)**: 2394–8.

McCahon S (1999) Faecal stomas. In: Porrett T & Daniel N (ed) *Essential Coloproctology for Nurses.* London: Whurr.

MacKeigan JM (1997) Stomas. In: Nicholls RJ & Dozois RR (eds) *Surgery of the Colon and Rectum.* London: Churchill Livingstone.

Mallender E (2006) Stoma care update. *The Tract.* Winter.

Miller GG, Gardner CM & Ripstein CB (1949) Primary resection of the colon in ulcerative colitis. *Canadian Medical Association Journal.* **60**: 584–5.

Nicholls RJ (1996) Surgical procedures. In: Myers C (ed) *Stoma Care Nursing: A Patient-centred Approach.* London: Arnold.

Nightingale JMD (2003) The medical management of intestinal failure: methods to reduce the severity. *Proceedings of the Nutrition Society.* **62(3)**: 703–10.

Norton C & Porrett T (2006) Wake up and smell the coffee. *Gastrointestinal Nursing.* **4(6)**: 12–14.

Parks AG, Nicholls RJ & Belliveau P (1980) Proctocolectomy with ileal reservoir and anal anastomosis. *The British Journal of Surgery.* **67(8)**: 533–8.

Perry-Woodford Z (2005) The link that improves care and practice. *Gastrointestinal Nursing.* **3(3)**: 20–4.

Porrett T (1996) Extending the role of the stoma care nurse. *Nursing Standard.* **10(27)**: 33–5.

Rush B & Cook J (2006) What makes a good nurse? Views of patients and carers. *British Journal of Nursing.* **15(7)**: 382–5.

Shollenberger D, Spirk M & Small CC (2000) Gastrointestinal care. In: Holmers HN (ed) *Nursing Procedures.* 3rd edn. Pennsylvania: Springhouse Corporation.

Skingley S (2006) Community nurses' understanding of the community stoma care nurse. *British Journal of Nursing.* **15(2)**: 83–9.

Stephenson BM, Myers C & Phillips RKS (1995) Minimally raised end colostomy. *Colorectal Disease.* **10**: 232–3.

Taylor-Mahood E (1982) Magnetic colostomy system. In: Broadwell DC & Jackson BS (eds) *Principles of Ostomy Care.* London: The CV Mosby Co.

Thomas S (2007) Spotlight on: nurse specialists. *RCN Magazine.* Spring.

Wallace M (2002) *Competencies in Nursing: Caring for People with Colorectal Problems.* London: Royal College of Nursing and Coloplast.

Webster P (1985) Special babies. *Community Outlook.* July. 19–22.

Williams J & Ebanks A (2003) Types of stoma and associated surgical procedures. In: Elcoat C (ed) *Stoma Care Nursing.* London: Hollister.

Williams J, Porrett T, Fillingham S & MacLeod E (2007) A computer-based interactive educational resource for stoma care nursing. *Gastrointestinal Nursing.* **5(8)**: 14–20.

Yeo G (1995) *Nursing at Bart's.* Gloucestershire: Alan Sutton Publishing Ltd.

Chapter 2

Anatomy and Physiology of the Urinary and Gastrointestinal System

Jennie Burch

Introduction

This chapter aims to give a broad explanation of the body systems and their functions. The chapter will focus upon the gastrointestinal (GI) tract and the urinary system and how these may influence stomas and stoma function. There is also a discussion on the skin and abdominal muscles to provide an explanation of the way in which the body usually functions. We will start at the abdominal wall, with the skin, and work through to the internal organs related to the GI tract and urinary system.

The skin

The skin is the largest organ of the body (see Figure 2.1), providing about 10 per cent of the body mass (Butcher & White 2005). The layers of the skin are the epidermis (the outer layer), the dermis (Watson 2002) and beneath these lies the subcutaneous layer (hypodermis). The skin has many functions including:

- body temperature regulation;
- excretion of waste products;
- awareness of surroundings;
- defence against bacteria entry;
- protection from the sun (melanocytes – pigmented cells);
- synthesis of vitamin D (keratinocytes – keratin producing cells);
- secretion of sebum;
- sensation – nerve endings.

(Hess 2005; Thibodeau & Patton 2007)

Appendages

- sweat glands
- hair
- nails
- sebaceous glands.
      (Hess 2005)

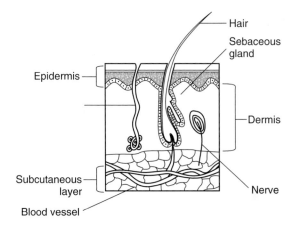

Figure 2.1   Cross section of the skin.

Sweat glands secrete water, salts and a trace of other waste products onto the skin surface. Sweat is produced at a rate of approximately 500–600 ml daily (Watson 2002). This fluid volume can be critical when planning care for patients with high output stomas. Sweat glands are present all over the body but are more abundant in areas such as the palms of the hands. Excessive sweat production can be problematic for adhering stoma appliances.

Hairs grow from the hair follicles, through the dermis and epidermis (Hess 2005). Hair is formed from modified epithelium. Hair, if too profuse, can reduce the adhesion of stoma appliances and may require shaving or trimming.

Nails are also modified epithelium and protect the tips of the digits. The nails are continuous with the epithelium and keep bacteria out.

Sebaceous glands are found throughout the body, except for the palms of the hand and the soles of the feet and are generally associated with hair follicles (Butcher & White 2005). Sebaceous glands secrete sebum, an oily substance that lubricates the skin and hair, reducing the risk of breakage. However, as the sebum collects dirt, the hair and skin requires cleaning. Careful cleaning of the peristomal skin is important to remove dirt and excess oil, but care needs to be taken to prevent damage to the skin.

The epidermis

The epidermis is non-vascular and consists of stratified epithelial cells, varying in thickness from 0.1 mm to 2 mm (Butcher & White 2005). There are several types of epithelial cells; keratinocytes, melanocytes and Langerhans cells. Keratinocytes make up more than 90% of the epidermal cells and form the principal structure of the outer skin. Cells are filled with a fibrous protein called keratin and are arranged in distinct strata (layers). Melanocytes contribute to skin colour and reduce ultraviolet light penetration. These cells can be absent in certain conditions. The

Langerhans cells are antigen-presenting cells (APCs). Their role is to find markers (antigens) on invading cells such as bacteria and present them for recognition and destruction to other immune system cells (Thibodeau & Patton 2007). The epidermis can be broken down into two layers, namely the horny zone and the germinative zone (Watson 2002).

The horny zone is the hard, keratinised outer layer of the skin and can be further divided into three layers:

- horny layer (*stratum corneum*);
- clear layer (*stratum lucidum*);
- granular layer (*stratum granulosum*).

The germinative zone is made from:

- prickle cell layer (*stratum spinosum*);
- basal cell layer (*stratum basale*).

The lifespan of a skin cell is about 28 days from germination to shedding. The epidermis originates at the base of the germinative zone in the stratum basale and works upwards to the surface at the horny layer. The stratum basale is a single cell thick and here the epidermal cells start to divide (Burr & Penzer 2005). As cells mature they migrate upwards and take on different characteristics. In the final phase a protein called keratin reinforces the cells forming a hard, waterproof coating to the cell wall (Watson 2002). Eventually these cells shed and are replaced. The outer surface of the skin (stratum corneum) is robust and provides a protective barrier (Tortora & Derrickson 2006) and is without blood supply. However, disruption of the epidermis can expose the cells beneath to potential infection.

The dermis

The dermis is 15 to 20% of the human weight and varies from 1 to 5 mm in thickness (Butcher & White 2005). The dermis anchors the epidermis to the underlying subcutaneous tissue and consists of nerve fibres, collagen fibres, lymph vessels, sweat glands and blood vessels (Lyon & Smith 2001). The dermis is predominantly made from fibrous proteins, collagen and elastic and is known as connective tissue. This provides the skin with its tensile strength and elastic recoil, which degenerates with age and exposure to ultraviolet radiation.

Subcutaneous tissue

Subcutaneous tissue contains fat and connective tissue with larger blood vessels and nerves. The thickness of this layer varies throughout the body and each person will be different.

The skin is slightly acidic with a pH of 4.0–5.5 (Newton & Cameron 2003). The urine usually has a pH of 4.0–8.0 (Fillingham & Douglas 2004) and faeces are alkaline. If stoma appliances are not well fitting the urine or faeces touching the skin can cause a chemical reaction and result in broken skin.

Wound healing process

There are four main stages of wound healing:

- haemostasis;
- inflammation;
- proliferation;
- maturation.
    (Hess 2005)

Haemostasis occurs immediately a wound is formed. There may be blood to flush away debris and bacteria. Haemostasis commences with the blood vessels constricting (Cutting & Tong 2003) and platelets clotting to prevent further bleeding (Ovington & Schultz 2004). Platelets also release cytokines that gather cells required in later phases of healing (Hess 2005).

The inflammatory phase may also be termed the defensive or reaction phase and typically lasts for four to six days (Hess 2005). Histamine is released from the damaged cells and the leukocytes that destroy bacteria migrate into the wound. Vaso-dilation allows engorgement of the wound with macrophages that clean the wound of cellular debris and bacteria (Kindlen & Morison 1999). Macrophages also convert macromolecules into amino acids and sugars that are required for wound healing. The physical characteristics of the inflammatory phase are pain, heat, redness and tissue oedema (Lyon & Smith 2001).

The proliferation phase is also known as the fibroblastic, regenerative or connective tissue phase and normally lasts for several weeks. Open wounds form granulation (connective) tissue as red granules (Hess 2005). The granulation tissue consists of macrophages, fibroblasts, blood vessels and immature collagen (Kindlen & Morison 1999); the latter is produced as a result of fibroblast stimulation (Ovington & Schultz 2004).

New tissue forms across the wound providing a framework (stroma) that supports the epithelial cells that migrate across and fill the open area. As the wound fills with granulation tissue the edges also pull together, decreasing the wound surface (Tortora & Derrickson 2006). During epithelisation the keratinocytes migrate from the wound margins and close the wound, resulting in a scar.

Maturation or the remodelling phase can last from 21 days to several years. During this phase the collagen fibres reorganise, remodel, mature and gain tensile strength (Kindlen & Morison 1999). This phase continues until the scar tissue has regained a maximum of about 80% of the skin's original tensile strength (Hess 2005). This is true of the midline scar and the mucocutaneous junction of the stoma, thus there is a risk of herniation. A scar is formed from a dense fibrous mass (Thibodeau & Patton 2007).

There are a number of factors that can adversely affect wound healing. With increased age, skin becomes more friable, less elastic and the blood circulation is impaired. Other factors affecting wound healing may include vitamin C deficiency, protein starvation, hypovolemia, tissue hypoxia, obesity, chronic diseases, infection and foreign bodies in the wound (Tortora & Derrickson 2006). Drugs such as steroids used by patients with

Crohn's disease, for example, may affect post-operative healing by repressing the natural inflammatory process required for healing.

The abdominal wall

Beneath the skin is the superficial fascia (Ellis 2004) consisting of fibrous connective tissue and variable quantities of superficial fat (Monkhouse 2005). Below this are the muscles of the abdomen.

Muscles

The muscles of the anterior abdominal wall are:

- internal obliques;
- external obliques;
- transverse abdominus;
- rectus abdominus;
- pyramidalis although this is not always present.

(Faiz & Moffat 2002)

Muscles (see Figure 2.2) protect the viscera by their contraction, produce movement and increase the intra-abdominal pressure for defaecation and coughing for example. Stomas are generally sited through the rectus muscle to try and minimise problems such as parastomal hernias, although there is inconclusive evidence supporting this.

The external oblique muscle travels from the outer surface of the lower eight ribs to the iliac crest and forward to the anterior superior spine. The external and internal oblique muscles are used to flex the spine, for side flexion and rotation of the trunk (Snell 2004). The transverse abdominus pulls in and flattens the abdomen (Tortora & Derrickson 2006). The rectus sheath enables the pelvis to tilt backwards and encloses the rectus abdo-

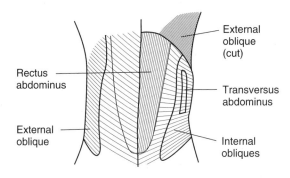

(Tortora & Derrickson 2006)

Figure 2.2   Abdominal muscles.

minus. The rectus abdominus muscle runs from the ribs to below the umbilicus and pelvis (Faiz & Moffat 2002).

The peritoneum

The peritoneum is a large, fine serous membrane (Richards 2005). The peritoneum also carries the blood vessels, nerves and lymphatics to the organs and the lymphatic nodes used to fight infection (Watson 2002). The peritoneum lines the walls of the entire abdominal cavity (parietal layer) and forms the serous outer coating of the organs (visceral layer), preventing friction (Thibodeau & Patton 2007). The peritoneum encloses some of the intra-abdominal organs, attaching many to the abdominal wall. The peritoneum encapsulates the bowel with some retro (behind), some areas of the peritoneum are fixed while other parts are free and mobile. Fixed areas will require mobilisation during stoma formation. The peritoneal cavity is sterile, but contains bowel that is bacteria laden. Thus, if there is an anastomotic leak following a bowel resection, it could lead to severe sepsis or possibly death. Mobilisation of the bowel may be problematic if previous abdominal surgery has resulted in adhesions. The area of peritoneum that lines the abdominal wall is the parietal portion and the visceral portion covers the organs (McGrath 2005). The two layers contact each other and the space between is called the peritoneal cavity, consisting of the greater and lesser peritoneal sac (omentum).

The greater omentum is a double fold of peritoneum, hanging on to the bowels like an apron and descends from the lower stomach to the transverse colon. The greater omentum provides protection, as it can attach itself to bowel perforations, enclosing any infection.

The lesser omentum extends to the liver from the stomach and duodenum.

The mesentery is a wide, fan-shaped fold of parietal peritoneum connecting the small intestine to the posterior abdominal wall. The mesentery encloses the jejunum and ileum, allowing free movement of the bowel but preventing strangulation (Thibodeau & Patton 2007). The transverse mesocolon, a smaller fold of peritoneum, attaches the transverse colon to the posterior abdominal wall.

The gastrointestinal tract

The GI tract/alimentary canal is a continuous, muscular digestive tube running from the mouth to the anus. The GI tract is about nine metres long and under the control of the autonomic nervous system (McGrath 2005).

The organs of the GI tract are the mouth, pharynx, oesophagus, stomach, small intestine, large intestine and anus (see Figure 2.3). There are also accessory organs associated with digestion, such as the teeth, tongue, gallbladder, salivary and other digestive glands, liver and pancreas (Marieb 1998). The function of the GI tract is to ingest and digest food by mechanical and chemical means, absorb and utilise ingested foods and finally pass the waste (Black & Hyde 2005).

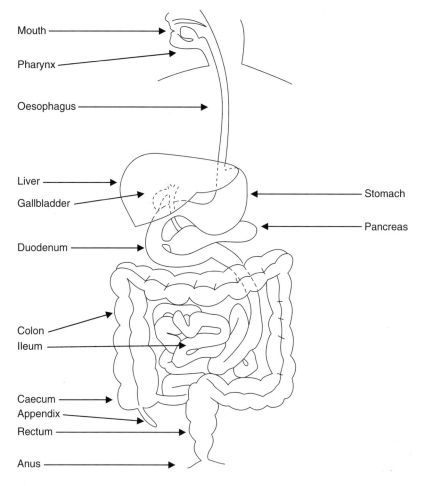

Figure 2.3   The gastrointestinal tract.

The digestive process

Digestion is basically the processing of food into nutrients for the body to use. The six steps of digestion are briefly discussed and then elaborated upon later on.

- *Ingestion* – the process of taking food and liquids into the body, usually via the mouth.
- *Secretion* – the cells within the walls of the GI tract and the accessory organs secrete about seven litres of fluid into the bowel lumen to assist in the digestion process (Tortora & Derrickson 2006).
- *Propulsion* – moves food along the GI tract. Swallowing is initiated voluntarily and peristalsis is involuntary, continuing the propulsion of food. Peristalsis is a wavelike ripple of the muscles, propelling

forward. Peristalsis can cease, for example following surgery (paralytic ileus). Segmentation is a back and forth action that breaks apart and mixes the food bolus (Thibodeau & Patton 2007).

- *Digestion* – mechanical and chemical digestion.
- *Absorption* – occurs when the nutrients pass from the bowel lumen to the blood or lymph.
- *Defaecation* – the elimination from the body of the waste/faeces, through the anus or stoma.

The bowel wall

To further examine the GI tract, it is important to review the bowel itself (see Figure 2.4). There are four layers to the bowel wall; the mucosa, submucosa, muscularis and serosa (adventitia) layers (McGrath 2005).

The mucosa is the layer closest to the bowel lumen and consists of three layers:

- epithelium;
- lamina propria;
- muscularis mucosa.

The mucosa has the functions of:

- secretion of mucus, hormones and digestive enzymes;
- protection;
- absorption into the blood.

The epithelium in the mouth, pharynx, oesophagus and anal canal is protective (McGrath 2005). Epithelium within the stomach and intestine has the function of secretion and absorption. The mucosa is formed from epithelial cells and secretory glands. The epithelial cells of the stomach and intestine rapidly renew every five to seven days and are then shed and passed in the faeces (Tortora & Derrickson 2006).

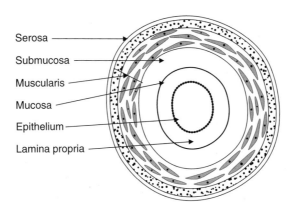

Figure 2.4 Cross section of the bowel wall.

The lamina propria lies below the epithelium and is loose areolar, connective tissue. The lamina propria consists of neutrophils, eosinophils and plasma cells (Jewell *et al.* 1992). The capillaries absorb the digested nutrients and provide nourishment to the epithelium (Marieb 1998).

The mucosa also has a very thin muscle layer called the muscularis mucosa (McGrath 2005). The muscle allows movement and expansion of the bowel surface. The mucosa is able to absorb the products of digestion and secrete mucus, digestive enzymes and hormones (Marieb 1998).

The submucosa is made from dense connective tissue to bind the mucosa to the deep muscle layer. There is also blood, lymphatic and nerve supply called the submucosal or Meissner's plexus (McGrath 2005). The regulation of secretion and movement is hormonal and achieved via the autonomic nervous system (Hinchliff 1981). The parasympathetic nerves generally increase digestive secretions and the sympathetic nerves decrease secretions.

The muscularis is smooth muscle from the end of the upper third of the oesophagus downwards. The muscle layer helps transportation of food/waste by involuntary peristalsis in wavelike contractions. There are also several sets of sphincters to prevent backflow (Richards 2005).

The serosa is the protective outer layer only present where there is mesentery surrounding or suspending the bowel. The serosa is a serous membrane of connective tissue (Richards 2005), with a single layer of epithelial cells covering it and carries the blood, lymph vessels and nerves to the bowel (McGrath 2005).

Blood supply

The blood vessels related to the GI tract include the coeliac artery that gives rise to the splenic, gastric, hepatic, inferior mesenteric and superior mesenteric arteries. The superior mesenteric artery (SMA) and inferior mesenteric artery supply oxygenated blood to the GI tract. The SMA runs between the layers of the mesentery and sends branches to the jejunum and ileum. These then pass through smaller arteries, the arterial arcades and finally the vasa recta (Moore & Agur 2002). Occlusion of the vasa recta by thrombi can result in ischemia of the small bowel. If ischaemia becomes necrosis a small bowel resection may be necessary. It is therefore important to ensure the blood supply to the bowel is not damaged during surgery. If the SMA infarcts it may necessitate an extensive small bowel resection.

Venous blood from the GI tract, containing nutrients, predominantly drains into the hepatic portal vein. This passes to the liver, where metabolism of the nutrients occurs. The liver and lymphatic system is also important when considering metastatic bowel cancer.

Lymphatic supply

The lymphatic drainage of the anterior abdominal wall is in four quadrants. Lymph drains superiorly to the left and right axillary nodes and inferiorly to the left and right inguinal nodes (Monkhouse 2005).

Mouth

In the mouth the food is ingested. The teeth mechanically break down the food by mastication; saliva is added to lubricate the food and turn it into a bolus. Saliva is produced in three pairs of salivary glands:

- parotid gland (in front of and below the ears);
- submandibular gland (below the mandibular angle);
- sublingual gland (anterior to the submandibular gland).

(Tortora & Derrickson 2006)

The salivary glands produce approximately 1–1.5 litres of saliva daily (Black & Hyde 2005). Saliva is an alkaline substance containing mainly water and some enzymes to soften and moisten the food. The enzyme salivary amylase (previously called ptyalin) breaks down cooked starch into maltose and dextrin and begins chemical digestion (Richards 2005). Saliva also cleanses and protects the teeth and mouth and keeps the soft parts supple.

In swallowing (deglutition) the tongue voluntarily propels the food bolus to the pharynx (oral stage) (Fox & Lombard 2004). To prevent aspiration of food and drinks when swallowing, the tongue closes the back of the mouth, the soft palate blocks the nasal passage (nasopharynx stage) and the epiglottis covers the larynx (pharyngeal stage) (Black & Hyde 2005). The final phase (oesphageal stage) is involuntary contractions to move the food bolus to the stomach. The swallowing reflex can be affected, for example, following a cerebrovascular accident or loss of consciousness.

Oesophagus

The oesophagus is a muscular tube about 25 cm in length (Forbes *et al.* 2005). The oesophagus is composed of two layers: the outer longitudinal layer and the inner circular muscle layer (Fox & Lombard 2004). There is striated muscle in the upper portion, which is under voluntary control, gradually changing to involuntarily controlled smooth muscle (Tortora & Derrickson 2006).

The oesophagus connects the oral cavity to the stomach with the vagus nerve responsible for peristalsis. The food is propelled down the oesophagus to the stomach (Aspinall & Taylor-Robinson 2002) in four to eight seconds (Richards 2005) and enters the stomach via the cardiac sphincter.

Stomach

The stomach is a J-shaped pouch about 25–30 cm long and the width about 10–15 cm (Black & Hyde 2005). The function of the stomach is to store food, mix it with gastric juices and pass chyme. The stomach consists of the cardia that joins the oesophagus to the stomach, the fundus (upper part), the body of the stomach and the antrum, extending to the pyloric sphincter (Tortora & Derrickson 2006). Within the stomach the gastric secretions mix with the food and change it by chemical breakdown to chyme (Aspinall & Taylor-Robinson 2002). The gastric secretions are hydrochloric acid (HCl), pepsin and intrinsic factor. Hydrochloric acid is secreted from the parietal cells of the gastric glands and the enzyme pepsin is secreted as the non-active pepsinogen and converted by hydrochloric acid. Pepsin is a protease that catalyses the breakdown of specific peptide bonds and therefore breaks down proteins. The chief cells (or zymogenic cells) of the gastric glands secrete intrinsic factor (Thibodeau & Patton 2007). Acid secretion in the stomach activates the digestive enzymes and hydrochloric acid also kills any ingested bacteria (Fox & Lombard 2004).

About three litres of gastric juice is produced daily (Black & Hyde 2005) and secreted before and during the ingestion of food (Watson 2002). Gastric secretion occurs in three phases:

- cephalic;
- gastric;
- intestinal.

The cephalic phase is stimulation by the sight, smell, taste or thought of food. Vagus nerve impulses stimulate production of gastrin. Endocrine G cells in the gastric mucosa stimulate the gastric secretions that secrete the hormone gastrin.

The gastric phase is instigated by protein foods in the pyloric area of the stomach. This stimulates the release of gastrin from the bowel mucosa to the blood system, resulting in an increase in secretions of gastric juice. Furthermore food within the stomach causes distension that stimulates release of gastrin, leading to activation of local and parasympathetic reflexes in the pylorus.

The intestinal phase occurs when the duodenal mucosa secretes gastric inhibitory peptide (GIP), secretin and cholecystokinin (CCK) that inhibit gastric secretions. This may be as a result of fat, carbohydrates and/or acid being present in the duodenum (Thibodeau & Patton 2007). It is important to consider these large volumes of gastric secretions in the management of patients with a short bowel. These gastric secretions may be lost before re-absorption occurs, resulting in a high faecal output. Also in the gastric juices is intrinsic factor, which is required for the absorption of vitamin B_{12} in the terminal ileum. Absence of vitamin B_{12} results in pernicious anaemia.

The digestion of protein and the absorption of alcohol occur in the stomach (Tortora & Derrickson 2006). Very little else is absorbed in the stomach (Richards 2005).

The three main functions of the stomach are storage of food (about 1500 ml in adults), breakdown of food to chyme and the controlled release of chyme to the small intestine (Snell 2004). Food spends about three to four hours in the stomach, depending upon the food type taken (Thibodeau & Patton 2007). For example, meals that are more fluid leave the stomach faster than dry foods. Thus for those with a high faecal output it can be advisable to discourage drinking at meal times to increase the length of time the food remains in the stomach.

The pyloric sphincter is generally closed, except to release at a rate of 20 seconds the chyme into the duodenum, under nervous and hormonal control. Fats and other nutrients in the duodenum stimulate release of the hormone GIP from the intestinal mucosa to the bloodstream. Gastric inhibitory peptide as the name suggests inhibits the gastric muscle and therefore slows passage into the duodenum. The nervous control that regulates the release of chyme is as a result of receptors in the duodenal mucosa that responds to distension and acid. The sensory and motor fibres in the vagus nerve cause a reflex inhibition of gastric peristalsis, called the enterogastric reflex (Thibodeau & Patton 2007).

Small intestine

The small intestine consists of the duodenum, jejunum and ileum. The length varies from 2 m (Richards 2005) to about 10 m in length, with an average of 6.5 m (Ellis 2004). The diameter is approximately 2.5 cm (McGrath 2005). Thus during bowel surgery it is important to note the bowel remaining and not that resected to assist in planning care.

Duodenum

Chyme passes from the stomach to the duodenum via the pyloric sphincter to prevent regurgitation (Watson 2002). The duodenum is shaped like the letter C and is about 25 cm long (Snell 2004), curving around the head of the pancreas.

Chyme enters the duodenum approximately 30 minutes after eating a meal. About 6–10 ml of chyme enter the duodenum every minute, emptying the stomach usually four to five hours after a meal (Richards 2005).

The common bile duct and the pancreatic duct empty into the mid section of the duodenum, through the sphincter of Oddi, at the ampulla of Vater (McGrath 2005). These secretions help to neutralise the acidic gastric contents making them more alkaline (Aspinall & Taylor-Robinson 2002). The enzyme-rich secretions aid digestion of carbohydrates, fats and proteins. In the duodenum the absorption of calcium, magnesium, iron, protein, fats and starch occurs (Hinchliff 1981).

Jejunum and ileum

The jejunum is the upper two-fifths (2.5 m) of the small intestine (Thibodeau & Patton 2007). The lower three-fifths (3.6 m) is the ileum (Watson 2002), although there is no sharp demarcation between the two sections of small intestine (Forbes *et al.* 2005). The jejunum begins at the duodenojejunal (DJ) flexure and gradually changes into ileum, ending at the ileocaecal junction. The jejunum allows further digestion of proteins, fats and carbohydrates.

The main function of the small intestine is to absorb nutrients via the many folds in the intestinal mucosa that increase the surface area about three times. The folds also force the chyme to move around the bowel lumen, mixing with intestinal juices and slowing down its passage to increase absorption (Richards 2005). It can be seen that following an extensive small bowel resection (where less than one metre remains) it may not be possible to reabsorb sufficient nutrients to maintain life.

The structure of the small bowel is ideally suited for absorption as there are five million small villi that project into the bowel lumen (Stevens & James 2003). The villi are about one millimetre in height and each villus has about 1000 microvilli, named the brush border, increasing the surface area more than 20 fold (Aspinall & Taylor-Robinson 2002). The brush border produces some intestinal juice (peptidase) that breaks down protein. Each epithelial cell (enterocyte) in the small intestine has about 600 microvilli (Ellis 2004). Villi require rapid replacement and have a very high rate of mitosis. The villi may be replaced every 36 hours and worn-out cells are shed and excreted in the faeces (Hinchliff 1981). The mucosa of the small intestine secretes about two litres daily of a slightly alkaline substance (pH 7.5–8.0). The villi rapidly reabsorb the secretions and use them as a transporter for the absorption of nutrients from the chyme (Richards 2005). Patients with a high faecal output may lose bowel secretions in addition to nutrients.

In starvation the enterocytes shrink and the villi can decrease in size by up to half; this reduces the absorptive capability of the small intestine. This generally reverses when enteric feeding recommences. Damage to enterocytes also occurs in coeliac disease, Crohn's disease or due to radiation, for example (Richards 2005).

When the body absorbs glucose and sodium from the ileum the luminal water is also drawn across the epithelium (Aspinall & Taylor-Robinson 2002). This is particularly important if rehydration therapy is required, for example by patients with a short bowel or diarrhoea. Rehydration therapy is more effective if it contains sodium and glucose in the water, as glucose is required for sodium uptake. The villi in the small intestine absorb almost all of the proteins, carbohydrates and fats. Proteins and carbohydrates as amino acids and simple sugars respectively are absorbed via the capillaries to the portal vein and liver. Fats as fatty acids and glycerol pass into the lymph within the villi and are drained into the lymphatic capillaries (Watson 2002). The proximal ileum absorbs vitamins, monosaccharides and disaccharides. The terminal ileum absorbs sodium, potassium, chloride, bicarbonate, bile salts and vitamin B_{12} (Stevens & James 2003). Considerable volumes of water are absorbed throughout the ileum.

Within about three to six hours the chyme will reach the ileocaecal valve (Richards 2005). CCK is thought to regulate the release of chyme and is secreted by endocrine cells in the intestinal mucosa when chyme is present, altering peristalsis (Thibodeau & Patton 2007). The ileum empties about 1.5 litres daily into the colon (McGrath 2005), having absorbed five to six litres in the jejunum and about two litres in the ileum. The various sites through which absorption of nutrients occurs can be important if that part of the bowel is resected during surgery and may therefore affect absorption of various dietary nutrients.

Large intestine

The large intestine extends from the ileum to the anus and consists of the caecum, appendix, ascending colon, transverse colon, descending colon, sigmoid colon, rectum and anal canal. The large intestine is attached to the posterior abdominal wall by visceral peritoneum (mesocolon) and frames the ileum (Richards 2005).

The colon is generally 1.5 m in length (Stevens & James 2003) with a diameter of 7 cm at the caecum, reducing to 2.5 cm at the sigmoid (McGrath 2005). The primary function of the colon is absorption of excess water and electrolytes, transforming semi-liquid stools into firmer formed faeces. Ninety per cent of the water absorption occurs in the small intestine, but the colon absorbs about one litre daily, which reduces the volume that enters the rectum to about 100–200 ml (Tortora & Derrickson 2006). The colon then stores the waste material prior to expulsion.

The gastro-ileal reflex occurs as a result of taking food into the stomach, initiating contractions of the duodenum and the small bowel (Watson 2002). Peristalsis does occur in the colon but less frequently than in the ileum. A very strong peristaltic wave occurs three to four times daily, moving faeces into the sigmoid colon. This is usually strongest in the first hour after breakfast (Richards 2005) and is when most people open their bowels.

The longitudinal muscles of the colon are gathered into three thick bands called taeniae coli. The taeniae run the length of the colon, gathering it into pouches called the haustra (Stevens & James 2003). The contraction of the circular muscles constricts the lumen and this segmental movement is called haustration (Pocock & Richards 2006).

Bacterial fermentation plays an important part in the digestion and production of vitamin K (Tortora & Derrickson 2007) as well as being potentially harmful. During surgery, if the barrier of the bowel is breached, there is a risk of infection due to translocation of the bacteria (Banning 2006). The colonic bacterial flora can also be affected by some medications such as antibiotics like cefuroxime. Antibiotics may eradicate some of the bacteria that are required by the body, allowing other species that are usually in low volumes to proliferate and may cause clostridium difficile diarrhoea.

The colonic bacteria ferment carbohydrates and release gas, such as methane (McGrath 2005). The volume of flatus passed is about 500 ml daily (Richards 2005), increasing with consumption of high fibre foods. The odour associated with flatus is due to the gases produced, such as hydrogen sulphide. Flatus can be very problematic for colostomates.

Caecum

The caecum is a blind-ended pouch, about 6 cm in length (Snell 2004). The ileocaecal valve prevents backflow to the ileum. The vermiform appendix joins the caecum and is up to 20 cm in length, although usually about 9 cm (Watson 2002).

Ascending colon

The ascending colon is approximately 13 cm in length (Snell 2004). As the faeces pass through the ascending colon the faecal output becomes thicker as a result of water absorption. Sodium, potassium, chloride and glucose are also absorbed in the ascending colon (Hinchliff 1981).

Transverse colon

The faeces travel from the ascending colon and move through the hepatic flexure to the transverse colon. The transverse colon is 50 cm in length (Watson 2002) and mobile. The faeces are thicker and mucus is secreted from the goblet cells in the epithelium (Richards 2005) in the transverse colon to lubricate the bowel mucosa (Hinchliff 1981). The mucus also protects against bacterial products that may be irritating and acidic.

Descending colon

Nine to ten hours following ingestion the faeces pass from the transverse colon through the splenic flexure to the descending colon. The descending colon is 25 cm in length (Snell 2004).

Sigmoid colon

The faeces then pass into the sigmoid colon. The sigmoid colon is about 40 cm in length and lies within the lesser pelvis (Watson 2002) and is mobile.

Rectum

The faeces move to the rectum, which is about 17–20 cm in length (Thibodeau & Patton 2007). The rectum gives the body the signal to pass the faeces from the body. The faeces are usually in a solid form at this stage and may take several days from ingestion to leave the body (McGrath 2005). The rectum can hold about 400 ml of faeces (Black & Hyde 2005). The longer the faeces are in the colon, the more water is absorbed and the drier the faeces will become.

Anal canal

The anal canal is about 3 cm in length (Marieb 1998) finishing at the anus. The anal canal has two sphincters, the involuntary internal anal sphincter and the voluntarily controlled external sphincter, which are usually closed unless defaecation occurs (Tortora & Derrickson 2006). The function of the sphincter muscles in the process of faecal continence and defaecation will be discussed in Chapter 6 on continence. Faeces are passed at a rate of about 100–150 g daily (Mañas *et al.* 2003). The solid part of faeces is a similar percentage of cellulose, indigestible matter from the diet and dead bacteria (Watson 2002).

Accessory organs associated with the GI tract

The liver

The liver is the largest organ in the body, with a left and a larger right lobe (Ellis 2004). The liver weighs 1.3–1.5 kg depending on age and sex (Black & Hyde 2005), which is about 2% of the total adult body weight (Forbes *et al.* 2005). It is situated in the upper right part of the abdominal cavity, fitting under the diaphragm. The hepatic portal vein brings deoxygenated blood via the GI tract to the liver and the hepatic artery brings oxygenated blood (Watson 2002). The functions of the liver are:

- metabolic
- storage
- secretory.

Metabolism by the liver of the ingested foods includes the breakdown of stored fat for energy (desaturation) and excess amino acids into urea, the detoxication of drugs and poisons, the synthesis of carotene from vitamin A and the conversion of excess carbohydrates to fat for storage. The amino acids from digested foods are absorbed by the villi and transported to the liver by the portal vein; some pass into the blood supply, while others are used to synthesise plasma proteins. Excess protein is broken up in the liver for body fuel. Worn out cells are broken down into uric acid and urea, the latter excreted via the kidneys.

The liver also synthesises prothrombin and fibrinogen from amino acids and manufactures antibodies, antitoxins and heparin (Watson 2002). The liver is also the main heat-producing organ in the body. There are a number of drugs that affect liver metabolism including cimetidine, warfarin and St John's wort.

Storage

- vitamin A;
- vitamin D;
- anti-anaemic factor;
- iron from diet;
- worn out blood cells;
- glucose is stored as glycogen (and converted back to glucose in the presence of glucagon).

(Watson 2002)

The alkaline bile secreted by the liver cells is a thick yellowish green fluid. Approximately one litre of bile is secreted daily (Tortora &

Derrickson 2006), consisting of water, bile salts and bile pigments (Watson 2002). The bile salts contain cholesterol, the main ingredient of typical gallstones. The bile pigments are derived from haemoglobin, as part of the worn out blood cells. The bile when excreted from the body provides the faeces with its normal brown colour (McGrath 2005). The function of bile is to:

- emulsify fats to fatty acids, monoglycerides and glycerol in the ileum, by the lecithin and bile salts (Thibodeau & Patton 2007);
- stimulate peristalsis, thus acting as a natural laxative;
- excrete toxic substances, poisons, alcohol, drugs and the by-products of red blood cells (Black & Hyde 2005);
- act as a deodorant for the faeces, although this may be incidental (Watson 2002).

The gallbladder

The gallbladder is usually a pear-shaped sac about 8–10 cm in length and situated under the liver (Forbes *et al.* 2005). The gallbladder concentrates unused bile secreted by the liver and can store 30–60 ml. When fatty foods enter the duodenum the bile duct sphincters relax and the bile from the gallbladder is released into the duodenum (Black & Hyde 2005). The intestinal hormone CCK stimulates contraction of the gallbladder (Thibodeau & Patton 2007).

The pancreas

The pancreas is about 12–15 cm in length, with a head, body and tail and is situated behind the stomach, with the head attached to the duodenum and its tail towards the spleen (Forbes *et al.* 2005). The pancreas is made of lobules, each consisting of tiny vessels that lead to the main duct and ending in several alveoli (Watson 2002). The pancreatic duct and common bile duct enter the duodenum at the ampulla of Vater (Tortora & Derrickson 2006).

The function of the pancreas is both exocrine and endocrine (Fox & Lombard 2004). The exocrine acinar cells secrete up to 1.5 litres daily of pancreatic juice containing enzymes, trypsinogen, amylase and lipase (Black & Hyde 2005). The pancreatic secretions are released as a result of stimulation by hormones such as secretin released by the intestinal mucosa. Trypsinogen is used to break down protein. The amylases hydrolyse polysaccharides to disaccharides (Thibodeau & Patton 2007). The lipases digest fat. Within the pancreas are cells, the islets of Langerhans, which secrete hormones into the bloodstream (Watson 2002). The endocrine function is the secretion of glucagon when blood sugar falls. In response to raised blood glucose after a meal the pancreas secretes insulin, which it has produced, to stimulate conversion from glucose to glycogen for storage and cellular uptake.

The spleen

The spleen is a large nodule of lymphoid tissue situated in the upper left quadrant behind and below the stomach (Watson 2002). The function of the spleen is to provide a source of fresh lymphocytes for the bloodstream and is where red blood cell destruction occurs. The spleen also assists fighting infections and it may help in the manufacture of antibodies.

Urinary system

The urinary system consists of the kidneys, ureters, bladder and urethra (see Figure 2.5). The three major functions of the urinary system are excretion, elimination and homeostasis of the blood plasma (McGrath 2005).

The kidneys

There are two kidneys situated in the posterior part of the abdomen, one either side of the spine, behind the peritoneum and with the right one slightly lower due to displacement by the liver (Tortora & Derrickson 2006). The kidneys are each 11 cm in length, 6 cm wide and 3 cm thick and embedded in perirenal fat (Watson 2002). The medial border is named the hilus and here the blood vessels, nerves and ureters enter and leave the kidney. If dissected in half vertically, the outer dark section is the cortex; the paler inner part is the medulla that leads to the renal pelvis that is a collecting space (see Figure 2.6). The kidneys receive about 20–25% of the total cardiac output, which is about 1.2 litres per minute (Mirpuri & Patel 2000). The blood from the renal artery is under high pressure allowing passage via the nephron into the kidney.

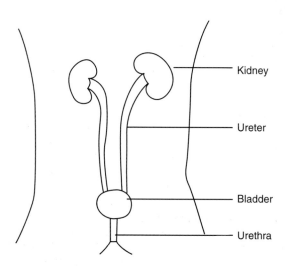

Figure 2.5 The urinary system.

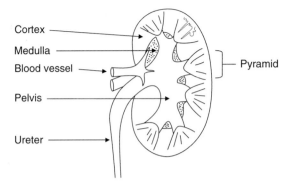

Figure 2.6   The kidney.

Kidney function

The function of the kidneys is to maintain homeostasis of body fluids, sodium, blood pressure and to produce urine. Homeostasis is achieved by keeping the composition and volume of the body fluids at a constant level (McGrath 2005) by regulating the water content, mineral composition and acidity of the body. This is achieved by secreting substances as required to maintain extra-cellular concentrations and blood levels within normal limits. Metabolic waste and foreign chemicals such as drugs and food preservatives are eliminated from the blood. The kidneys also secrete hormones to metabolise vitamin D and control sodium levels, for example (Mirpuri & Patel 2000). The waste products of metabolism are excreted as urine. The process of urine production is in three stages:

- glomerular filtration
- tubular reabsorption
- tubular secretion.

Glomerular filtration occurs from the glomerulus to the glomerular capsule. The walls are permeable to water and small molecules, but blood and protein are not passed via non-diseased kidneys. The fluid is called glomerular filtrate and is similar to plasma in composition, as it contains glucose, amino acids, fatty acids, salts, urea and uric acid (Watson 2002). From the 600 ml of blood passed each minute through the glomerulus 125 ml becomes glomerular filtrate. The majority is reabsorbed and the remainder passed as urine.

Tubular reabsorption occurs selectively with about 99% of the filtered fluid and many useful solutes reabsorbed (Tortora & Derrickson 2006). In health all the glucose is reabsorbed. Reabsorption of fluids back to the bloodstream occurs in the distal convoluted tubule of the nephron and is variable. The secretion of anti-diuretic hormone (ADH) by the pituitary gland controls reabsorption (Watson 2002).

Materials such as waste, drugs and excess ions are secreted into the renal tubule fluid. Finally, tubular secretions pass through the collecting duct from the tubule and duct cells (Tortora & Derrickson 2006).

The nephrons

Within the kidney are over a million tiny tubules called nephrons (McGrath 2005). Each nephron consists of a renal corpuscle, which filters the blood plasma, and a renal tubule, where the filtered fluid passes. The renal corpuscle (see Figure 2.7) consists of the glomerulus, the network of capillaries and the glomerular (Bowman's) capsule, a cup surrounding the capillaries (Tortora & Derrickson 2006). After the glomerular capsule the filtered blood plasma is transferred down the proximal convoluted tubule, before leaving the renal cortex and passing into the loop of Henle (within the renal medulla) and back to the kidney cortex via the distal convoluted tubule, into the straight collecting duct (Fillingham & Douglas 2004).

Medulla

The inner portion of the kidney, the medulla consists of straight collecting ducts into which the convoluted tubules in the cortex empty (Watson 2002). The function of the medulla is to collect the urine secreted in the cortex and transport it to the kidney pelvis. The pyramids of the medulla are 10 to 18 triangular structures that project into the kidney pelvis (Fillingham & Douglas 2004). At the apex of each of the pyramids are the mouths of fine collecting tubules that pour the urine into the kidney pelvis.

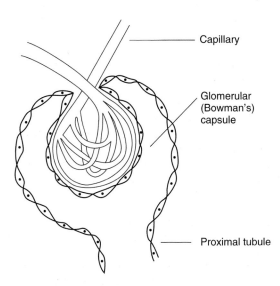

Capillary

Glomerular
(Bowman's)
capsule

Proximal tubule

Figure 2.7   Renal corpuscle.

Kidney pelvis

The pelvis of the kidney is an irregular, branched cavity (Watson 2002). The branches are the calyces of the pelvis and each branch receives one of the medulla pyramids to transfer the urine into the ureter.

The ureters

The two ureters are muscular tubes about 30 cm long and 3 mm in diameter (McGrath 2005). The ureters transport urine from the kidneys to the bladder. The muscle layer of the ureter also has peristaltic contractions that occur four or five times a minute (Watson 2002).

The bladder

The bladder is a reservoir for urine. The bladder when empty is within the lesser pelvis, moving upwards and forwards into the abdominal cavity as it fills. The bladder is lined with smooth muscle, known as the detrusor muscle (Mirpuri & Patel 2000). At the base of the bladder the ureters enter and the urethra leaves (Fillingham & Douglas 2004). To prevent back flow there are two bands of oblique muscle fibres close to the ureteric openings.

To allow expansion of the bladder there is an inner mucous coat with rugae (when empty). The bladder is lined with transitional epithelial tissue that also allows expansion (Fillingham & Douglas 2004). The desire to pass urine is usually felt when there are 200–400 ml of urine in the bladder, although it can hold over 500 ml with discomfort (Tortora & Derrickson 2006).

The urethra

The urethra runs from the bladder to the external urethral orifice. In females the urethra is about four centimetres, in males the length is 20 cm (McGrath 2005). In the male the urethra serves as a passage for both urine and the reproductive system, in the female only the urinary system.

There are muscle bundles to the sides of the urethra to form the involuntary controlled internal urethral sphincter. Slightly further down the urethra is the external sphincter (Mirpuri & Patel 2000), which is under voluntary control. Urinary continence (see Chapter 6 on continence) is not possible in infancy or with some nerve damage (Watson 2002).

Urine

Normal urine is an amber-coloured fluid. The normal quantity of urine secreted is one to two litres daily (Tortora & Derrickson 2007), although this varies on intake, exercise and sweating for example. Urine has a specific gravity of 1015–1025 and the normal urine acidity is a pH of about 7.4 and is virtually protein free (Watson 2002). Urine consists of:

- water (95%);
- salts (sodium chloride, phosphates and sulphates);
- the waste products of protein:
  ○ urea (two per cent);
  ○ uric acid;
  ○ creatinine.

This brief overview of the skin, abdomen, GI tract and the urinary system should assist in the understanding of the alterations that a stoma makes.

References

Aspinall RJ & Taylor-Robinson SD (2002) *Mosby's Color Atlas and Text of Gastroenterology and Liver Disease*. London: Mosby.

Banning M (2006) Bacteria and the gastrointestinal tract: beneficial and harmful effects. *British Journal of Nursing*. **15(3)**: 144–9.

Black PK & Hyde CH (2005) *Diverticular Disease*. London: Whurr.

Burr S & Penzer R (2005) Promoting skin health. *Nursing Standard*. **19(36)**: 57–66.

Butcher M & White R (2005) The structure and function of the skin. In: White R (ed) *Skin Care in Wound Management: Assessment, Prevention and Treatment*. Aberdeen: Wounds UK Publishing.

Cutting KF & Tong A (2003) *Wound Physiology and Moist Wound Healing*. London: Medical Communications UK Ltd.

Ellis H (2004) *Clinical Anatomy. A Revision and Applied Anatomy for Clinical Students*. Oxford: Blackwell Science.

Faiz O & Moffat D (2002) *Anatomy at a Glance*. Oxford: Blackwell Science.

Fillingham S & Douglas J (2004) *Urological Nursing*. 3rd edn. London: Baillière Tindall.

Forbes A, Misiewicz JJ, Compton CC, Levine MS & Quraishy MS *et al.* (2005) *Atlas of Clinical Gastroenterology*. 3rd edn. London: Elsevier Mosby.

Fox C & Lombard M (2004) *Gastroenterology*. 2nd edn. London: Mosby.

Hess CT (2005) *Clinical Guide: Wound Care*. 5th edn. London: Lippincott Williams & Wilkins.

Hinchliff SM (1981) The normal function of the alimentary tract. In: Breckman B (ed) *Stoma Care*. Buckinghamshire: Beaconsfield Publishers.

Jewell DP, Chapman RGW & Mortensen N (1992) *Ulcerative Colitis and Crohn's Disease*. London: Churchill Livingstone.

Kindlen S & Morison M (1999) The physiology of wound healing. In: Morison M, Moffatt C, Bridel-Nixon J & Bale S (eds) *A Colour Guide to the Nursing Management of Chronic Wounds*. 2nd edn. London: Mosby.

Lyon CC & Smith AJ (2001) *Abdominal Stomas and Their Skin Disorders*. London: Martin Dunitz.

McGrath A (2005) Anatomy and physiology of the bowel and urinary systems. In: Porrett T & McGrath A (eds) *Stoma Care*. Oxford: Blackwell Publishing.

Mañas M, De Victoria EM, Gil A, Yago M & Mathers J (2003) The gastrointestinal tract. In: Gibney MJ, Macdonald IA & Roche HM (eds) *Nutrition and Metabolism*. Oxford: Blackwell Publishing.

Marieb EN (1998) *Human Anatomy and Physiology*. 4th edn. California: Benjamin/Cummings Science Publishing.

Mirpuri N & Patel P (2000) *Renal and Urinary Systems*. London: Mosby.

Monkhouse S (2005) *Clinical Anatomy: A Core Text with Self Assessment*. London: Churchill Livingstone.

Moore KL & Agur AMR (2002) *Essential Clinical Anatomy*. 2nd edn. London: Lippincott Williams & Wilkins.

Newton H & Cameron J (2003) *Skin Care in Wound Management*. London: Medical Communications UK Ltd.

Ovington LG & Schultz GS (2004) The physiology of wound healing. In: Morison MJ, Ovington LG & Wilkie K (eds) *Chronic Wound Care: A Problem-based Learning Approach*. London: Mosby.

Pocock G & Richards CD (2006) *Human Physiology: The Basis of Medicine*. 3rd edn. Oxford: Oxford University Press.

Richards A (2005) Intestinal physiology and its implications for patients with bowel stomas. In: Breckman B (ed) *Stoma Care and Rehabilitation*. London: Elsevier Churchill Livingstone.

Snell RS (2004) *Clinical Anatomy for Medical Students*. 7th edn. London: Lippincott Williams & Wilkins.

Stevens P & James P (2003) Anatomy and physiology associated with stoma care. In: Elcoat C (ed) *Stoma Care Nursing*. London: Hollister.

Thibodeau GA & Patton KT (2007) *Anatomy and Physiology*. 6th edn. Missouri: Mosby Elsevier.

Tortora GJ & Derrickson B (2006) *Principles of Anatomy and Physiology*. 11th edn. New Jersey: John Wiley & Sons, Inc.

Tortora GJ & Derrickson B (2007) *Introduction to the Human Body and Essentials of Anatomy and Physiology*. 7th edn. New York: Wiley.

Watson R (2002) *Anatomy and Physiology for Nurses*. 11th edn. London: Baillière Tindall.

Chapter 3

Colorectal Cancer and Adjunct Therapy

Deep Tolia-Shah

Introduction

The significant effect of the diagnosis of cancer needs careful consideration. A number of studies state that every patient will feel some fundamental fear on contracting this disease with such a reputation. Some of the fears highlighted are:

- *Fear of alienation*: the patient may feel abandonment, rejection and isolation and as the treatment continues these fears are reinforced.
- *Fear of mutilation*: cancer will be a threat to the integrity of the body. The images of the effects of treatment (surgery, chemotherapy, radiotherapy) are often too much to comprehend.
- *Vulnerability*: no matter what the prognosis, the patient will feel life has a time limit.
- *Fear of the loss of control*: the reputation of this disease gives rise to the feelings of loss of control and of instability. The implications of balance, usefulness and autonomy that are acquired in adulthood come under threat.

Incidence

Cancer remains high on the list for improving outcomes. A government audit in 1995 by Calman/Hine highlighted that all cancer care should be regulated and standardised throughout the United Kingdom. The introduction of the fast track system by the Department of Health (DOH) meant that patients who showed any signs or symptoms of suspected colorectal cancer (CRC) were to be seen in hospital within two weeks. As part of the two-week rule initiative (DOH 1997), it is felt that colorectal cancer care should be delivered through a multidisciplinary approach (NHS Executive 1997).

Colorectal cancer is the second most common cancer in England and Wales (Langman & Boyle 2002). There are approximately 30 000 new cases diagnosed each year and approximately 20 000 deaths from the disease per annum (Scholefield & Steel 2002). Of the 30 000 people affected with colorectal cancer, 10 000 are diagnosed with rectal cancer and 20 000 with

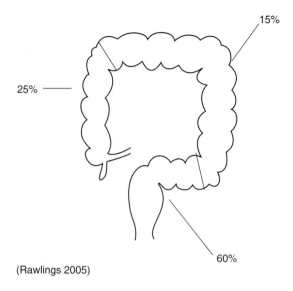

15%

25% ———

(Rawlings 2005)

60%

Figure 3.1   Distribution of colorectal cancer.

colon cancer (see Figure 3.1). The overall numbers are almost identical in men and women. The average age of developing colorectal cancer is between 55 and 70 years. The incidence of developing colorectal cancer under the age of 45 is about two per 100 000 (Steel 1998).

Possible causal factors

Hereditary influences

Increases in lifestyle pressures and other factors have led to a corresponding increase in the incidence of colorectal cancer in the past 25 years. However, death rates from the disease have fallen. This could be due both to early detection and the fact that treatments have improved.

Approximately 90% of colorectal cancers are sporadic (Acheson & Scholefield 2002). In these cases evidence of a long-standing disease such as ulcerative colitis, that may predispose the patient to developing colorectal cancer, is not apparent.

Other factors that may predispose a patient to colorectal cancer are hereditary factors, such as familial adenomatous polyposis (FAP) and hereditary non-polyposis colorectal cancer (HNPCC).

The risk of developing colorectal cancer can be seen in Table 3.1.

Environmental factors

The impact of environment factors must not be underestimated when identifying their effect on colorectal cancer. They are known to influence the development of the disease in approximately 70–80% of all individuals

Table 3.1   Lifetime risk of colorectal cancer

Risk of colorectal cancer	Lifetime risk (%)
General population	5
Personal family history of CRC (tubulovillous adenomas, etc.)	15 to 20
Inflammatory bowel disease	15 to 40
Hereditary non-polyposis colon cancer mutation (HNPCC)	70 to 80
Familial adenomatous polyposis	95

Source: adapted from Swan 2005.

who develop cancer. Lifestyle, social and cultural factors may play a large part in the incidence of colorectal cancer. For example, within the Japanese population in the USA the risk of developing colorectal cancer is three to four times higher than for those in Japan (Boyle & Langman 2001).

Dietary factors

It is generally believed that animal fat and meat intake may account for 80% of large bowel cancer (Cummings & Bingham 1998). It is thought to lead to an increased synthesis of the bile salts that may act as a carcinogenic agent that affects the lining of the colon and gut flora.

Dietary fibre, fruit and vegetables have been linked to faecal bulk and transit time. It is thought that this has a protective influence on the bowel lining. Studies show that fruit and vegetables may contain more protective factors within them as cereal fibre alone. The presence of free radicals (harmful molecules that the body produces) can increase the risk of bowel cancer. Antioxidants, vitamins A, C and E, present in fruit and vegetables will deactivate these free radicals. The importance of this was recognised by the Department of Health, hence the 'five-a-day' campaign, launched in 2004.

Smoking and alcohol

Regular intake of cigarette smoke with the combination of increased alcohol intake may also contribute to the risk of developing colorectal cancer.

Lifestyle issues

There is evidence to suggest that physical activity offers some protective influence against colonic but perhaps not rectal cancer. Regular physical activity has been shown to reduce the occurrence of large adenomas in the distal colon. Generally, increasing dietary fibre will allow less time for potential carcinogens to have contact with the gut. Obesity is on the increase and currently the links between obesity and colorectal cancer remain unclear. However, there is evidence to suggest that there may be some links with obesity and adenomas and most bowel cancers arise from pre-existing adenomas.

Diagnosis and staging investigations

Even in the twenty-first century discussing one's bowel habit causes great embarrassment and distress to patients. However, those that experience persistent progressive or sinister symptoms must not delay in presentation to their general practitioner (GP).

Twenty per cent of patients with colorectal cancer are diagnosed incurable and 20% present as emergencies (Mella *et al.* 1997). It is hoped that the continued efforts by health care professionals and voluntary organisations will help reduce this and break down prejudice.

Symptoms and clinical presentations

When questioning patients it is essential to get a detailed history. Therefore it is important to understand the possible manifestations of colorectal cancer in order to address them. However, it is also important to remember that further investigation is needed to help give a complete diagnosis for the patient in order to plan the appropriate investigations and treatments.

The site of the tumour in the colon often determines the clinical presentations. The different sites of cancer will be explained in more detail as three different areas, namely right-sided, left-sided and rectal cancers.

Right-sided cancers

The signs and symptoms of right-sided cancers include:

- anaemia
- occasional diarrhoea
- palpable mass
- weight loss: often a late feature.

Patients with right-sided cancers including within the caecum may have the clinical manifestations of fatigue, palpitations, tiredness or weakness. These symptoms are due to the lesions that bleed easily into the bowel, causing iron deficiency anaemia (Crawford 1999). However, we must remember that anaemia alone is not a diagnosis. Weight loss may also feature, along with a palpable mass on physical examination. Diarrhoea may also be a feature although this is not so common. Obstruction rarely occurs unless the ileocaecal valve is involved.

Left-sided cancers

The signs and symptoms of left-sided cancer are:

- altered bowel habit
- abdominal pain

- possible rectal bleeding
- weight loss
- palpable mass: often a late feature.

Alterations in bowel habit, diarrhoea and intestinal obstruction are typical signs of lesions in the left side of the colon. It is important to remember, however, that within the population bowel frequency varies from three times a day to once every three days. With this in mind it is important to remember to establish the 'norm' for each individual prior to any investigation.

Altered bowel habit (this can mean either diarrhoea, constipation or a combination of the two, also a change to the patient's normal bowel habit) may also be accompanied by rectal bleeding. Left-sided cancers are most likely to bleed due to their location in the bowel. Passing dark blood either mixed in, on the stool or alone may be associated with cancer especially if accompanied by a change in bowel habit and abdominal pain. This may give rise to symptoms of obstruction (Neugut *et al.* 1993). Weight loss and a palpable mass are both late features. Bright red blood on the toilet paper or dripping into the toilet is more than likely to be associated with anal bleeding e.g. haemorrhoids or fissures (Forde & Waye 1989).

Rectal cancers

The signs and symptoms of a rectal cancer are:

- rectal bleeding
- altered bowel habit
- tenesmus
- mucus discharge
- weight loss
- pain.

Bleeding, tenesmus and a change in bowel habit are most common with rectal cancers. Ninety-seven per cent of the population have some form of rectal bleeding (Thompson *et al.* 2003). It is therefore not surprising that haemorrhoids are assumed to be the main cause of bleeding.

Rectal bleeding in rectal cancer is bright red and may be seen with stool or post defaecation. An altered bowel habit is also a feature of rectal cancer. Faeces can also be accompanied by mucus, slime or blood. It is therefore important that this is investigated fully to establish a cause.

Another significant symptom for rectal cancers is tenesmus; this is an unpleasant and uncomfortable symptom giving patients the feeling of incomplete or unsatisfactory evacuation. This can be associated with tumours low in the rectum. Weight loss and pain are usually late features. Weight loss can be associated with patients being afraid to eat due to their altered bowel habit and tenesmus as well as the disease process. Pain in rectal cancers is not common; however this may occur due to obstruction of the bowel.

Anal carcinomas

Cancers of the anus or anal canal are rare. Their features are similar to those of rectal cancer; however, histologically they often show as a skin cancer. The common way to manage these lesions is with radiotherapy alone. Patients will be referred to the oncologist for further management.

Assessment, staging investigations and the multidisciplinary team

This section of the chapter covers a number of investigations used to help diagnose colorectal cancer. Access to specialist services, as mentioned earlier, has been given high priority by the DOH (1997) in conjunction with the Calman/Hine policy. Since July 2000, specialists have been required to see patients whose GP suspects a high risk of colorectal cancer within two weeks of the referral; this is known as the fast-track system or two-week wait (NHS Executive 1997).

GPs have guidelines for referral to follow (Association of Coloproctology of Great Britain and Ireland 2001). These guidelines highlight specific persistent features and symptom combinations to help identify the patients who need referral/reviewing within two weeks.

Assessment

Following referral to the outpatients department, a physical examination takes place after a detailed clinical history. This includes inspection of the abdomen for distension; abdominal masses and any other abdominal scarring that may be present. Palpation may identify any tenderness and the presence or absence of ascites. Digital examination helps identify any masses present in the rectum; 40–80% of patients with a rectal cancer present with a palpable mass in the rectum.

Faecal occult blood testing (FOBT)

The faecal occult blood test is not a diagnostic test specific to colorectal cancer. This test picks up any sign of bleeding in the gastrointestinal tract, e.g. stomach or gums, and therefore cannot be relied upon to diagnose colorectal cancer.

Rigid sigmoidoscopy

This examination is usually carried out in the outpatients setting with the specialists. Rigid sigmoidoscopy allows close inspection of the mucosa to identify any abnormalities, mucus or blood. A proctoscope reaches up to about 10 cm in the rectum and a sigmoidoscope reaches up to 20 cm.

Flexible sigmoidoscopy

If facilities are available within the outpatients department, a flexible sigmoidoscopy can be performed there. The main advantage of this is that it can go beyond 20 cm up to 60 cm. Biopsies can be performed following an enema bowel preparation.

Colonoscopy

Colonoscopy allows the complete examination of the colon. When concerned about the possibility of colorectal cancer the majority of patients will undergo a colonoscopy. This allows visualisation of the entire bowel up to the caecum. It has a high sensitivity of more than 95% of all lesions (Winawer *et al.* 1997). However, colonoscopy does carry a risk of perforation of one in 1000 (Smith & Nivatongs 1975).

Other investigations

Some other investigations useful for colorectal cancers that may not be so common include the following.

Barium enema (double contrast barium enema)

The barium enema is a technique that uses barium, a radio-opaque liquid with a high sensitivity and specificity to cancers of the colon. The barium is given rectally, removed and then gas is inserted. The bowel is then examined with an x-ray.

Computed tomography (CT) colonography/virtual colonoscopy/CT pneumocolon

This investigation is a relatively new procedure and is now being used more often in most Trusts. CT scans produce three-dimensional images of the abdomen. The data produced are similar to those of a colonoscopy. It gives a cross-sectional view of the colon and can reliably pick up lesions more than 6 mm in size. It has the ability to identify lymph nodes and liver involvement (Halligan & Fenlon 1999). This is an ideal investigation for those patients who are frail and elderly and may not be able to tolerate a colonoscopy. However, it is important to remember that this investigation does not give a tissue diagnosis, as biopsies are not possible.

Capsule endoscopy

This new technique to predominantly investigate the small bowel has been developed in the last few years. Not many centres have facilities for this at present, but it should be more common in the future. This method of investigation is where a patient swallows a capsule that contains a transmitter. A receiver belt and electrodes are attached to the patient. The capsule and receiver belt collect data from the patient's gastrointestinal tract. This can take up to eight hours in which time the patient continues to eat and drink as normal. Once this information has been gathered, the receiver is attached to a computer that downloads all the information. This can detect any abnormalities within the GI tract. The advantage of this is that the capsule can reach areas of the GI tract that an ordinary endo-scope cannot.

Multidisciplinary team

Once histological evidence has confirmed a carcinoma then a treatment plan should be determined. As part of the Calman/Hine (1995) and DOH (1997) initiative it was felt that colorectal cancer care should be delivered through a multidisciplinary team (MDT) approach. The aim of the MDT approach is to unite health care professionals who are caring for colorectal cancer patients. This allows a team decision and implementation of a therapeutic strategy to help in the management of these patients. Team members may vary; however, they usually consist of the core members – the colorectal surgeon, oncologist, radiologist, pathologist and specialist nurse. The MDT makes decisions using a multi-faceted approach on the patient's diagnosis and treatment plan.

Pre-operative staging

Staging or determining the extent of the disease is important in its manage-ment. The pre-operative staging investigations for colonic and rectal cancers vary. Blood tests are part of the routine investigations. Tests include the measurement of the carcinogen embryonic antigen (CEA), a protein that is produced by the carcinoma. The CEA measurement is used as a 'tumour marker'. The staging classification will be discussed later.

Computed tomography (CT) scan

The CT scan is used to determine the presence of metastases, mainly in the liver and lungs. Although the liver can be looked at with the use of an ultrasound scan, a CT scan is more sensitive to lymph node enlargement. This may indicate a possible deposit and can identify disease extension beyond the bowel wall. However, it must be noted that it cannot distin-guish the layers of the rectal wall; this is determined by MRI.

Magnetic resonance imaging (MRI)

MRI is used in the assessment of the local spread of rectal tumours. An MRI can identify the lower edge of the tumour and helps determine whether the CRM (circumferential resection margin) is threatened. Enlarged nodes can be identified, which helps in the staging of rectal tumours. This also determines whether any pre-operative chemo-radiation treatment may be of benefit to the patient.

Endoanal ultrasound scans

Some centres occasionally use this method of investigation. This is where a probe is placed into the anus through to the rectum. It looks at the tumour status within the rectum. This can offer good sensitivity to stage early rectal cancers.

Ultrasound scan (USS)

If a CT scan shows liver metastases or a suspicious area within the liver that needs closer inspection, USS can play a pivotal role. This can be used to diagnose the spread of distant disease or in conjunction with a CT scan.

Positron emission tomography (PET) scan

Although principally not used to diagnose primary cancers, it is used to determine local or recurrent disease. It is commonly used when other imaging shows doubt. It is only available in certain cancer centres throughout the country.

Surgery

Treatment for colorectal cancer is primarily surgical. Curative surgery involves the complete removal of the tumour to prevent local recurrence (Williams 1996). The surgical treatment for both colonic and rectal cancers will be considered separately in this section. The treatment for colonic cancers has relatively standard procedures, whereas rectal cancer tumours require multiple considerations to ensure the best treatment. Pre-operative combination of chemotherapy and radiotherapy plays an important role on the impact of the cancer surgically.

Colon cancer

Right hemicolectomy

A right hemicolectomy (see Figure 3.2) is considered for tumours affecting the caecum, ascending colon, hepatic flexure and proximal part of the transverse colon. This also entails the removal of 5–10 cm of the terminal ileum. The blood supply to this segment, including the lymph nodes and lymphatics, is also removed. The anastomosis joins the ileum and the transverse colon (end to end or end to side).

Extended right hemicolectomy

An extended right hemicolectomy (see Figure 3.3) is used where tumours of the transverse colon and splenic flexure are located. It involves the removal of the right colon, transverse colon and occasionally part of the descending colon.

Surgery to resect right-sided cancers is very unlikely to require a covering stoma, as there is enough bowel to allow for safe anastomosis. However

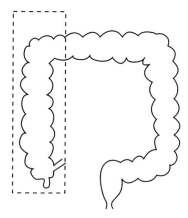

Figure 3.2   Right hemicolectomy.

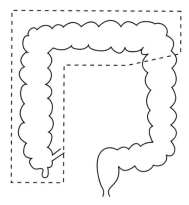

Figure 3.3   Extended right hemicolectomy.

in cases of obstruction, bypass surgery may be required to divert away from the tumour. This would be considered as a palliative procedure.

A referral to the stoma specialist nurse is essential whenever a stoma formation is considered.

Left hemicolectomy

A left hemicolectomy (see Figure 3.4) is mainly performed for tumours of the descending colon, splenic flexure and sigmoid colon. This entails the removal of the mid transverse colon to below the sigmoid colon. The associated arteries and lymph nodes are also removed. The transverse colon is anastomosed to the upper rectum. Usually a defunctioning stoma is not required to protect the anastomosis.

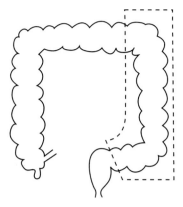

Figure 3.4　Left hemicolectomy.

Sigmoid colectomy

This technique is less radical than the left hemicolectomy and is used to remove cancers of the sigmoid colon. The sigmoid colon is removed including any lymph nodes. Patients may require a covering stoma therefore an appropriate referral to a stoma specialist nurse is needed prior to surgery.

Emergency surgery

The Hartmann's procedure is mainly used for patients who present as an emergency with intestinal obstruction; 8–9% of patients with colon cancer present in this way. The procedure consists of a standard left hemicolectomy (Borwell 2005) with a covering end colostomy fashioned at surgery. Due to the nature of the admission/surgery it is not always possible for the stoma specialist nurse to see these patients pre-operatively. The rectal stump can be closed with a purse string suture and then attached to the inside of the abdominal wall. In some centres the rectal stump is brought out at the end of the laparotomy scar creating a mucous fistula. This stoma is non-functional. The mucous fistula in itself can have some management problems that need specialist advice. However this is not as commonplace as in previous years.

A Hartmann's procedure allows the patient to have their stoma reversed in the future. However, a third of these patients will not have this done due to surgical morbidity.

Rectal cancer

Surgical treatment for rectal cancer is more complex. When localised it is treatable and curable. New surgical techniques have been developed to spare the anal sphincters. Using a low, stapled anastomosis allows intestinal continuity and preserves continence. Tumours as low as two centimetres can now have sphincter saving procedures carried out on them, thus avoiding a permanent colostomy.

For most rectal cancers, pre-operative neoadjuvant chemo radiotherapy may be used to help shrink the tumours as a precursor to the surgery. It must be noted, however, that the core members of the team, following the MRI review, make the neoadjuvant treatment plan.

Abdominoperineal excision of the rectum (AP/APR/APER)

For many decades an APER (see Figure 3.5) was considered to be the treatment for all rectal cancers. Since 1985 (Keighley & Williams 1993) this has reduced by two-thirds. This surgical procedure is performed:

- on cancers that are within 5 cm of the anal verge;
- on cancers of the anus, which have had a poor response to chemotherapy and/or radiotherapy;
- to achieve effective surgical clearance of the cancer, which involves complete removal of the rectum.

Surgery involves the removal of the rectum and anal canal, using an abdominal and perineal approach, leaving the patient with a permanent end colostomy. The patient will have a perineal wound which will also need management. Due to the nature of the pre-operative treatment of these cancers, there may be some delay in wound healing that will need discussing with the patient prior to treatment both by the oncologist and the stoma specialist nurse. There is significant risk of urinary dysfunction and sexual impairment, as well as the issues around a permanent stoma that need to be dealt with in a timely manner by the stoma specialist nurse.

Anterior resection

This operation can be classed as two different techniques, high anterior resection and low anterior resection.

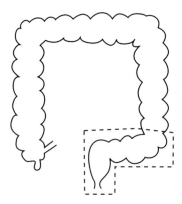

Figure 3.5 Abdominoperineal resection of the rectum.

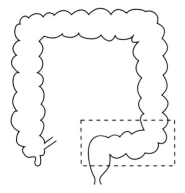

Figure 3.6   Anterior resection.

High anterior resection

A high anterior resection (see Figure 3.6) is considered for tumours of the upper third of the rectum, approximately 12 cm above the anal verge. In these cases patients do not undergo pre-operative chemo radiation due to the height of the cancer within the rectum. The higher the cancer is within the radiotherapy field, the more likely the involvement of the small bowel and other organs during treatment.

The sigmoid colon and part of the rectum are removed. The descending colon and the remaining part of the rectum are anastomosed. To protect the anastomosis, a temporary covering loop ileostomy may be required.

Low/ultra low anterior resection

The majority of patients undergoing a low/ultra low anterior resection may be given pre-operative chemo radiation. The sigmoid colon and the entire rectum are removed. The descending colon and anal canal are anastomosed. Patients undergoing this technique will require a covering temporary loop ileostomy to defunction the anastomosis. The anastomosis is about 5–6 cm from the anal verge. For some patients a coloanal pouch may be formed by the surgeon to mimic the rectum; this is described briefly below. Careful assessment of the patient's sphincter control may be needed before creating the coloanal pouch. It is also important to discuss with patients that the pouch does not replace the rectum and its function can be quite different.

Coloanal pouch

Reconstructive surgery following rectal cancer surgery is becoming more favourable now. The coloanal pouch is the formation of a reservoir to help store faeces to improve continence and faecal urgency. The colonic pouch (Parc *et al.* 1986) is favoured by many to be the surgical technique of choice as the restorative procedure for rectal cancer.

Histopathology

The overall outcome of colorectal cancer is dependent on staging. This indicates the extent of disease and therefore the prognosis and outcome. Histopathology is the microscopic evidence of the cancer after resection. To this day Dukes' (1930) staging remains the most used classification system:

Dukes' classification

Stage A   Invasion not beyond the muscularis propria, no lymph node metastases

Stage B   Invasion beyond the muscularis propria, no lymph node metastases

Stage C1   Regional lymph node metastases, without apical node involvement

Stage C2   Regional lymph node metastases, with apical node involvement

Stage D   Distant metastases (not commonly used)

However, the UICC Committee, International Union against Cancer developed a system for *all* tumours, the TNM staging system: Tumour/Node/Metastases

- T relates to tumour size and extent of the invasion of the various layers of the bowel wall;
- N is number of lymph nodes invaded by cancer cells;
- M relates to any metastases.

TNM classification for colorectal cancer adapted from UICC

T   Primary tumour
Tx   Primary tumour cannot be assessed
T0   No evidence of primary tumour
T1   Tumour invades submucosa
T2   Tumour invades muscularis propria
T3   Tumour invades through muscularis propria into subserosa or into non-peritonealised pericolic or peritoneal tissues
T4   Tumour directly invades other organs or structures and/or perforates visceral peritoneum

N   Regional lymph nodes
Nx   Regional lymph nodes cannot be assessed
N0   No regional lymph node metastases
N1   Metastases in one to three pericolic or perirectal lymph nodes
N2   Metastases in four or more pericolic or perirectal lymph nodes
N3   Metastases in any lymph node along the course of a named vascular trunk

M   Distant metastases
Mx   Presence of distant metastases cannot be assessed
M0   No distant metastases
M1   Distant metastases

Both pathological staging systems are used jointly in describing the grading of colorectal cancer in histological reporting.

Adjuvant chemotherapy

Chemotherapy refers to 'drug therapy'. In terms of cancer 'cytotoxic chemotherapy' refers to drug therapy used to 'kill' cancer cells. The aim of adjuvant chemotherapy is to improve long-term survival outcomes and to help reduce tumour recurrence.

The decision to treat is discussed at the MDT meeting with the support of the oncologist. The use of chemotherapy is indicated following tumour staging. In broad terms this decision is made dependent on lymph node involvement and the extent of tumour growth within the bowel wall. It is also important to take into account any other vascular involvement, i.e. if an apical node is involved or there is vascular involvement.

Cytotoxic chemotherapy for colorectal cancer can be given orally or intravenously. Intravenous administration can consist of either a bolus dose or given via a peripherally inserted central catheter (PICC) line or Hickman line, dependent on the regimen. There are many different types of chemotherapy, and studies show the benefits of 5 fluorouracil (5FU) in an adjuvant setting (Laurie *et al.* 1989).

Adjuvant chemotherapy for colorectal cancer is given in a cyclical regimen to maximise its effectiveness. This can be over a period of six months or approximately 24 weeks; however, the length of time that treatment is given is dependent on the type of treatment. The type of chemotherapy drug determines its administration and can vary from weekly to once every three weeks. This is determined with the histology and oncologists' expertise.

5FU was the only active drug available in the management of colorectal cancer for the past 40 years (Ferns 1999). 5FU is usually prescribed in combination with a vitamin called Folinic Acid (FA) to help enhance the action of 5FU, thus increasing its effectiveness. It is also now available in a tablet form, Capecitibine/Ufotral. The benefits of this are that the patients can administer the medication at home and thus reduce their hospital and outpatient stay.

As there are many trials and even more in the pipeline, it is important to mention the most common drugs used in adjuvant chemotherapy treatment for colorectal cancer. Other drugs, often used in clinical trials, are Oxaliplatin and Irinotecan. They may be used in combination with 5FU. Patients will receive individual information on their specific chemotherapy regimens from the chemotherapy team prior to commencing treatment.

There are some associated side effects linked with chemotherapy administration. The most common associated with 5FU include:

- fatigue;
- diarrhoea (constipation with Capecitibine);
- mucositis;
- nausea;
- palmar/plantar – soreness of the palms of hands and soles of feet (mainly associated with Capecitibine);
- pancytopenia.

Oxaliplatin used in combination with 5FU can also be given for advanced colorectal cancer in the presence of liver metastases. Oxaliplatin is administered intravenously via a PICC/Hickman line/Portocath. Some of the side effects associated with this chemotherapy are:

- peripheral neuropathy: numbness or tingling sensation in the hands and feet; this can be long lasting for some patients and even permanent; this is of particular significance to those patients with stomas and the management of them;
- diarrhoea;
- nausea;
- fatigue;
- neutropenia.

Irinotecan is often given in the presence of aggressive cancers and/or metastases or where the other chemotherapy regimens have had no impact. This is given either as an infusion or via a central or PICC line or Portocath. Some of the common side effects with Irinotecan are:

- diarrhoea;
- neutropenia;
- fatigue;
- nausea;
- loss of appetite;
- hair loss.

It is important to note that due to the effects of chemotherapy on wound healing and lowering of the immunity most oncologists, dependent on treatment regimens, do not like an interruption to the chemotherapy cycle. Therefore those patients with temporary stomas generally do not have their stomas reversed until after completion of their chemotherapy.

Ulcers on the surface of the stoma can occur as a result of chemotherapy treatment. Ulcers may also form on the parastomal skin. Stoma powder can be useful if used sparingly on the ulcers in either location. It can also be useful to advise very gentle pouch removal if the ulcers are on the skin, as the chemotherapy weakens the skin.

Effects of chemotherapy on stomas

The side effects associated with chemotherapy include nausea and vomiting that can disrupt eating and drinking, this and the chemotherapy may lead to constipation in the colostomate (Earhart *et al.* 1998). There may, however, be diarrhoea, if this does occur an anti-diarrhoeal medication and plenty of oral fluids should be taken. If diarrhoea persists throughout the chemotherapy then a drainable appliance might be more appropriate for the colostomate to empty.

In respect to the stoma itself there may be increased bleeding of the stoma. Pressure from a soft cloth will usually stop the bleeding and very gentle cleansing is required at appliance changes. There may be mouth and stoma sores; those on the actual stoma require no treatment and will heal without treatment. The stoma may become slightly swollen and the aperture in the appliance may need to be enlarged. The peristomal skin may become irritated, requiring review by the stoma specialist nurse and gentle care. Additionally there can be a decreased libido and immunosuppression that may predispose the ostomate to infections, peristomal or elsewhere.

Radiotherapy

Radiotherapy is rarely used post-operatively to the pelvis, as the majority of those patients would have had some form of pre-operative treatment prior to their surgery. Post-operative radiotherapy can be used if histopathology indicates and the patient has not been irradiated previously in the pelvic region.

The effects of radiotherapy on the stoma

Patients that require radiotherapy may experience skin reactions. These need careful assessment prior to initiating therapy. It may be more suitable for the colostomate to wear a two-piece appliance during therapy and for a few weeks after treatment is completed. It may be beneficial to discontinue the use of soaps or ointments used within the radiation area (Earhart *et al.* 1998). There can also be a decrease in libido and some perineal discomfort. Stomal oedema and ulcerations can occur and generally heal without additional therapy after the radiation treatment finishes. Wearing natural fibres can reduce the chances of skin reactions, which include the skin becoming pink and itchy, similar to the effects of sunburn. Showers may be more comfortable than bathing.

Palliative chemotherapy

Chemotherapy in the palliative setting can be used for advanced colorectal cancers. It is used when surgery is not an option in the presence of advanced disease, with the aim to palliate the disease rather than a curative intent. The benefits of this must be weighed against the possible treatment toxicities and the effects on quality of life.

Surveillance and follow-up

There is no single definitive strategy for follow-up for those patients who have undergone curative resection for colorectal cancer. Patients will be followed up for the next five to seven years, depending on the surgeon's preference and the intensity of the follow-up varies throughout the UK. In general terms, however, follow-up includes the investigation of the patient's tumour markers, e.g. CEA, regular colonoscopy and CT scans at various intervals throughout the follow-up period.

The FACS trial is run by the National Cancer Research Network, part of the National Can-up. Recruitment ends in 2011. The government along with the Association of Coloproctology of Great Britain and Ireland (2001) have recommended guidelines to follow. However, intensity varies from clinician to clinician.

Screening

Health promotion has led to the introduction of a national bowel cancer screening programme. The Cancer Research Institute is currently running a randomised control trial to assess follow-up (Twite 2007). This includes a faecal occult blood test and explanation in different languages for those over 60 years old.

Conclusion

Cancer care will remain high on the government's agenda. Improvements and efficiency in the way cancer care is managed not only improves outcome but also helps streamline diagnosis, treatment and long-term gain for both the patient and the professional.

The management and diagnosis of cancer can be complex and all-consuming. It provokes feelings of fear, loss of control and the possibility of death. However, with psychological support and comprehensive information and education about the disease and treatment pathway, the journey can be made manageable for patients and their carers. As nurses we are in the ideal position to help support patients and their carers through this time of diagnosis and throughout their treatment pathway.

However, it is important to remember that the treatment of colorectal cancer is multifocal and multi-professional in order to provide the best care for the individual based on their individual diagnosis. The aim of a multidisciplinary team is to treat patients in line with national protocols and guidelines as well as help support them in making choices in their treatment.

Further information and websites

Information for professionals, patients and their carers comes in a variety of forms. Increasingly information is available over the Internet, but some of it might not be accurate or the amount may be overwhelming. Below are a few recommended organisations, telephone numbers and/or websites that may be helpful:

Beating Bowel Cancer – provides information and support for patients and professionals about the symptoms and diagnosis of bowel cancer.
Website: http://www.beatingbowelcancer.org
Advisory line: 020 8892 1331

Bowel Cancer UK (formerly Colon Cancer Concern) – provides fact sheets, support and information online and via the telephone on all aspects of bowel cancer and raising awareness.
Website: http://www.coloncancer.org.uk
Telephone helpline: 0870 850 60 50

Cancerbackup – provides information, support and practical advice on all aspects of cancer, specifically for patients, their families and carers, with cancer questions and answers available online.
Website: http://www.cancerbackup.org.uk
Telephone helpline: 0808 800 1234

CancerHelp: an information service about the diagnosis and treatment of cancer, accessible for people with cancer and their families, provided by Cancer Research UK.
Website: http://www.cancerhelp.org.uk

DIPex: personal experiences of health and illness – DIPex provides a wide variety of personal experiences of health and illness. You can watch, listen to or read their interviews, find reliable information on treatment choices and where to find support.
Website: http://www.dipex.org.uk

Macmillan Cancer Support – working to ensuring every patient diagnosed with cancer has ready access to the best information, treatment and care. Helping people cope with cancer includes funding medical and nursing cancer experts, information leaflets and patient grants.
Website: http://www.macmillan.org.uk
Information line: 0808 8082020

References

Acheson AG & Scholefield JH (2002) What is new in colorectal cancer? *Surgery.* **20(10)**: 244–8.

Association of Coloproctology of Great Britain and Ireland (2001) *Guidelines for the Management of Colorectal Cancer.* London: ACPGBI.

Borwell B (2005) *Bowel Cancer Foundations for Practice.* London: Whurr.

Boyle P & Langman JS (2001) In: Kerr D, Young AM & Hobbs FDR (eds) *ABC of Colorectal Cancer.* London: BMJ Publications.

Calman K & Hine D (1995) *A Policy Framework for Commissioning Cancer.* London: Department of Health.

Crawford JM (1999) The gastrointestinal tract. In: Cotran RS, Kumar V & Collins T (eds) *Robbins' Pathological Basis for Disease.* 6th edn. Philadelphia: WB Saunders.

Cummings JH & Bingham SA (1998) Diet and the prevention of cancer. *British Medical Journal.* **317**: 1636–40.

Department of Health (1997) *The New NHS – Modern, Dependable.* London: Department of Health.

Dukes CE (1930) The spread of cancer of the rectum. *British Journal of Surgery.* **17**: 643–8.

Earhart K, Mueller V & Murray D (1998) Stoma care during cancer therapy: special people/special needs. *WCET Journal.* **18(3)**: 21–2.

Ferns H (1999) Campto: effective chemotherapy for advanced colorectal cancer. *International Journal of Palliative Nurses.* **5**: 6.

Forde KA & Waye JD (1989) Is there a need to perform full colonoscopies in middle age person with episodic bright red blood per rectum and internal haemorrhoids? *American Journal of Gastroenterology.* **84**: 1227–8.

Halligan S & Fenlon HM (1999) Virtual colonoscopy. *British Medical Journal.* **319**: 1249–52.

Keighley MRB & Williams NS (1993) *Surgery of the Anus, Rectum and Colon.* London: WB Saunders.

Langman M & Boyle P (2002) Colorectal epidemiology. In: Cunningham D, Topham C & Miles A (eds) *The Effective Management of Colorectal Cancer*, 2nd edn. London: Aesculapius Medical Press.

Laurie JA, Moertel CG & Fleming TR (1989) Surgical adjunct therapy of large bowel carcinoma: an evaluation of levamisole and the combination of levamisole and fluorouracil. *Journal of Clinical Oncology.* **7(10)**: 1447–56.

Mella J, Biffin A, Radcliff AG, Stamatakis JD & Steele RJ (1997) Population based audit of colorectal management in two UK health regions. *British Journal of Surgery.* **84(12)**: 1731–6.

Neugut AI, Garbowsk GC, Waye JD, Forde KA, Treat MR *et al.* (1993) Diagnosis yield of colorectal neoplasia with the use of abdominal pain, change in bowel habit and rectal bleeding. *American Journal Gastroenterology* **88(8)**: 1179–84.

NHS Executive (1997) *Improving Outcomes in Colorectal Cancer. Guidelines on Commissioning Cancer Services.* London: Department of Health.

Parc R, Tiret E, Frileux P, Moszkowsi E & Loygue J (1986) Resection and coloanal anastomosis for rectal carcinoma. *British Journal of Surgery.* **73(2)**: 139–41.

Scholefield JH & Steele RJ (2002) British Society for Gastroenterology. Association of Coloproctology for Great Britain and Ireland. Guidelines for follow up after resection of colorectal cancer. *Gut.* **51 (3–5)**: Suppl 5.

Smith LE & Nivatongs S (1975) Complications in colonoscopy. *Diseases of the Colon and Rectum.* **18(3)**: 214–20.

Steel R (1998) Colonic cancer. In: Phillips RKS (ed) *Colorectal Surgery.* London: WB Saunders.

Swan E (2005) *Colorectal Cancer.* London: Whurr.

Thompson MR, Heath I, Ellis BG, Swarbrick ET, Wood LF *et al.* (2003) Identifying and managing patients at low risk of bowel cancer in general practice. *British Medical Journal.* **327(7409)**: 263–5.

Twite S (2007) Public health and the national bowel cancer screening programme. *Gastrointestinal Nursing.* **5(6)**: 20–4.

Williams NS (1996) *Colorectal Cancer.* Churchill Livingstone: Singapore.

Winawer SJ, Fletcher RH, Miller L, Godlee F, Stolar MH *et al.* (1997) Colorectal cancer screening: clinical guidelines and rationale. *Gastroenterology.* **112(2)**: 594–642.

Further reading

Berrenberg J (1989) Attitude towards cancer as a function of experience with the disease: a test of three models. *Psychology and Health.* **3**: 233–43.

Cairns S & Scholefield A (1992) Guidelines for colorectal cancer screening in high risk groups. *Gut.* Supplement. Nova. **51**: 1–2.

Cancer Research Campaign (1993) *Cancer of the Large Bowel.* Fact sheet 18. London: CRC.

Cancer Research UK (2003) *Colorectal Cancer Fact Sheet*. London: Office of National Statistics.

Chauhan G & Long A (2000) Communication is the essence of nursing care 2: Ethical foundations. *British Journal of Nursing*. **9(15)**: 979–84.

Daniels N & Porrett T (1999) *Essential Coloproctology for Nurses*. London: Whurr.

Dent OF, Goulston KJ, Zubrzychi J & Chapius PH (1986) Bowel symptoms in the apparently well population. *Diseases of Colon and Rectum*. **29**: 243–7.

Department of Health (1999) *Saving Lives: Our Healthier Nation*. London: Department of Health.

Department of Health (2000) *The NHS Cancer Plan*. London: Department of Health.

Effective Health Care (1997) *The Management of Colorectal Cancer NHS Centre for Reviews and Dissemination*. York: University of York.

Ellis BG, Baig KM, Senapati A, Flashman K, Jaral M *et al.* (1999) Common modes of presentation of colorectal cancer patients. *Colorectal Disease*. **1 (supp)**: 24.

Goiligher J (1984) *Surgery of the Anus, Rectum and Colon*. London: Baillière Tindall.

Groenwald SL, Frogge MH, Goodman M & Yarbro CH (1997) *Cancer Nursing Principles and Practice*. 4th edn. London: Jones & Bartlett.

Guex P (1994) *An Introduction to Psych-oncology*. London: Routledge.

Holmes S (1996) *Cancer Chemotherapy: A Guide for Practice*. 2nd edn. Dorking: Asset Books Ltd.

National Cancer Guidance Group (2004) *Improving Outcomes in Colorectal Cancer: Updated Manual*. London: NICE.

NHS Executive (1997) *Improving Outcomes in Colorectal Cancer: The Research Evidence*. London: Department of Health.

Nicholls RJ & Glass R (1985) *Coloproctology: Diagnosis and Outpatient Management*. Berlin: Springer-Verlag.

Rawlings B (2005) The biological basis of bowel cancer. In: Borwell B (ed) *Bowel Cancer Foundations for Practice*. London: Whurr.

Robinson L (ed) (2000) Health promotion and cancer nursing. *European Journal of Oncology Nursing*. **4**: 3.

Royal College of Nursing (1998) *Specialists in Nursing*. London: RCN.

Royal College of Surgeons of England (1996) *Guidelines for the Management for Colorectal Cancer*. London: RCSE.

Chapter 4

Inflammatory Bowel Disease

Jennie Burch

Introduction

Inflammatory bowel disease (IBD) is an umbrella term for two main diseases, Crohn's disease and ulcerative colitis (UC) (Black 2000). IBD is described as inflammation of the gastrointestinal tract. Ulcerative colitis affects only the colon compared to Crohn's disease that affects any part of the gastrointestinal tract from the mouth to the anus. Inflammatory bowel disease should not be confused with irritable bowel syndrome (IBS), which is not discussed. People with indeterminate colitis display features of both UC and Crohn's colitis. Differentiation between the two diseases may not be possible in up to 10% of patients (Campbell & Travis 2004). The incidence may be two in 100000 with a prevalence of 27 in 100000 (Travis *et al.* 2005). This chapter will cover the common treatments used for IBD and also identify the surgical interventions available, which may result in a stoma formation.

Crohn's disease

Crohn's disease was first described early last century. Crohn's disease is a chronic condition and can affect any part of the gastrointestinal tract from the mouth to the anus, but most commonly the terminal ileum (Jewell *et al.* 1992) and is often relatively rectal sparing (Nightingale 2004). The disease can affect different segments of the intestine simultaneously and there are often areas of normal bowel between the inflamed sections termed skip lesions (Hall *et al.* 2007a). Crohn's disease can affect the full thickness of the intestinal wall (transmural). Patients experience periodic and often unpredictable symptomatic flare-ups with periods of remission where they are symptom free (Fow & Grossman 2007) but Crohn's disease is currently incurable.

Ulcerative colitis

Ulcerative colitis was first discussed in the mid-nineteenth century (Forbes 2001). UC affects only the colon. Inflammation and ulceration starts at the rectum and extends proximally in continuity (Jewell *et al.* 1992). Unpredictable episodes of remission and relapse can occur with UC.

Inflammatory bowel disease statistics

In the Western population, Crohn's disease affects more than 1 in every 1000 people (Rampton & Shanahan 2006) and incidence appears to be rising. Crohn's disease is more common in the western world than in Africa, Asia or South America. However, incidence of Crohn's disease is increasing as the developing countries become more Westernised. Crohn's disease is reported in woman slightly more commonly than men (Campbell & Travis 2004) with onset often in early adulthood.

Ulcerative colitis can develop at any age, but is most common in young adults aged 20–40 years (Jewell *et al.* 1992). Generally there are slightly more men affected than women (Campbell & Travis 2004). In the Western population the prevalence of UC is approximately 15 in 10000 and increasing (Rampton & Shanahan 2006).

Signs and symptoms for ulcerative colitis

The anatomical extent of the disease is the distance from the anus that the inflammation reaches:

- proctitis – inflamed rectum only;
- left sided colitis – inflammation up to the splenic flexure;
- extensive – colitis extending from the hepatic flexure;
- pan/total colitis – the whole colon is inflamed and possibly backwash ileitis involving the terminal ileum.

The common symptoms of UC are:

- rectal bleeding
- diarrhoea
- rectal mucus
- faecal urgency.
  (Rowlinson 1999a)

The mucosal lining of the colon contains numerous goblet cells that secrete mucus when the colon is irritated. Additionally electrolytes and water move into the colon by osmosis (Donnelly 2003), resulting in diarrhoea; both characteristics of UC. Stools of 20 or more daily can be reported. Acute disease flares may cause anaemia, low blood albumin levels and an electrolyte imbalance (Ward & Stanford 2003).

Fulminant colitis

The patient with fulminant colitis is systemically unwell with a distended and tender abdomen, pyrexia, tachycardia and severe bloody diarrhoea mixed with pus (Smith & Watson 2005). These patients should be in hospital and treated often with intravenous steroids. However, as treatment with steroids can mask some of these symptoms the patient requires a daily review by a specialist and x-ray monitoring. Surgery that includes a temporary stoma formation needs to be discussed at this stage, as there is a high chance of this being required.

Toxic megacolon

When there is severe or fulminant disease there is a risk of colonic perforation. Emergency surgery may be required to prevent bowel perforation from occurring as this leads to higher morbidity. It is imperative never to use antimotility drugs for patients with a toxic megacolon.

Crohn's disease: signs and symptoms

Crohn's disease occurs at different sites with varying frequency and can be classified into:

- colonic (20%);
- perianal (65%);
- small bowel (80%);
- ileocolonic (50%);
- gastroduodenal disease.
  (Smith & Watson 2005)

Colonic disease is associated with rectal bleeding, diarrhoea, abdominal discomfort, general malaise, anorexia and weight loss. Perianal disease can include local abscess formation, perianal fistulation or an anal fissure. Small bowel disease presents with colicky abdominal pain, malabsorption, weight loss, diarrhoea and abdominal mass (Jewell *et al.* 1992). Gastroduodenal disease affects less than 5% and symptoms include epigastric pain, nausea and postprandial vomiting.

The different sites of active Crohn's disease are associated with different symptoms most commonly:

- diarrhoea (70 to 90% of patients);
- abdominal pain (50% of patients);
- rectal bleeding (33% of patients);
- anorexia;
- malaise;
- fever;
- nausea and vomiting;
- weight loss;
- obstructive symptoms;
- persistent mouth ulcers;
- perianal problems:
  - fistulae – abnormal passage between the gut and skin;
  - abscesses;

○   fissures – a break in the skin lining the anal canal causing pain and/or bleeding during defaecation;
○   anal skin tags.

(Rampton & Shanahan 2006)

The inflammation and fibrosis associated with Crohn's disease predispose the patients to bowel strictures. These tight areas within the bowel are often due to scarring or the disease process. Strictures can cause obstructive symptoms, such as vomiting, severe abdominal pain and lack of bowel motions (Nightingale 2004). Alternatively they may lead to local perforation of the bowel wall and abscess formation (Rampton & Shanahan 2006).

The signs of Crohn's disease when examined endoscopically include aphthoid ulceration, deep fissuring ulcers, typical cobble-stoning, fibrosis, stricturing and fistulation (Rampton & Shanahan 2006). Crohn's disease can involve the mucosal, muscular and serosal layers of the bowel. Within the mucosal layer can be seen ulceration, both aphthous (small ulcers on the mucous membrane) and serpiginous (snakelike) can occur. Strictures can occur within the muscle layer. Finally fistulae, masses and abscesses can occur in the serosal layer.

Aetiology of IBD

The pathogenesis of IBD is unclear, but a number of factors appear to be involved (see Figure 4.1). These will be discussed under the headings of environmental issues, genetic, abnormal immune response and response to bacteria.

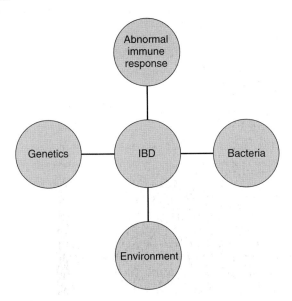

Figure 4.1 Potential causal factors for IBD.

Environmental issues

There are a number of environmental issues associated with Crohn's disease. Smoking increases the risk of developing Crohn's disease and doubles the risk of recurrence after surgery (Kamm 1999) and is associated with more severe disease (Smith & Watson 2005). Furthermore unidentified environmental factors may be important such as diet (Mason 2001).

Predisposing factors for UC include environmental factors, such as diet (Smith & Watson 2005). Additionally, the incidence of UC is highest in non-smokers, suggesting that smoking is protective against the development of UC, although smoking cannot be recommended.

Genetics

There is a genetic influence (caspase-activating recruitment domain CARD 15 gene formerly called the NOD 2 gene) in Crohn's disease. There is about a 10–15% familial incidence occurring predominantly in first-degree relatives (Jewell *et al.* 1992).

Abnormal immune response

The most generally accepted hypothesis relates to abnormal immune responses (Smith & Watson 2005) which fails to down regulate or 'switch off' leading to tissue destruction and IBD symptoms (Rayhorn & Rayhorn 2002a). This may occur for a number of reasons: one theory is a dysfunctional CARD 15 gene (Cunliffe 2005). If down regulation of the immune response fails, the inflammatory response will continue and result in chronic uncontrolled inflammation and intestinal tissue damage.

Response to bacteria

The gastrointestinal immune system response to bacteria is not fully understood. It is, however, generally very effective as we are exposed to bacteria from our diet or our own natural bowel flora on a daily basis (Cunliffe 2005) and we are able to tolerate non-sterile foods without becoming ill. However in active IBD the concentrations of the colonic bacteria are altered compared to normal and there may also be altered bacterial recognition (Hart *et al.* 2002).

Diagnosing IBD

A diagnosis of Crohn's disease is usually made based on the symptom history, the presenting clinical features, supporting serological markers and histology is essential. Endoscopy is important for diagnosis, prognosis, monitoring of therapy and occasionally for stricture dilation (Sachar 2007). The blood results may include a high C-reactive protein (CRP), raised erythrocyte sedimentation rate (ESR), elevated platelet count and low plasma albumin levels (Nightingale 2004). Imaging the bowel with barium

Table 4.1 Categorisation of ulcerative colitis

Feature	Mild	Moderate	Severe
Daily motions	Less than four	Four to six	More than six
Rectal bleeding	Small	Moderate	Large volumes
Temperature (°C)	Apyrexial	Intermediate	More than 37.8
Pulse (per minute)	Normal	Intermediate	More than 90
Haemoglobin (g/dl)	More than 11	Intermediate	Less than 10.5
ESR (mm/h)	Less than 30	Intermediate	More than 30

studies can also be useful. However, computed tomography (CT) scans or magnetic resonance imaging (MRI) can be useful to evaluate alterations in the bowel wall structure (Shen 2007) and for evaluating perianal disease.

When assessing Crohn's disease an activity index (CDAI) score can be useful in research contexts but is rarely used in clinical practice, as it is impractical. This includes a combination of scores related to the patient's recent disease including the number of liquid or very soft stools for the last week, presence of an abdominal mass and weight. This score can then be used to classify the severity of the disease. Mild disease activity scores under 150, moderate scores 150–250 and severe disease is above 250 (Smith & Watson 2005).

To consider UC an endoscopy, to examine the anatomical extent and severity of the colonic inflammation, is generally advocated (Kamm 1999). Endoscopic findings include inflammation uniformly along the colon wall with the rectum always affected, unless rectal therapy is used. An x-ray is also recommended and will show any dilated bowel and mucosal oedema, but strictures are uncommon. The severity of the inflammation associated with UC can be categorised with the worst cases being severe and progressing to fulminant colitis (Kamm 1999). Disease severity can be categorised using Truelove and Witts (1955), see Table 4.1.

Medical therapy for IBD

Currently the first line therapy for the treatment of IBD is 5-ASAs (5-aminosalicylic acid compounds) and often steroids to gain remission. The second line of therapy is immunosuppression and finally the third line of drug options is the biologicals. There are also other drugs used in IBD such as thalidomide, antibiotics and apheresis. The aims of therapy are to induce and maintain remission.

5-ASAs (5-aminosalicylic acid compounds)

5-ASAs are anti-inflammatory drugs that act locally on the bowel mucosa. These drugs contain salicylate bonded to various carrying agents that are transported to the colon and then absorbed (Rayhorn & Rayhorn 2002b). 5-ASAs have some benefit in the treatment of those with acute mild to moderate disease (Nightingale 2004) and can be useful to maintain remission in UC (Gisbert *et al.* 2002). There are a number of drugs within this category including:

- sulphasalazine
- mesalazine
- asacol
- pentasa
- olsalazide
- balsalazide (colazide).

Most of the 5-ASA compounds are licensed for use in UC; additionally asacol is also indicated for use in Crohn's disease. However these drugs are commonly used for both conditions. Sulphasalazine is a 5-ASA linked to sulphapyridine (the carrier molecule) and has been the standard treatment of UC since being developed in the 1950s (Rowlinson 1999b). Many patients cannot tolerate it due to the high incidence of side effects, one of which is rare but reversible oligospermia (a reduced sperm count). Alongside oral mesalazine are rectal preparations available as suppositories and enemas (foam and liquid) that are useful for left-sided disease. The newer 5-ASAs do not contain sulphur and are therefore better tolerated. Balsalazide is the newest 5-ASA therapy.

Patients with mild to moderate Crohn's disease are generally treated with 5-ASAs (Fow & Grossman 2007). 5-ASAs can be useful to treat and maintain remission in those with colonic Crohn's disease (Kamm 1999) particularly post surgery (Gisbert *et al.* 2002).

Side effects of 5-ASAs include haematological abnormalities and nephrotoxicity; therefore blood monitoring is essential.

Corticosteroids

The most commonly used drugs for an IBD flare are corticosteroids, such as prednisolone (Rowlinson 1999b). Corticosteroids have been used since the 1950s with good effect. Often a short, reducing course of oral prednisolone is highly effective for acute exacerbations. Steroids are not suitable to maintain remission and thus long-term usage should be avoided (Smith & Watson 2005). Corticosteroids do control symptoms but only 30% reach endoscopic remission (Truelove & Witts 1955). Some patients do not respond to steroids and others become steroid dependent and are unable to remain disease free without steroids, so less than 50% of patients benefit from corticosteroid therapy (Feagan 2007).

Hospitalisation and intravenous hydrocortisone may be used for severe episodes. Rectal steroid preparations may be useful for distal disease (Kamm 1999) with less risk of systemic reaction.

The common side effects of corticosteroids are weight gain, acne, fluid retention and mood swings. The patient also needs to be advised that sudden withdrawal of steroids can precipitate adrenal crisis and potentially death; thus a reducing dose is required. It is also necessary to consider the potential side effects including developing hypertension, osteoporosis, diabetes and there is also an increased risk of infections due to an altered immune response (Hall *et al.* 2007a). It is also advisable to prescribe calcium and vitamin D supplements when taking steroids (Rayhorn & Rayhorn 2002b).

Budesonide is a newer type of corticosteroid for treating mild to moderate Crohn's disease (Rayhorn & Rayhorn 2002b) that is effective in the terminal ileum and right colon and has fewer side effects (Nightingale 2004). The efficacy of the budesonide enemas with fewer associated side effects for distal UC is also encouraging (Marín-Jiménez & Peña 2006).

Immunosuppressant therapy

Immunosuppressant therapy includes azathioprine, methotrexate, 6-mercaptopurine (6MP) and ciclosporin (Rowlinson 1999b). These drugs are useful for refractory Crohn's disease, helping to achieve and maintain clinical remission and avoid surgery. However, although these drugs are prescribed for patients with steroid dependent or resistant disease the data to support this practice is sparse (Feagan 2007). These types of medication probably work by decreasing the uncontrolled immune response associated with IBD, but more than four months of therapy are required to obtain a benefit (Rayhorn & Rayhorn 2002b). 6-mercaptopurine is an azathioprine metabolite and is effectively the same drug. Azathioprine and 6-mercaptopurine are very useful for patients, who have failed, were intolerant to or who have frequent relapses despite the use of 5-ASA and steroids and can also be effective maintenance treatment.

Azathioprine and 6-mercaptopurine are beneficial in about a third of patients, but take up to 12 weeks for a clinical response (Buckton 2003). Azathioprine is most commonly used for maintaining long-term remission. These medications are associated with some rare but serious side effects, including leucopaenia (low white cell count), that necessitate careful screening and regular blood monitoring. Other side effects include nausea, vomiting, flu-like symptoms, bone marrow suppression, pancreatitis and hepatitis. An increased cancer risk is a possibility of long-term therapy, but risks are very low (Rampton & Shanahan 2006).

Methotrexate is a cytotoxic agent and is an effective option for patients with moderate refractory, steroid dependent or resistant Crohn's disease. Methotrexate is used where azathioprine and 6MP are not tolerated or are ineffective. Methotrexate can be given as a subcutaneous injection or taken orally. Side effects include rash, nausea, diarrhoea and/or stomatitis (Nightingale 2004). Methotrexate as an adjunct with infliximab is useful for patients with moderate to severe, active Crohn's disease. However, methotrexate should not be used in pregnancy or when breast-feeding. In fact pregnancy should be avoided for three to six months following cessation of methotrexate as it is teratogenic. Regular blood monitoring is required while on treatment. The effectiveness of methotrexate remains controversial for UC (Buckton 2003). Intravenous ciclosporin is used to treat severe acute UC that does not respond to intravenous steroids (Rayhorn & Rayhorn 2002b).

Biological therapy

Biological therapies licensed for IBD are Remicade (infliximab) and Humira (adalimumab). Infliximab is a monoclonal chimeric (mouse/human) antibody that binds to and blocks the action of the pro-inflammatory cytokines TNF-α that causes inflammation (Bard 2003). Infliximab was the first of this drug type to be licensed in the UK in 1999. Infliximab is designed to suppress inflammation and thus symptoms and to maintain remission without the need for steroids (Rayhorn & Rayhorn 2002b). Infliximab is given as an intravenous infusion, initially at weeks zero, two and six and if responding every eight weeks. Infliximab has been associated with healing in moderate to severe active Crohn's disease and perianal fistula closure (Rayhorn & Rayhorn 2002b), shown in a variety of studies (Hanauer *et al.* 2002; Lichtenstein *et al.* 2005). Repeated infusions seem to maintain clinical response and remission, but long-term safety is uncertain. It should be remembered that as the immune system is suppressed these patients are at risk of infections and therefore patients require regular assessment prior to infusions.

Infliximab has been shown in studies to be useful in treating UC (Rutgeerts *et al.* 2005). There are also suggestions that new drugs natalizumab and visilizumab are likely to be effective for treatment of severe ulcerative colitis (Feagan 2007).

Adalimumab is a fully humanised IgG anti-TNFα monoclonal antibody, given by subcutaneous injection. There have been a variety of trials carried out on adalimumab for Crohn's disease (Colombel *et al.* 2007; Hanauer *et al.* 2006; Papadakis *et al.* 2005; Sandborn *et al.* 2004; Sandborn *et al.* 2007a; Sandborn *et al.* 2007b). Initial dosing is 160 mg at week zero, 80 mg at week two and then an injection of 40 mg on alternate weeks (Hanauer *et al.* 2006). There is some evidence that if there is a loss of response the drug can be increased to weekly injections to maintain efficacy. Adalimumab received licensing in the UK in 2007.

Biological compounds are expensive but if surgery and other hospitalisation are prevented this should be also considered (Lichtenstein 2007).

Apheresis

Another therapy for UC is apheresis, which is a type of centrifuge removal of leukocytes from the blood. It is associated with few side effects but efficacy is yet to be proven (Sandborn 2006).

Thalidomide

Thalidomide has received bad press previously and pregnancy needs to be avoided. However it has been shown to be an effective short-term treatment in Crohn's disease. There are a number of side effects which limit its use (Bariol *et al.* 2002), these include peripheral neuropathy and drowsiness.

Antibiotics

Antibiotics such as metronidazole and ciprofloxacin are useful for patients with perianal Crohn's disease, such as fistulae and abscesses (Hall *et al.*

2007a). Metronidazole can be useful to fight coexisting infection and anti-biotics also exert immunomodulating effects (Rayhorn & Rayhorn 2002b).

Other medication

Antidiarrhoeal agents including loperamide and codeine phosphate are used sparingly and with caution to decrease gastrointestinal motility (Rayhorn & Rayhorn 2002b). In the presence of active inflammation or infection they are contraindicated due to the risk of toxic bowel dilation and potentially perforation. Antidiarrhoeal medication should be generally avoided in those with UC.

Non-steroidal anti-inflammatory drugs such as ibuprofen, should not be used as pain relief for patients with Crohn's disease, the rationale being that these types of drugs have been shown to exacerbate bowel symptoms (Rayhorn & Rayhorn 2002b).

Dietary therapy for IBD

For children and adolescents growth may be retarded if there is inadequate nutrition (Kamm 1999). Liquid diet can be very beneficial either taken orally or via a nasogastric tube.

Oral liquid diets as the only source of nutrition improve Crohn's disease activity (Kamm 1999). These can include polymeric diets that are simple proteins or elemental diets that consist of amino acids. Additionally polymeric feeds are generally better tolerated and seem to be as effective as elemental diets. The exact mechanisms of the action are uncertain, but may be due to anti-inflammatory effects (Nightingale 2004). Remission rates are comparable to those of steroids, especially in children (Rayhorn & Rayhorn 2002b). Typically symptoms will recur rapidly when diet is re-introduced.

It is thought that fish oils can also be anti-inflammatory. Good general nutrition is important to try and achieve, particularly with the risk of malabsorption with Crohn's disease.

There is evidence to support the use of probiotics for mild or moderate ulcerative colitis (Fedorak 2007). Probiotics are live bacteria ingested to improve health (Hart 2003). Studies report maintaining remission with probiotics (Ishikawa *et al.* 2003) and inducing remission in UC (Tursi *et al.* 2004). Currently there is no strong evidence for the efficacy of probiotics in Crohn's disease (Fedorak 2007).

There are limited data on prebiotics, which are carbohydrates that encourage the growth of beneficial colonic bacteria in the effective treatment of Crohn's disease (Lindsay *et al.* 2006). Studies currently on the use of prebiotics and probiotics are limited but some patients do report a benefit.

Surgery for Crohn's disease

There are a number of indications for surgery in patients suffering from Crohn's disease, however surgery is generally reserved for complicated or severe disease of limited extent. Within ten years of diagnosis almost half of the patients have had an intestinal resection, rising to more than 75% within 20 years of onset and 90% within 30 years (Rayhorn & Rayhorn 2002b). For those having surgery 40% will need further surgery within ten years (Kamm 1999). It is recognised that there is a need to minimise resections due to the risk of a short bowel resulting from this. One method of achieving this is to perform a strictureplasty rather than a resection for strictures. This preserves bowel length by opening and resuturing the stricture to widen the lumen without removing the area of bowel. Surgery can include a temporary or permanent stoma.

The indications for surgery in patients with Crohn's disease are:

- abscesses that do not respond to radiological or percutaneous drainage;
- bowel obstruction that does not respond to medical or endoscopic therapy;
- a limited segment of diseased bowel that is not responding to maximum medical therapy and causing severe symptoms;
- perianal infection that requires drainage with a seton stitch (a stitch that remains in situ in the perianal area to allow drainage of infection);
- strictures that cause obstruction and are not responding to medical therapy.

(Kamm 1999)

Surgery for ulcerative colitis

Of patients with UC, 30–40% will have surgery (Nicholls 1997) and about 25% of patients will have a colectomy within the first ten years of diagnosis. Situations that may lead to surgery are:

- an acute, severe disease flare;
- failed medical therapy;
- toxic dilation of the colon;
- bleeding;
- pre-cancerous changes in the colon;
- bowel perforation (which is associated with a high mortality rate).

There are three surgical options:

- restorative proctocolectomy (RPC) and ileoanal pouch (performed in up to three operations);
- pan-proctocolectomy and permanent ileostomy;
- sub-total colectomy and ileorectal anastomosis.

There are benefits and complications associated with each procedure that need to be discussed in detail with the patient for them to make an informed choice on the best option for them (see Chapter 10 on intestinal pouches).

Ishikawa H, Akedo I, Umesaki Y, Tanaka R, Imaoka A *et al.* (2003) Randomized controlled trial of the effect of bifidobacteria-fermented milk on ulcerative colitis. *Journal of the American College of Nutrition.* **22(1)**: 56–63.

Jewell DP, Chapman RGW & Mortensen N (1992) *Ulcerative Colitis and Crohn's Disease.* London: Churchill Livingstone.

Kamm MA (1999) *Inflammatory Bowel Disease.* 2nd edn. London: Martin Dunitz.

Kurina LM, Goldacre MJ, Yeates D & Gill LR (2001) Depression and anxiety in people with inflammatory bowel disease. *Journal of Epidemiology and Community Health.* **55(10)**: 716–20.

Lichtenstein GR (2007) Medical management of Crohn's disease in 2006: what's on the horizon? *American Journal of Gastroenterology.* **102(S1)**: S2–S6.

Lichtenstein GR, Yan S, Bala M, Blank M & Sands BE (2005) Infliximab maintenance treatment reduces hospitalisations, surgeries, and procedures in fistulizing Crohn's disease. *Gastroenterology.* **128**: 862–9.

Lindsay JO, Whelan K, Stagg AJ, Gobin P, Al-Hassi HO *et al.* (2006) Clinical, micro-biological, and immunological effects of fructo-oligosaccharide in patients with Crohn's disease. *Gut.* **55(3)**: 348–55.

Mahadevan U, Sandborn WJ, Li D-K, Hakimian S, Kane S *et al.* (2007) Pregnancy outcomes in women with inflammatory bowel disease; a large community-based study from northern California. *Gastroenterology.* **133(4)**: 1106–12.

Marín-Jiménez I & Peña AS (2006) Budesonide for ulcerative colitis. *Revista Espanola de Enfermedades Digestivas.* **98(5)**: 362–73.

Mason I (2001) Inflammatory bowel disease. *Nursing Times.* **97(9)**: 33–5.

Metcalf C (1994) Effects of pregnancy on ulcerative colitis and Crohn's disease. *Professional Nurse.* **9(10)**: 685–8.

Nicholls RJ (1997) Ulcerative colitis. In: Phillips RKS (ed) *Colorectal Surgery. A Companion to Specialist Surgical Practice.* London: W.B. Saunders.

Nightingale A (2004) An overview of the diagnosis and management of Crohn's disease. *Gastrointestinal Nursing.* **2(4)**: 31–9.

Papadakis KA, Shaye OA, Vasiliauskas EA, Ippoliti A, Dubinsky MC *et al.* (2005) Safety and efficacy of adalimumab (D2E7) in Crohn's disease patients with an attenuated response to infliximab. *American Journal of Gastroenterology.* **100**: 75–9.

Rampton DA & Shanahan F (2006) *Fast Facts: Inflammatory Bowel Disease.* 2nd edn. Oxford: Health Press.

Rayhorn N & Rayhorn DJ (2002a) Inflammatory bowel disease: symptoms in the bowel and beyond. *The Nurse Practitioner.* **27(11)**: 13–27.

Rayhorn N & Rayhorn DJ (2002b) An in-depth look at inflammatory bowel disease. *Nursing.* **32(7)**: 36–43.

Rowlinson A (1999a) Inflammatory bowel disease 1: aetiology and pathogenesis. *British Journal of Nursing.* **8(13)**: 858–62.

Rowlinson A (1999b) Inflammatory bowel disease 2: medical and surgical treatment. *British Journal of Nursing.* **8(14)**: 926–30.

Rowlinson A (1999c) Inflammatory bowel disease 3: importance of partnership in care. *British Journal of Nursing.* **8(15)**: 1013–18.

Rutgeerts P, Sandborn J, Feagan BG, Reinisch W, Olsen A *et al.* (2005) Infliximab for induction and maintenance therapy for ulcerative colitis. *New England Journal of Medicine.* **353(23)**: 2462–76.

Sachar DB (2007) What is the role of endoscopy in inflammatory bowel disease. *American Journal of Gastroenterology.* **102**: S29–S31.

Sandborn WJ (2006) Preliminary data in the use of apheresis in inflammatory bowel disease. *Inflammatory Bowel Diseases.* **12(suppl 1)**: S15–S21.

Sandborn WJ, Sutherland L, Pearson D, May G, Modigliani R *et al.* (1998) Azathio-prine or 6-mercaptopurine for induction of remission in Crohn's disease. *Cochrane*

Database of Systematic Reviews. Issue 3. Art. No.: CD000545. DOI: 10.1002/14651858. CD000545.

Sandborn WJ, Hanauer S, Loftus Jnr EV, Tremaine WJ, Kane S *et al.* (2004) An open-label study of the human anti-TNF monoclonal antibody adalimumab in subjects with prior loss of response or intolerance to infliximab for Crohn's disease. *American Journal of Gastroenterology.* **99**: 1984–9.

Sandborn WJ, Hanauer SB, Rutgeerts PJ, Fedorak RN, Lukas M *et al.* (2007a) Adalimumab for maintenance treatment of Crohn's disease: results of the CLASSIC II trial. *Gut.* **56(9)**: 1232–9.

Sandborn WJ, Rutgeerts P, Enns R, Hanauer SB, Colombel J-F *et al.* (2007b) Adalimumab induction therapy for Crohn's disease previously treated with infliximab – a randomised trial. *Annals of Internal Medicine.* **146(12)**: 829–38.

Shen B (2007) Endoscopic, imaging and histologic evaluation of Crohn's disease and ulcerative colitis. *American Journal of Gastroenterology.* **102(S1)**: S41–S45.

Smith G & Watson R (2005) *Gastrointestinal Nursing.* Oxford: Blackwell Publishing.

Travis SP, Ahmad T, Collier J & Steinhart AH (2005) *Pocket Consultant Gastroenterology.* 3rd edn. Oxford: Blackwell Publishing.

Truelove SC & Witts LJ (1955) Cortisone in ulcerative colitis. *British Medical Journal.* **2**: 1041–8.

Tursi A, Brandimarte G, Giorgetti GM, Forti G, Modeo ME *et al.* (2004) Low-dose balsalazide plus a high-potency probiotic preparation is more effective than balsalazide alone or mesalazine in the treatment of acute mild-to-moderate ulcerative colitis. *Medical Science Monitor.* **10(11)**: PI126–31.

Von Roon AC, Reese G, Teare J, Constantinides V & Darzi AW (2007) The risk of cancer in patients with Crohn's disease. *Diseases of the Colon and Rectum.* **50**: 839–55.

Walters S (2000) *National Association for Colitis & Crohn's Disease (NACC) Audit of IBD.* West Sussex: Aeneas Press.

Ward J & Stanford E (2003) Conditions that may require surgery involving a stoma. In: Elcoat C (ed) *Stoma Care Nursing.* London: Hollister.

Younge L & Norton C (2007) Contribution of specialist nurses managing patients with IBD. British Journal of Nursing. **16(4)**: 208–12.

Chapter 5

Familial Adenomatous Polyposis

Jacquie Wright and Kay Neale

Introduction

Familial adenomatous polyposis (FAP) is a genetically inherited disease, predominantly of the gastrointestinal tract and specifically the colon and rectum. FAP results in the formation of hundreds to thousands of colorectal polyps (adenomas) (see Figure 5.1) and affected patients have a 100% risk of developing bowel cancer if left untreated. FAP is caused by a fault on the APC (adenomatous polyposis coli) gene, which is situated on the long arm of chromosome 5. In a hospital specialising in the care of patients with this condition, it has been possible to maintain a registry dedicated to detection of the disease, to promote the health of those affected and to support these patients and their families.

The Polyposis Registry and research

The Polyposis Registry began as The St Mark's Hospital Polyposis Register in 1924 with the registration of three families by J.P. Lockhart-Mummery (Consultant Surgeon), Cuthbert Dukes (Pathologist) and H.J.R. Bussey (at that time, a pathology technician). There are now 730 families with known polyposis syndromes registered at St Mark's and over 800 patients attending clinics. This includes patients with other rare polyposis syndromes, such as Peutz-Jeghers syndrome and juvenile polyposis syndrome (JPS); also Cowden's disease, which is a rare variant of JPS affecting the skin, intestine, breast and thyroid gland; and MYH associated polyposis (MAP), the only known recessive polyposis syndrome at this time. The majority of patients, however, have FAP.

Cuthbert Dukes' work researching the adenoma-carcinoma sequence initiated investigation of polyposis and the decision to keep a register. By the 1940s the inheritance pattern of FAP had been established so that it was possible to predict which people in a family with the condition were at risk of inheriting it. By 1958 a system for warning people who were at risk had been put into place and prophylactic surgery introduced with such success that Dr Dukes stated:

It would be difficult to find a more promising field for the exercise of cancer control than a polyposis family because both diagnosis and treatment are possible in the precancerous stage and because the results of surgical treatment are excellent. (St Mark's Hospital Polyposis Registry)

Polyposis families continue kindly to consent to participate in research trials and studies. The Polyposis Registry assists in identifying which patients may be suitable for a particular study, but performs a protective function to prevent what might feel like harassment to members of this much-studied group. Due to their personal knowledge of their patients the Registry nursing staff are able to advise research fellows of any patients who may be unhappy to participate, or where difficult personal circumstances should preclude their being approached.

Diagnosing FAP

Dr Dukes and his assistant, H.J.R. Bussey, made a habit of close examination of the colectomy specimens at St Mark's. By the 1960s strict criteria for a clinical diagnosis of FAP had been established and depended upon visualising at least one hundred, but usually hundreds or thousands, of adenomas throughout the colon and rectum (see Figure 5.1). Any person at risk of inheriting FAP would be invited to enter a bowel-screening programme. Bodmer *et al.* (1987) identified the location of the causative gene on the long arm of chromosome 5, later to become known as the APC gene. By 1996 genetic testing via a blood test became available on the NHS to patients at St Mark's. This enables people with FAP to have their blood taken for DNA analysis. If a genetic mutation is found within that family, a blood test is available for relatives who may be at risk, and the need for

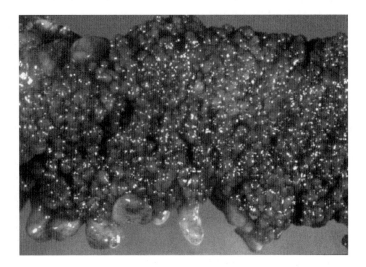

Figure 5.1 Colonic specimen.

regular colonoscopy (and its attendant risks) to detect whether FAP has been inherited is avoided in those testing negative. However, the need for careful genetic counselling and obtaining informed consent prior to any gene testing is of paramount importance, to explain the implications of both a positive and a negative result (a negative result for FAP does not exclude bowel cancer in the future, as that patient remains at population risk and should be advised to contact their GP with any concerns regarding rectal bleeding or change in bowel habit).

FAP is inherited as autosomal dominant and affects male and female offspring equally. This means that the risk to each child of a parent who is affected with FAP is, therefore, 50% of inheriting the disease. At around the age of 12–14, children of affected parents whose genetic mutation has been identified are offered genetic testing. This age has been set as it is known that, at this stage, there is very little chance of any polyps having made much progression. Any child who develops symptoms earlier than this should, of course, be investigated. However, cancer of the bowel has been found at 17 years of age in two patients who were referred to St Mark's and described in a nine-year-old child (Eccles *et al.* 1997). All of these patients had reported rectal bleeding. Testing is not, however, generally performed earlier than 12 years of age and children who are gene positive are rarely symptomatic at this age. The age at which colectomy is recommended will depend on the severity of the polyposis but is usually between the ages of 15–20 and planned to coincide with the school/college/university/work timetable. Also, it is advisable to discuss screening and possible surgery and implications of FAP with adolescents while they are still under the care and control of their parents. Once they have left home, encouraging them to come to hospital for surveillance and treatment may become problematic and, indeed, they may become lost to follow-up and be at a great risk of developing colorectal cancer. Conversely, earlier screening of children could be traumatic and risk alienation, making further surveillance difficult, especially as surgery would not normally be planned for some years.

The initial consultation for gene testing for children at St Mark's Hospital is often done in a dedicated paediatric clinic. The consultation is with a consultant paediatrician who is a specialist in polyposis syndromes. A polyposis specialist nurse, who is able to give genetic counselling, will accompany the paediatrician.

A negative genetic result would mean that the child had not inherited FAP and so could be discharged from follow-up (while being advised of the population risk of developing bowel cancer). A positive result would necessitate dye-spray colonoscopy to determine the number, size and distribution of polyps present to enable planning for a prophylactic colectomy.

Aside from children who attend for genetic testing, there are also the adult relatives of people who are considered to have 'new mutations', i.e. they are the first people in their family to develop FAP – and have no family history of FAP. It is estimated that approximately 20% of new FAP patients seen in clinic have no family history of the disease. Again, if a genetic mutation can be detected in the first affected person (the 'index case'), a blood test may be offered to the rest of the family.

Bowel screening of relatives 'at-risk'

In the event that no genetic mutation has been found in a family (and that is currently the position for approximately 15% of FAP families) bowel screening is the only option. The protocol for screening at-risk relatives of polyposis patients is constantly being reviewed and updated at The Polyposis Registry, as a result of ongoing research and experience (The Polyposis Registry 2006). It is currently recommended that bowel screening for at-risk relatives should take place in the form of flexible sigmoidoscopy at the age of 14. If polyps are seen, a dye-spray colonoscopy should be performed and the number of polyps and histological analysis taken into account in deciding when prophylactic surgery should take place. If no polyps are seen, dye-spray colonoscopy will be planned at five-yearly intervals from the age of 20 years, with annual flexible sigmoidoscopy in the intervening years. The screening continues until any polyps are seen (when surgery may be considered) or, if no polyps are seen, indefinitely.

The risk of being diagnosed with FAP diminishes with age and negative endoscopy, but family history should be considered when contemplating reducing/discontinuing screening. Any person who is at risk of FAP who wishes to stop screening should, after counselling regarding their risk of bowel cancer, be advised to contact their GP/hospital in the event of rectal bleeding or a change in bowel habit. On average polyps become evident in the colon/rectum during adolescence; the practitioner should, however, be alert for onset after the age of 25, as the family may have attenuated FAP (a mild form of polyposis with later onset). A person with FAP, who is not surgically treated, would develop colorectal cancer on average by 39 years of age (Bussey 1975).

Surgery

Surgical treatment for FAP became possible with the increase in medical knowledge and is accessible to all with the advent of the NHS. At St Mark's in 1948, O.V. Lloyd-Davies pioneered the ileorectal anastomosis (IRA) for those with FAP, a turning point for these patients. An IRA obviates the need for a stoma and increases life expectancy and quality of life for those with FAP. The risk of rectal cancer remained but it was thought that as long as patients underwent regular rectal surveillance with removal of large adenomas all would be well; on the whole this was largely proved to be correct and the operation is still the operation of choice for many patients today. In 1977, Sir Alan Parks performed the first restorative proctocolectomy for FAP patients at St Mark's. At the time it was hoped that this would negate the need for follow-up as the colorectal cancer risk had been removed. With fewer people dying from colorectal cancer it soon became evident that those surviving presented with other problems.

There are three prophylactic surgical options that may be considered for these patients:

- colectomy with ileorectal anastomosis (IRA);
- restorative proctocolectomy (with formation of ileoanal pouch) – RPC;
- and, rarely, a total proctocolectomy (with permanent ileostomy) – TPC.

In some centres, these procedures may now be considered using laparoscopic techniques. Laparoscopic surgery is associated with less traumatic effect, improved cosmetic result and reduced recovery time (King *et al.* 2006).

Many centres now opt for the restorative proctocolectomy as first choice surgery. However, it is essential to consider what may be the best operation for the individual.

Colectomy with IRA

Colectomy with IRA is a low-risk operation with good functional results. It is indicated in young patients who have low-density phenotype (where fewer than 1000 polyps are visible) and where the genetic mutation, if known, indicates that the degree of polyposis will not be too severe (this is called a low-density genotype). An IRA is often considered where the young patient has not yet had a family, due to reduced female fertility/fecundity which may arise as a result of pouch surgery (Olsen *et al.* 2003). However, as the rectum is retained, the risk of developing rectal cancer remains high and the patient should attend for six-monthly flexible sigmoidoscopy to remove any polyps greater than 5 mm in size. Conversion to an ileoanal pouch may be necessary (but not inevitable) in the future. Where severe rectal polyposis develops and surgery is to be avoided (for instance, in the presence of pelvic desmoid disease), chemoprevention may be considered to reduce and regress polyps (Steinbach *et al.* 2000).

Restorative proctocolectomy

Restorative proctocolectomy removes the risk of colorectal cancer, although the risk of polyp recurrence at the anastomosis may depend on whether the pouch is stapled or hand-sewn at the anastomosis. An RPC is more likely to be the operation of choice in older, new patients (over 25 years old). An RPC may also be done as a conversion of an IRA if rectal polyps become too numerous or histologically worrying. It is likely that an RPC would be considered where there is a high-density phenotype or the genotype indicates that polyposis will be severe (high-density genotype) and is performed for some patients with colorectal cancer. It may also be considered where there is a family history of desmoid disease, where the aim would be to perform the minimum number of abdominal surgical interventions.

Flexible pouchoscopy is recommended on a yearly basis as it is recognised that, although it is constructed from a part of the small intestine which is not usually at risk in FAP patients, adenomas do arise in the body of the pouch and remaining rectal tissue at the pouch–anal anastomosis is susceptible to the formation of adenomas (Groves *et al.* 2005). Annual blood tests for haemoglobin, vitamin B_{12} and serum folate levels should also be performed. While RPC reduces the risk of colonic malignancy compared to an IRA, the disadvantages are that surgery is more complex with a higher complication rate, a temporary ileostomy is required (with the risk of permanent ileostomy) and there is a risk to fertility and fecundity, as previously mentioned. In addition there is a small, but identifiable, risk to sexual function in males.

Total/panproctocolectomy

A total or panproctocolectomy and formation of an end ileostomy is not generally considered. However in situations such as a low rectal cancer, where there is desmoid involvement, where there is anal sphincter deficiency or there is another technical reason that an RPC cannot be done, it may be required.

Upper GI disease

Colorectal cancer is the main cause of death in untreated patients with FAP. Once the risk of colorectal cancer is removed after colectomy/RPC, one of the main causes of death in patients with FAP is duodenal cancer. Approximately 90% of patients with FAP have duodenal adenomas by the age of 70 and of these 5–10% progress to duodenal cancer (Groves *et al.* 2002). Duodenal adenomas are more difficult to treat at endoscopy and a general anaesthetic is required for endoscopic therapeutic work.

Planned surveillance of the duodenum, using a side-viewing endoscope, commences at age 25, as it is known that upper GI disease is rarely problematic (although it may be present) before that age. A side-viewing endoscope is essential in order to visualise the ampullary region, which is particularly affected in FAP and not well visualised with standard forward-viewing endoscopy. The extent of duodenal disease and size of polyps (if any), along with the histology, indicates the severity of the disease and dictates the date at which the procedure should be repeated, calculated using the Spigelman staging system (see Table 5.1). The risk of duodenal cancer increases with a higher Spigelman staging score and at Spigelman Stage IV there is a 36% risk at 10 years of developing duodenal cancer (Groves *et al.* 2002).

Where Spigelman Stage III duodenal disease is diagnosed, chemoprevention may be considered in an attempt to regress and reduce polyp size and number (Phillips *et al.* 2002). An endoscopic ultrasound may be required to assess the ampullary region and if progression to Spigelman Stage IV duodenal disease occurs, the patient should be considered for surgery, currently in the form of prophylactic duodenectomy.

Table 5.1   (a) Spigelman staging system

Spigelman Stage	Points	Recommendation
0 & I	0–4	5-yearly endoscopy
II	5–6	3-yearly endoscopy
III	7–8	Annual endoscopy +/– endoscopic therapy. May benefit from chemoprevention
IV	9–12	Should be considered for surgery and/or endoscopic therapy and chemoprevention

(b) Calculating the Spigelman stage

No. of polyps	1–4	5–20	> 20
Size of polyps	1–4 mm	5–10 mm	>10 mm
Histology	Tubular adenoma	Tubulovillous adenoma	Villous adenoma
Dysplasia	Mild	Moderate	Severe
Points to be allocated	1	2	3

Box 5.1   Extra-colonic manifestations

Duodenal adenomas
Fundic gland polyps
Osteomas
Epidermoid cysts
Abnormal dentition
Desmoid tumours
Congenital hypertrophy of the retinal pigment epithelium (CHRPE)
Adrenal adenomas
Thyroid cancer
Hepatoblastoma
Increased risk of cancer in general

Extra-colonic manifestations (ECMs)

Patients with FAP may or may not present with other physical signs that are associated with the disease. These extra-colonic manifestations are listed in Box 5.1. ECMs are benign conditions; rarely, however, desmoid tumours and duodenal polyps may be problematic and occasionally life threatening. There is also an increased incidence of cancer outside of the GI tract; notably thyroid.

It can be sometimes noted that children of an affected parent may display signs of ECM prior to formal testing/screening. It is, however, by no means certain that a child with an osteoma or with abnormal dentition will prove to have FAP, as these are not uncommon in the general population, but it is more likely. Epidermoid cysts are extremely rare in children (Leppard & Bussey 1975) and so their appearance in the child of an affected parent is more likely to be of significance. Congenital hypertrophy of the retinal pigment epithelium (CHRPE) may be an indicator of the co-existence of FAP. However, only an ophthalmologist with specialised equipment can diagnose this. People not affected with FAP may have CHRPE and CHRPE is not always present in FAP and if a gene test is available for the child, eye testing is unnecessary. Fundic gland polyps (FGPs) are present in 50% of FAP patients (Domizio *et al.* 1990) and are visible when the upper gastrointestinal tract is examined. Although these are generally benign, if there is carpeting of FGPs, a gastric adenoma may go undetected; fortunately this is rare. However, FGPs on their own may not be considered an indicator of FAP as it is known that long-term proton pump inhibitor (PPI) use may result in their growth.

Desmoid disease

Desmoid tumours are non-metastasising, fibrous tumours (see Figure 5.2). There is an incidence of approximately 15% in people with FAP (Sturt *et al.* 2004) and they are more likely to occur in patients with a family history of desmoid disease. Desmoid tumours do occur in the general

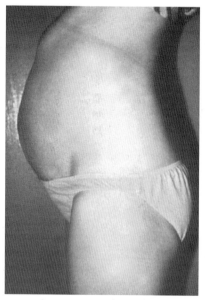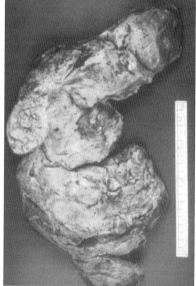

Figure 5.2 Desmoid tumour.

population, but with a much-reduced incidence. Approximately 70% of desmoids in patients with FAP are intra-abdominal or mesenteric, in contrast to sporadic desmoids, which are generally elsewhere on the body. Occasionally, it is a diagnosis of a desmoid tumour that may alert the clinician to the fact that the patient may have an underlying diagnosis of FAP. If a desmoid tumour is suspected, CT scanning is the imaging tool of choice to confirm the diagnosis. In patients known to have FAP a CT scan is not immediately necessary if the desmoid is not problematic as in the majority of cases, patients remain asymptomatic and desmoids do not necessarily progress; they may undergo cycles of progression and resolution or resolve completely.

It is known that, while a patient may have an inherited propensity to develop desmoid disease, surgery may stimulate growth (Clark *et al.* 1999). Therefore it is not uncommon to note the presence of an abdominal desmoid tumour on palpation of the abdomen of a patient who has undergone prophylactic colectomy eighteen months to two years earlier and who is susceptible to the disease. It is also sometimes possible, at the time of the primary surgery, that desmoid precursor lesions may be noted in the mesentery.

Although desmoids are benign tumours, once prophylactic colectomy and regular screening have removed the risk of colorectal cancer, desmoids are one of the major causes of FAP-related deaths, along with duodenal/ ampullary cancer (Clark & Phillips 1996). Desmoid tumours become problematic when they arise in the small bowel mesentery and continue to grow large. The pressure of the enlarging desmoid on the small bowel, ureters and major blood vessels can cause obstruction.

For intra-abdominal disease, currently the first line of treatment for potentially problematic, enlarging desmoids are non-steroidal anti-inflammatory drugs (NSAIDs) followed by inclusion of an anti-oestrogen. Surgical resection can be hazardous when desmoids arise in the mesentery, due to their vascular nature. If surgery is necessary it should be performed in specialist centres. Desmoids at extra-abdominal sites or in the abdominal wall should be considered for surgical resection as the first line of treatment. With all desmoid surgery recurrence is a major problem (Latchford *et al.* 2006).

The risk of desmoid disease is, therefore, always a major consideration when planning any abdominal surgery. Whether a primary colectomy, conversion of the IRA to an ileoanal pouch or the possibility of a duodenectomy, it is important to check whether there is any family history of desmoid disease or any desmoid palpable and if so, a CT scan should be performed.

An accessible expert centre

The Polyposis Registry employs specialist nurses to care for patients with polyposis syndromes. These patients have to contend with a rare, lifelong, life-threatening condition that may have already claimed the lives of many of their relatives. The patients' interests are served by having expert clinicians who can impart knowledge, reassure and support them. In addition to having in-depth knowledge of the condition the specialist nurses get to know the individual patients and their families and are able to build an understanding and professional relationship with them. They provide a point of contact for the patients, their families and their GPs. Specialist nurses are also a resource for medical and nursing staff within St Mark's Hospital and as a tertiary referral centre, they are able to offer help and advice to other health and social work professionals involved in caring for patients across the country, both attending St Mark's Hospital and being seen elsewhere. A helpline is available to patients and professionals alike. It is essential that heath care professionals are aware of this resource in order to provide optimum care for their patients with FAP.

Patients with FAP, wherever they are cared for, should be monitored regularly as described earlier, both endoscopically and in the outpatient clinic, to prevent malignancy. Most find it reassuring to be able to understand how monitoring is planned, histological progression of their polyps, why their endoscopic screening is increased, why specific drugs may be used and the need for other intestinal imaging and if necessary, for surgery. Patients should be able to be as informed as they wish and with the added provision of nursing time and encouragement many become 'expert patients' and conversant with most aspects of their care.

Equally, it is important that those patients who cannot or do not wish to face their diagnosis are not confronted with more information than they are willing to accept. There are many reasons why these patients may choose not to participate in their care. Inheriting a potentially fatal disease from a parent can (and often does) result in that parent being 'blamed' for passing on their 'bad gene'; parents feel guilty for their child inheriting a disease which may claim their lives prematurely; affected siblings may feel aggrieved that they and not their unaffected sibling have been afflicted and unaffected siblings may feel guilty that their brother/sister has FAP while they do not. Aside from guilt and blame there is fear for some that they have a disease that has resulted in the death of their parent/aunt/uncle/grandparent and fear that they may not be around for their own children as they grow and may also have to cope with the condition.

The Polyposis Registry is committed to the needs of these people. The nurse practitioner is employed to see patients with polyposis syndromes for their follow-up alongside each surgical consultant clinic in place of their regular doctor's appointment. Another specialist nurse is available to see any other patient with polyposis within the doctor's clinic. The nurse practitioner in endoscopy, specialising in polyposis also ensures continuity of care. This regular face-to-face contact helps the patients to feel comfortable in contacting the Registry with any worries. It also helps to reinforce the importance of attendance, enhancing the patients' understanding of the physical risks of non-compliance with screening. Rates of non-attendance have been reduced by the Registry's policy of determinedly persuading patients to attend. It is essential to consider that any patient lost to follow-up may have children who will not therefore be screened and who will be at risk of developing colorectal cancer when they grow older.

FAP is a complex condition and individual cases vary. Any health professional or patient requiring information is welcome to contact the Polyposis Registry at St Mark's Hospital.

References

Bodmer WF, Bailey CJ, Bodmer J, Bussey HJR, Ellis A *et al.* (1987) Localisation of the gene for Familial Adenomatous Polyposis on chromosome 5. *Nature.* **328(6131)**: 614–16.

Bussey HJR (1975) *Familial Polyposis Coli.* Baltimore: The Johns Hopkins University Press.

Clark SK & Phillips RKS (1996) Desmoids in familial adenomatous polyposis. *British Journal of Surgery.* **83(11)**: 1494–1504.

Clark SK, Neale KF, Landgrebe JC & Phillips RKS (1999) Desmoid tumours complicating familial adenomatous polyposis. *British Journal of Surgery.* **86(9)**: 1185–9.

Domizio P, Talbot IC, Spigelman AD, Williams CB & Phillips RKS (1990) Upper gastrointestinal pathology in familial adenomatous polyposis; results from a prospective study of 102 patients. *Journal of Clinical Pathology.* **43(9)**: 738–43.

Eccles DM, Lunt PW, Wallis Y, Griffiths M, Sandhu B *et al.* (1997) An unusually severe phenotype for familial adenomatous polyposis. *Archives of Disease in Childhood.* **77(5)**: 431–5.

Groves CJ, Saunders BP, Spigelman AD & Phillips RKS (2002) Duodenal cancer in patients with familial adenomatous polyposis (FAP): results of a 10 year prospective study. *Gut.* **50(5)**: 636–41.

Groves CJ, Beveridge G, Swain DJ, Saunders BP, Talbot IC *et al.* (2005) Prevalence and morphology of pouch and ileal adenomas in familial adenomatous polyposis. *Diseases of the Colon and Rectum.* **48(4)**: 816–23.

King PM, Blazeby JM, Ewings P, Franks PJ, Longman RJ *et al.* (2006) Randomized clinical trial comparing laparoscopic and open surgery for colorectal cancer within an enhanced recovery programme. *British Journal of Surgery.* **93(3)**: 300–8.

Latchford AR, Sturt NJH, Neale K, Rogers PA & Phillips RKS (2006) A 10-year review of surgery for desmoid disease associated with familial adenomatous polyposis. *British Journal of Surgery.* **93(10)**: 1258–64.

Leppard B & Bussey HJR (1975) Epidermoid cysts, polyposis coli and Gardner's syndrome. *British Journal of Surgery.* **62(5)**: 387–93.

Olsen KO, Juul S, Bulow S, Jarvinen HJ, Bakka A *et al.* (2003) Female fecundity before and after operation for familial adenomatous polyposis. *British Journal of Surgery.* **90(2)**: 227–31.

Phillips RKS, Wallace MH & Lynch PM (2002) A randomised, double blind, placebo controlled study of celecoxib, a selective cyclooxygenase 2 inhibitor, on duodenal polyposis in familial adenomatous polyposis. *Gut.* **50(6)**: 857–60.

Polyposis Registry (2006) *Protocol for the Management of Patients with Polyposis: A Guide for Medical Staff.* London: St Mark's Hospital.

Steinbach G, Lynch PM, Phillips RK, Wallace MH, Hawk E *et al.* (2000) The effect of celecoxib, a cyclooxygenase-2 inhibitor, in familial adenomatous polyposis. *New England Journal of Medicine.* **342(26)**: 1946–52.

Sturt NJH, Gallagher MC, Bassett P, Philp CR, Neale KF *et al.* (2004) Evidence for genetic predisposition to desmoid tumours in familial adenomatous polyposis independent of the germline APC mutation. *Gut.* **53(12)**: 1832–6.

Chapter 6

Continence

Julie Duncan and Christine Norton

Introduction

Bladder and bowel control is a social norm and therefore any deviation from this can lead to stigma and social isolation. Incontinence often invokes negative attitudes from society and even health care professionals. There are also incorrectly held beliefs about incontinence, for example, that it is only associated with older adults or those with disabilities. In reality incontinence transcends age, sex and race affecting approximately two per cent of the general population (faecal incontinence) and 8.5% for urinary incontinence. There are studies which report prevalence of lower urinary tract symptoms as approximately 40%; however, the majority of those affected do not report these symptoms as troublesome. Symptoms of incontinence have been shown to affect quality of life negatively and have harmful consequences physically, psychologically and socially.

This chapter will explore the mechanisms of urinary and faecal continence, the causes of incontinence and the resultant investigations and treatments, including conservative and surgical management. It is not meant as an extensive text but is aimed at providing an overview of the management of incontinence and giving the reader a basis for further reading and exploration.

Normal bladder and bowel control

Bowel and bladder control is normally achieved by the age of three through the development of physical maturation and socialisation. Continence is a subconscious, though largely voluntary, function. Normal bowel function is defined as anything between three times per day to three times per week. There are three important structures in bowel continence: the colon, rectum and anal sphincter muscles. Faeces move through the colon in peristaltic waves, where water is reabsorbed, forming a fairly solid matter by the time it reaches the sigmoid colon and rectum. The rectum is essentially a reservoir. As the rectum fills the rectal muscles relax to accommodate the increasing volume. This is termed rectal compliance. The anal sphincters are made up of two circles of muscle (internal and external anal sphincters) surrounding the anal canal. The internal anal sphincter (IAS) is composed of smooth, circular muscle that can maintain involuntary, tonic contraction for long periods of time. Thus the internal sphincter acts as a 'seal' to maintain continence. Disruption to the IAS can result in passive leakage of faeces or flatus incontinence. The external anal sphincter (EAS) is a fatigable striated muscle under voluntary control. Disruption or weakness of this muscle can lead to urgency and urge faecal incontinence. Failure in the function of the colon, rectum or sphincters can lead to bowel control issues either due to poor muscle control, diarrhoea, severe constipation, or inadequate rectal compliance.

Similarly the bladder relies on both voluntary and involuntary control. The bladder is a flexible sac of muscle (detrusor muscle) that stores urine. Urine is retained in the bladder by the urethral sphincter and pelvic floor muscles. There are essentially two phases of bladder function: filling and voiding. As the bladder fills with urine the urethral sphincters maintain a high pressure whilst the bladder itself relaxes and expands, creating a reservoir. When voiding, the urethral and pelvic floor muscles relax and a contraction of the detrusor muscle expels the urine. Stress urinary incontinence is the involuntary leakage of urine associated with exertion or actions such as coughing or sneezing and is most usually associated with weakness of the sphincter or pelvic floor muscles. Urge urinary incontinence is associated with, or preceded by, urgency which is difficult to defer. It is often (although not always) associated with an overactive detrusor muscle. 'Overactive bladder' is the preferred term for the syndrome of urinary frequency and urgency, with or without frank incontinence. 'Overflow' incontinence is secondary to incomplete bladder emptying and a volume of residual urine (e.g. with prostatic enlargement).

Both bladder and bowel control are also supported by the pelvic floor muscles and complex nerve pathways. Any disruption to these mechanisms can affect bladder and bowel function.

Risk factors for incontinence

For some there will be an obvious and straightforward cause for their incontinence but for others it will be multi-factorial and more difficult to determine. Table 6.1 lists some of these factors.

Obstetric trauma to the pelvic floor

Sultan *et al.* (1993) found evidence of new anal sphincter damage in one-third of women following their first vaginal delivery. The obstetric risk factors associated with faecal incontinence are thought to be:

- vaginal delivery;
- prolonged second stage of delivery;
- instrumental delivery (particularly forceps);
- large birth weight (over 4 kg);
- first baby;
- higher maternal age;
- abnormal presentation.

Table 6.1   Risk factors for incontinence

Urinary incontinence	Faecal incontinence
Pregnancy and delivery, multiparity, obstetric trauma, difficult or instrumented delivery	Vaginal delivery, multiparity, obstetric trauma, difficult or instrumented delivery
Functional impairment, e.g. immobility	Functional impairment, e.g. immobility
Urinary tract infection or bladder disease	Underlying bowel condition (e.g. inflammatory bowel disease) or anorectal pathology (e.g. prolapse, haemorrhoids)
Neurological disease or injury	Neurological disease or injury
Obesity	Obesity
Cognitive impairment	Cognitive impairment
Increasing age and frailty	Increasing age and frailty
Congenital abnormality	Congenital abnormality
Incomplete bladder emptying (e.g. prostatic enlargement)	Iatrogenic trauma (e.g. sphincterotomy)
Prolapse of uterus or bladder	Faecal impaction
Constipation and straining	Severe constipation in children
Medications (e.g. diuretics)	Medications with constipation or diarrhoea as side effects

The anterior portion of the pelvic floor may become detached from its attachments to the pelvic rim, leading to immediate or later urinary symptoms. Goldberg *et al.* (2003) found an association between multiple pregnancy and childbirth with faecal and flatus incontinence. In those surveyed 10% reported symptoms of faecal incontinence. This can be compared to population data that estimates prevalence of faecal incontinence in the general population to be approximately 2%. It has been shown that up to 30% of women have post partum urinary incontinence (Wilson *et al.* 1996).

Age

The incidence of both urinary and faecal incontinence has been shown to increase with age. It is thought this may not necessarily relate to the ageing process itself but may be as a result of multiple factors including menopause, polypharmacy, constipation, reduced mobility, cognitive impairment and underlying chronic conditions. Edwards & Jones (2001) report that older adults living at home have a prevalence rate of 3% for faecal incontinence and that 69% of those had co-existent urinary incontinence.

This prevalence has been shown to increase markedly in older adults living in institutions such as nursing homes.

Loening-Baucke (2007) retrospectively reviewed children aged 4–17 years old who had attended a primary care paediatric clinic. She found a 10.5% prevalence of urinary incontinence and 4.4% for faecal incontinence. This was strongly associated with constipation. All these studies highlight the complexity in assessing incidence, prevalence and causation for these conditions.

Investigations

In Table 6.2 are listed some of the investigations which *may* be required to assess urinary or faecal incontinence.

It is important to note that good clinical assessment including history taking (Norton & Chelvanayagam 2000) and physical assessment is the basis for a treatment pathway for this group of patients. The investigations listed in Table 6.2 have been listed as potential investigations rather than essential ones. It may be that a good clinical assessment and examination gives more than adequate information to treat a patient conservatively. The National Institute for Health and Clinical Excellence (NICE 2006; NICE 2007) is clear that the more invasive investigations of urinary or faecal incontinence such as MRI, ultrasound, anorectal physiology or urodynamic studies should not be performed routinely, or at least until after conservative management has been tried. Other investigations may be required to assess an underlying disease causing symptoms of incontinence, such as colonoscopy to assess the cause of diarrhoea or cystoscopy to exclude bladder stones or a tumour.

The porridge enema is a simple novel test to evaluate sphincter function prior to stoma closure particularly in those patients who have had a defunctioning stoma due to major anorectal surgery, sphincter injury or ileoanal pouch formation. Recently this test has been evaluated retrospectively and has been shown to be a positive predictor of continence post stoma closure (Páres *et al.* 2007).

Table 6.2 Investigations

Urinary incontinence	Faecal incontinence
Clinical assessment	Clinical assessment
Midstream urine (MSU) sample for culture and sensitivity analysis	Endoscopy (to assess underlying bowel disorder)
Post-void residual urine (bladder scan)	Barium studies
Urodynamic studies	Endoanal ultrasound scan
Bladder diary	Anorectal physiology studies
Cystoscopy	MRI scan
MRI/CT scans	Evacuation proctography

Treatment of incontinence

Conservative management

Following good assessment conservative management is likely to be the first line of approach to therapeutic intervention. There are a number of conservative therapies that may benefit those with incontinence. These are listed in Table 6.3.

Behavioural therapy (biofeedback)

The term 'biofeedback' refers to the use of immediate visual or auditory feedback on bodily functions not normally consciously controlled. In the management of bladder and bowel incontinence biofeedback may be used to teach pelvic floor exercises and other retraining techniques. It will normally take the form of computer aided biofeedback. An anal or vaginal probe attached to a computer is inserted into the patient. The patient and therapist view the computer screen. The patient is asked to squeeze their pelvic floor muscles and receives immediate feedback as to the strength, duration and co-ordination of pelvic floor contraction from the computer program. However, in practice, biofeedback is normally a package of care involving techniques such as bladder or bowel retraining, pelvic floor exercises, behavioural methods, electrical stimulation and practical management in addition to the computer aided biofeedback techniques. These services are normally nurse or physiotherapist led.

Table 6.3 Conservative management

Urinary incontinence	Faecal incontinence
Patient education	Patient education
Pelvic floor muscle training (stress incontinence and overactive bladder)	Pelvic floor muscle training (anal sphincter exercises)
Anti-muscarinic medication e.g. oxybutynin (overactive bladder)	Anti-diarrhoeal medication (e.g. loperamide)
Bladder retraining (urge resistance)	Bowel retraining (establish a routine with complete evacuation and urge resistance)
Behavioural (biofeedback) therapy	Behavioural (biofeedback) therapy
Electrical stimulation	Electrical stimulation
Caffeine reduction	Caffeine and dietary fibre modification
Practical management techniques (e.g. pads)	Practical management techniques (e.g. anal plugs)
Intravaginal oestrogen	Rectal irrigation
Intermittent self-catheterisation (for large residual urine volume)	Rectal evacuants (e.g. glycerine suppositories)

Biofeedback therapy is considered a useful management strategy for both bowel and bladder incontinence; however, methodological variations in research and practice make it difficult to fully evaluate. Approximately two-thirds of patients will respond to biofeedback therapy and benefits are largely maintained in the long term. However it is difficult to extrapolate which aspects of the therapy are important and useful. One study compared four levels of intervention in women with faecal incontinence in an attempt to answer this (Norton *et al.* 2003). It was hypothesised that biofeedback techniques would provide better results than standard care alone. However, 80% of patients responded and there were no statistical differences over the four groups. This led to a suggestion that issues of time, attention and therapeutic relationship are important factors in biofeedback therapy.

Pelvic floor muscle training

There is evidence that pelvic floor muscle training is an effective management strategy in the treatment of urinary incontinence although the evidence is not strong for faecal incontinence (NICE 2006; NICE 2007). This effect does not seem to be necessarily maintained in the longer term, possibly due to issues with compliance. Another difficulty with the evidence base is a lack of homogeneity in practice and research. There is a lack of consistency in the methods used in teaching pelvic floor exercises and the regimes used. This makes it difficult to fully evaluate the benefits of these minimally invasive therapies. Current recommendations of pelvic floor techniques can be found on the Continence Foundation website (www.continence-foundation.org.uk).

Oestrogen

There is some evidence that topical rather than systemic hormone replacement therapy may be of benefit to post-menopausal women with symptoms of overactive bladder. However, hormone replacement has not been recommended for general use in the treatment of urinary incontinence. There is also some, limited, evidence that hormone replacement may improve symptoms of faecal incontinence.

Practical management

The main focus of the management of bladder and bowel incontinence should be patient focused, symptomatic care. From a good assessment the clinician can establish what is bothersome to the patient and base their interventions accordingly. It is difficult to establish a 'one size fits all' care pathway for this group of patients as their symptoms can be diverse with multiple physical and psychological influences. Recent NICE guidelines for urinary and faecal incontinence have suggested treatment algorithms (NICE 2006; NICE 2007). However, these are merely *guidelines* and each patient's individual requirements need to be considered in their treatment plan. Decisions will need to be made accordingly with the patient.

A structured, stepwise approach is often helpful in clinical practice. For example:

- history taking and physical assessment;
- referral to medical colleague if indicated (e.g. alarm signs, such as rectal bleeding);
- explanation and patient teaching;
- treat underlying cause if relevant (e.g. polypharmacy);
- investigations if appropriate;
- conservative management:
  - bladder or bowel habit training;
  - diet and fluid modification if indicated;
  - pelvic floor muscle training;
  - biofeedback therapy;
  - medications;
  - practical advice;
- surgical or specialist referral.

There are a number of practical techniques that patients may find useful, most of which will be trial and error to see what suits the individual patient. Some patients with faecal incontinence may benefit from the use of rectal evacuants before they leave home, to give them confidence, so they are less likely to need a bowel action whilst out. This may be used in conjunction with anti-diarrhoeal medication. Rectal irrigation has been used in the treatment of constipation and faecal incontinence. It is effectively a large volume tap water enema. In patients with spinal injury it has been shown to improve symptoms of constipation, faecal incontinence, and quality of life compared to conservative bowel management (Christensen *et al.* 2006).

Anal plugs can be a useful adjunct though they are often poorly tolerated. Many patients will use them for particular activities only, such as swimming. Intermittent self-catheterisation can be considered if persistent urinary retention is causing symptoms of incontinence or infection. Caffeine reduction and modification of fluid or fibre intake can be helpful in both bladder and bowel management. A number of devices can be used to aid pelvic floor muscle training such as vaginal cones and home biofeedback units. Pads and toileting aids are widely available but are not considered a treatment in themselves. They should be used as a coping strategy during treatment or as a long-term management tool only after treatment options have been fully explored. However, in practice, many patients report difficulty in obtaining such products from their local continence service.

Surgical interventions

There are a number of surgical approaches that can be used in the treatment of bladder and bowel incontinence. Listed in Table 6.4 are some of the procedures that may be utilised.

Table 6.4 Surgical treatments of incontinence

Urinary incontinence	Faecal incontinence
Bio-injectable material for sphincter bulking	Anterior sphincter repair
Mid-urethral tape procedures (e.g. TVT, TOT)	Sacral nerve stimulation
Sacral nerve stimulation	Neo-sphincter e.g. dynamic graciloplasty or artificial bowel sphincter
Artificial urinary sphincter	Antegrade colonic enema (ACE)
Bladder wall injection (BotulinumA) (for severe overactive bladder)	Percutaneous endoscopic colostomy (PEC)
Colposuspension	Colostomy formation
Augmentation cystoplasty	
Urinary stoma formation	

Sacral nerve stimulation

Sacral nerve stimulation (SNS) is a minimally invasive surgical procedure that has been used for approximately two decades in the treatment of urinary and faecal incontinence. It is a two-stage procedure. First the potential efficacy is assessed using percutaneous nerve evaluation (PNE). This is assessment of the response to nerve stimulating needles placed percutaneously through the sacral foramen adjacent to the sacral nerves. Stimulation at that point produces an anal contraction, perineal 'bellowing' or flexion of the big toe. The patient wears an external stimulating device for a few weeks whilst maintaining a bladder or bowel symptom diary. The wires are then removed. If the trial has been successful the patient will proceed to the second stage, a permanent implantation. This involves subcutaneous tunnelling of a sacral electrode and an implantable pulse generator (a pacemaker type device) which is placed in a buttock.

Recent five-year prospective evaluation of the implant for patients with urinary incontinence, frequency and retention has demonstrated efficacy in approximately two-thirds (van Kerrebroeck *et al.* 2007). Similar results are reported in faecal incontinence (Dudding *et al.* 2007). It appears a safe method of management but is expensive and only available in specialist centres. Therefore it is only recommended for use in those who have proved refractory to medical and behavioural techniques.

Colostomy

Formation of a colostomy for faecal incontinence is generally reserved for those in whom all other medical, behavioural and surgical treatments have failed. Therefore, it is often seen as a 'last resort'. Norton, Burch & Kamm

(2005) evaluated 69 patients who had undergone colostomy formation for faecal incontinence. The majority had undergone many interventions prior to stoma surgery. Eighty-three per cent felt their stoma did not restrict their life. For those who did experience problems these appeared similar to reported experiences of faecal incontinence, for example, concerns related to being able to locate toilet facilities, worries about smells or leaks, or about travelling. Unsurprisingly those whose bowel control had been very poor prior to stoma formation were more likely to be satisfied with their stoma. Depending on the available treatment options locally, patients may be offered stoma formation as an early intervention. This will not be acceptable to all. However, with careful assessment and appropriate counselling, stoma formation can be a viable and successful treatment option for severe faecal incontinence.

Conclusion

In summary, bowel and bladder incontinence is socially debilitating, affecting all aspects of quality of life. It is important to take a good clinical history focussing on what is important to the patient and using this as a basis for a management plan. Conservative techniques should be the first line of therapy. There is a range of good surgical interventions if these measures fail.

Useful websites

http://www.bowelcontrol.org.uk
http://www.burdettinstitute.org.uk
http://www.continence-foundation.org.uk

References

Christensen P, Bazzocchi G, Coggrave M, Abel R, Hulting C *et al.* (2006) A randomised controlled trial of transanal irrigation versus conservative bowel management in spinal cord-injured patients. *Gastroenterology.* **131**: 738–47.

Dudding TC, Parés D, Vaizey CJ & Kamm MA (2007) Predictive factors for successful Sacral Nerve Stimulation in the treatment of faecal incontinence: a 10 year cohort analysis. *Colorectal Disease*: online early articles. Published online: 26 July 2007. Doi: 10.1111/j.1463-1318.2007.01319

Edwards NI & Jones D (2001) The prevalence of faecal incontinence in older people living at home. *Age and Ageing.* **30**: 503–7.

Goldberg RP, Kwon C, Gandhi S, Atkuru LV, Sorensen MS & PK (2003) Prevalence of anal incontinence among mothers of multiples and analysis of risk factors. *American Journal of Obstetrics and Gynaecology.* **189(6)**: 1627–31.

Loening-Baucke V (2007) Prevalence rates for constipation and faecal and urinary incontinence. *Archives of Diseases in Childhood.* **92**: 486–9.

National Institute for Health and Clinical Excellence (2006) *Urinary Incontinence: The Management of Urinary Incontinence in Women. NICE Clinical Guideline 40.* London: NICE.

National Institute for Health and Clinical Excellence (2007) *Faecal Incontinence: The Management of Faecal Incontinence in Adults. NICE Clinical Guideline 49.* London: NICE.

Norton C & Chelvanayagam S (2000) A nursing assessment tool for adults with fecal incontinence. *Journal of Wound, Ostomy & Continence Nursing.* **27**: 279–91.

Norton C, Chelvanayagam S, Wilson-Barnett J, Redfern S & Kamm MA (2003) Randomised controlled trial of faecal incontinence. *Gastroenterology.* **125**: 1320–9.

Norton C, Burch J & Kamm MA (2005) Patients' views of a colostomy for fecal incontinence. *Diseases of the Colon and Rectum.* **48**: 1062–9.

Parés D, Duncan J, Dudding T, Phillips RKS & Norton C (2007) Investigation to predict faecal incontinence in patients undergoing reversal of a defunctioning stoma (Porridge enema test). *Colorectal Disease,* online early articles. Published article online: 16 August 2007. Doi:10.1111/j.1463-1318.2007.01333.x.

Sultan AH, Kamm MA, Hudson CN, Thomas JM & Bartram CI (1993) Anal sphincter disruption during vaginal delivery. *New England Journal of Medicine.* **329**: 1905–11.

van Kerrebroeck PEV, van Voskuilen AC, Heesakkers JPFA, á Nijholt L, Siegal S et al. (2007) Results of sacral neuromodulation therapy for urinary voiding dysfunction: outcomes of a prospective, worldwide clinical study. *Journal of Urology.* **178**: 2029–34.

Wilson PD, Herbison RM & Herbison G (1996) Obstetric practice and the prevalence of urinary incontinence three months after delivery. *British Journal of Obstetrics and Gynaecology.* **103**: 154–61.

Chapter 7

Other Conditions Leading to Stoma Formation

Jennie Burch

Introduction

There are a number of conditions that may lead to the formation of a stoma that have already been discussed in detail. Various other conditions or diseases may result in stoma-forming surgery. Some of these diseases or conditions affect infants and children, while others occur in later life.

Congenital malformations/anomalies

There are a number of congenital anorectal anomalies that can occur. The following will be discussed separately:

- anorectal malformations
- atresia
- bladder exstrophy
- cloacal exstrophy
- imperforate anus (proctatresia).

Anorectal malformations

Anorectal malformations range from anterior displacement of the anus at the mild end of the spectrum to caudal regression (absence of the sacrum) and sirenomelia (where there is a fusion of the legs). All of these are generally detected shortly after the birth of the infant (Lindley *et al.* 2006). Mild irregularity may not require treatment, while other malformations may require surgery that can include stoma formation.

For some anorectal malformations a colostomy can be formed to decompress an obstructed colon, to prevent faecal contamination of the urinary tract or to protect a future operation on the perineum (Pena *et al.* 2006). A study of children with anorectal malformations found their bowel function not to be as good as their peers, but their quality of life was not significantly worse (Goyal *et al.* 2006).

A further study that reviewed the quality of life in adults with anorectal malformations found that less than 10% had a stoma. However, approximately 85% reported faecal incontinence, with more incontinence reported in older patients. Those with a permanent stoma reported deterioration in

their quality of life over time and those with more severe anorectal malformations reported the worst quality of life (Hartman *et al.* 2007).

Atresia

Atresia of the gastrointestinal (GI) tract is the absence of continuity along
the tract. Atresia may occur at all levels of the GI tract and may be single
or multiple and is more common in the upper GI tract (Klostermann 1982).
The infant will rarely require a stoma formation as an anastomosis is
usually possible.

Bladder exstrophy

Exstrophy of the bladder is the failure of the abdominal wall to fuse and
results in an exposed, everted bladder (Jeter 1982). Although it is possible
to reconstruct the bladder, this was previously associated with significant
problems such as urinary tract infections. However with improved surgical techniques it should be possible to provide normal voiding, without
the need for a stoma (Mitchell 2005). If bladder reconstruction is not possible a permanent urinary diversion may be required (Ward & Stanford
2003).

Cloacal exstrophy

A cloacal exstrophy is a developmental abnormality in the foetus where
there is a defective abdominal wall that does not close, thus exposing the
intestinal and urinary organs (Jeter 1982). The baby is often born prematurely and therefore may not even survive (Ward & Stanford 2003). Surgery
may include formation of a faecal and urinary stoma, which is generally
required immediately. In a small study of 22 patients, 10 received an ileostomy, 7 a colostomy, 3 had no stoma and 2 died before surgery. Half of
the colostomates were re-operated on due to complications and given an
ileostomy (McHoney *et al.* 2004). These patients are likely to have a lifelong
stoma.

Imperforate anus

Imperforate anus is an absence of an anal orifice (Jeter 1982). This can vary
from anal stenosis to rectal atresia (absence). Imperforate anus is generally
accompanied by other anomalies such as cardiac problems (Klostermann
1982). A high imperforate anus may result in faecal incontinence (Johnson
1992). The treatment depends upon the location of the atresia and a
temporary stoma may be required, which may occasionally need to be
permanent.

Cystic fibrosis

Cystic fibrosis is a disease affecting various organs in the body, resulting
in production of very thick mucus. In the infant this mucus can block

various ducts and in particular the digestive enzymes from the pancreas are not released. This results in pancreatic damage and the meconium is not broken down. The meconium may then cause intestinal obstruction and colonic perforation. Surgery can include formation of a temporary ileostomy to relieve problems, which is generally reversed later (Ward & Stanford 2003).

Diverticular disease

Diverticular disease encompasses diverticulosis and diverticulitis (Black & Hyde 2005). Diverticulosis is the presence of diverticula (small pockets that protrude from the colon). Diverticula form due to a weakened bowel wall and are most commonly found in the sigmoid colon (Hyde 2003). Diverticulosis affects more than half of the over 50s in the UK (Ingram *et al.* 2004) and has been linked with low fibre diets, constipation and colonic hypermotility (Ward & Stanford 2003). Despite this, many people live symptom free with their diverticular disease.

Diverticulitis is inflammation of the diverticula leading to clinical symptoms. The acute signs and symptoms of diverticulitis include distension, bloody diarrhoea, abdominal pain and fever. Conservative treatment includes increasing dietary fibre, anti-spasmodic drugs and/or softening laxatives (Hyde 2003), which can be effective and prevent the symptoms associated with diverticular disease. Occasionally surgery is required and this may be emergency surgery, such as a Hartmann's procedure, which results in a colostomy formation (William & Ebanks 2003). There have been recent suggestions that a primary anastomosis and a defunctioning stoma are preferable to a Hartmann's procedure in those without other complications (Constantinides *et al.* 2007).

Ehlers Danlos

Ehlers Danlos syndrome is a hereditary connective tissue (collagen) disorder, with several disease variations. Type IV Ehlers Danlos syndrome has the unique complication of colonic rupture often associated with bleeding and poor wound healing. Surgery is discouraged for those with Ehlers Danlos, except in the emergency situation where a colonic rupture may necessitate a colectomy and possibly the formation of an ileostomy (Pepin *et al.* 2000).

Gynaecological tumour

A gynaecological cancer may also involve the bowel. This may result in the formation of an unplanned temporary or permanent stoma.

Hereditary non-polyposis colon cancer (HNPCC)

Hereditary non-polyposis colon cancer is a familial form of colonic cancer (Kirkwood 2006). Children of parents who had a cancer diagnosis when they were under the age of 45 are at an increased risk. Screening for this population occurs from the age of 30. There also seems to be an associated risk of breast and gynaecological cancer in this group. Surgical treatment is the removal of the affected bowel, which may result in the formation of a temporary stoma.

Hirschsprung's disease

Hirschsprung's disease or congenital aganglionic megacolon (de Lagausie *et al.* 1998) is a disease of the colon. The characteristics are an absence of ganglion cells in the rectum and recto-sigmoid and in some individuals longer bowel segments or small bowel involvement can also occur. This means the nerves in the bowel are incomplete and ineffectual (Ward & Stanford 2003). The incidence is approximately one in 5000 births (Hanneman *et al.* 2001) and is predominant in males (Telander & Brennom 1997). Aetiology is unknown but there is a 7% familial incidence (Fitzpatrick 1996).

The symptoms include constipation, abdominal distension or intestinal obstruction from birth that can lead to a megacolon (Fitzpatrick 1996). The surgical options in infancy are a colostomy that is formed in ganglionic bowel, which may be a life-saving procedure. Alternatively a pull-through operation is performed, such as a Duhamel (Huddart 1998), generally in childhood (Telander & Brennom 1997). This procedure involves removal of the ineffective bowel and the remaining bowel is pulled through the anus to retain intestinal continuity. Long-term incontinence and constipation is common with Hirschsprung's disease regardless of the extent of the aganglionosis (Ludman *et al.* 2002). Thus patients and parents need to be advised of this and sometimes a permanent colostomy is required.

Interstitial cystitis

Interstitial cystitis is a rare bladder condition. The signs and symptoms are recurring pain or discomfort in the bladder. There can also be urgency and frequency associated with passing urine. The cause of interstitial cystitis is unknown but irritation of the bladder may result in scarring, which can reduce the bladder capacity and may lead to an increased frequency of micturition. There are a number of options that are effective for interstitial cystitis such as drug therapy that can include analgesia to relieve symptoms. In severe cases when all therapy has failed, surgery may be indicated which can be a cystectomy and ileal conduit formation.

Intussusception

Intussusception is when one part of the bowel telescopes into an adjacent section. This can lead to colonic obstruction, which may require surgical formation of a stoma to relieve symptoms.

Irradiation damage

There may be late complications associated with radiation therapy for a cancer, which can follow treatment for a gynaecological or bladder tumour. Initial presentation of irradiation damage may be diarrhoea or abdominal cramps. These symptoms may be due to stenosis, perforation or a fistula (rectovaginal or rectovesical). Surgical treatment if medical therapy fails may result in a temporary or even permanent stoma formation.

Ischaemic bowel

Bowel ischaemia may be the result of a bowel infarct, most commonly of the superior mesenteric artery. Ischaemia can occur if there is a compromised blood supply and gangrene may develop within a few hours (Ward & Stanford 2003). The area of bowel that is affected will depend upon which blood vessels are damaged. The causes of a bowel infarction include embolus. An ischaemic bowel may result in an extensive resection of the bowel to remove the dead or necrotic tissue. Surgery often results in a stoma, sometimes two. In some situations there is a risk of further ischaemia occurring, so both ends of the bowel may be exteriorised as either a double-barrelled stoma or a stoma and a mucous fistula. Although bowel ischaemia is rare the consequences can be devastating. Re-joining the bowel may be possible but an anastomosis is not always achievable, resulting in a permanent stoma. Large resections of the bowel, in multiple operations, can also result in a short bowel and potentially the formation of a high-output stoma (for further information see Chapter 16).

Meconium ileus

Meconium ileus is a state of intestinal obstruction that is caused by inspissation (thickening of fluids) of abnormal meconium in neonates, particularly those with cystic fibrosis. This causes mid-ileal distension and obstruction (Klostermann 1982). Mortality is high and a stoma may be required to relieve the obstruction.

Megarectum

The aetiology for megarectum is unknown but may be related to neuromuscular or behavioural factors. Megarectum is associated with functional idiopathic constipation and may require a stoma formation (Nicholls 1996). There appears to be a problem emptying the rectum, which can create a slow colonic transit time. Treatment can include laxatives to manage the constipation, biofeedback and/or psychotherapy. Biofeedback is behavioural retraining of the bowel that improves symptoms in most patients with idiopathic megarectum (Mimura 2002). Surgery should be reserved as the last option for functional constipation and a stoma is occasionally indicated to resolve intolerable constipation or evacuation problems.

Necrotising enterocolitis

Necrotising enterocolitis (NEC) is rare and occurs in the premature neonate. Necrotising enterocolitis is characterised by ischaemia of the gastrointestinal system that can progress to necrosis and death (Delanty 1997). The cause is unclear but the signs and symptoms are rectal bleeding, diarrhoea, abdominal distension, bile-stained vomiting and pyrexia (Fitzpatrick 1996). First-line treatment is conservative with insertion of a naso-gastric tube, intravenous fluids and antibiotics; if this does not resolve the symptoms then surgery may be required. The most commonly affected area of the bowel is the terminal ileum, which will require resection and a temporary ileostomy formation (Jeter 1982).

Necrotising fasciitis

Necrotising fasciitis is a rare but life-threatening infection that affects the fascia and subcutaneous tissue (Jallali 2003) and rapidly progresses. In very rare situations the perianal area can be damaged to such an extent that a temporary colostomy may be required to allow the area to heal.

Obstruction

Large bowel obstruction that presents as an emergency is most commonly the result of a colonic tumour. The obstruction may also be the result of diverticular disease, a volvulus or adhesions, although adhesions are more likely to cause small bowel obstruction. In infants obstruction may be the result of an imperforate anus or Hirschsprung's disease (Nicholls 1996). For patients with an obstructing tumour the general condition of the patient may dictate the surgery required, as presentation is often late in the elderly. If a tumour is resected often a Hartmann's procedure is undertaken. Although the colostomy should only be temporary, for various reasons, such as co-morbidity, many are not reversed.

Perforated bowel

A bowel perforation is potentially very serious as faecal peritonitis can occur and death rates are high. Bowel perforation may be the result of a perforated colonic tumour, diverticular disease or trauma for example. If a carcinoma perforates there is a high risk of peritoneal involvement by the tumour and treatment will only be palliative (Nicholls 1996). Surgery may include a stoma formation and possibly resection of the perforated bowel. Peritoneal cavity lavage is also required to reduce the risk of sepsis.

Solitary rectal ulcer

Solitary rectal ulcer syndrome is a rare disorder characterised by erythema and ulceration of the rectal wall. There is also disturbed defaecation behaviour with the passage of blood and mucus (Vaizey *et al.* 1998). Conservative therapy should be the first line of treatment, such as biofeedback therapy (Vaizey *et al.* 1997). Dietary changes may also be useful, such as to increase the fibre intake. It is also important for patients to stop digital rectal evacuations to enable the ulcer to heal. Surgery such as a resection should be performed only if other therapy fails, but it has disappointing success rates (Sitzler *et al.* 1998). I have nursed one patient with a colostomy for a solitary rectal ulcer, which was deemed necessary due to the large blood loss from the ulcer and failure of other treatment.

Spina bifida

Spina bifida is a defect in the central nervous system. The foetus develops with a gap in the spinal column and the spinal canal can protrude through. This often leads to urinary dysfunction due to a neurogenic bladder and bowel problems. Treatment may include intermittent self-catheterisation, if urinary retention is a problem. Surgical resolution of urinary incontinence may result in a urostomy formation (Ward & Stanford 2003). A colostomy is generally only considered if all other medical therapy fails.

Spinal cord injury

Following a spinal cord injury bowel dysfunction can result. If this occurs it can be a significant problem for the patient and reduces their quality of life. If conservative treatment fails, such as medication, the surgical options include sacral nerve stimulation or stoma formation, most commonly a colostomy (Branagan *et al.* 2003).

Trauma

Trauma to the abdomen such as stabbing injury, road traffic accident, self-harm or gunshot wounds may require emergency surgery. The site of the injury dictates the treatment required; when the bowel is involved a stoma formation may be necessary (Steele 2006). Anal or rectal trauma can occur from inserted foreign objects. Trauma may result in a stoma to either allow healing or if the damage is irreparable, such as extensive damage to the anal sphincters, a permanent colostomy may be required.

Visceral myopathy

Visceral myopathy is rare and is also classified as chronic intestinal pseudo-obstruction. Patients will have the signs and symptoms of intestinal obstruction without any mechanical blockage (Nightingale 2003). Visceral myopathy is due to damage of the smooth muscle in the bowel that leads to ineffective intestinal propulsion or intestinal obstruction. Investigations include an x-ray to exclude mechanical obstruction.

If there is small bowel bacterial overgrowth antibiotics may be required. Small bowel overgrowth can lead to diarrhoea and malabsorption. Treatment is required to overcome the abdominal pain, vomiting and diarrhoea, although constipation is more common in the early stages (Nightingale 2003). Malnutrition may occur which may require the patient to have supplemental feeding possible intravenously. Surgery may be needed to form a stoma but this may not totally resolve symptoms.

Volvulus

A volvulus is a twist in the bowel on its mesentery (Ward & Stanford 2003). This is most common in the elderly or those with a long bowel. A volvulus may present in an emergency situation as a bowel obstruction. It will depend upon which part of the bowel has twisted to what treatment is required. A volvulus may resolve with conservative therapy, for example decompression of the bowel using an endoscope. If this does not resolve the problem, surgery may be needed. If gangrene is suspected then surgery is certainly indicated; this may be a Hartmann's procedure with a colostomy formation.

Conclusion

Many of the problems discussed in this chapter are rare, so nurses are unlikely to encounter a stoma formed for many of these reasons. A stoma for diverticular disease is probably the most commonly seen from this chapter. However, understanding why the stoma was formed can help in planning the care for the patient.

References

Black PK & Hyde CH (2005) *Diverticular Disease*. London: Whurr.

Branagan G, Tromans A & Finnis D (2003) Effects of stoma formation on bowel care and quality of life in patients with spinal cord injury. *Spinal Cord*. **41**: 680–3.

Constantinides VA, Heriot A, Remzi F, Darzi A, Senapati A *et al.* (2007) Operative strategies for diverticular peritonitis. *Annals of Surgery*. **245(1)**: 94–103.

de Lagausie P, Bruneau B, Besnard M, Jaby O & Aigrain Y (1998) Definitive treatment of Hirschsprung's disease with a laparoscopic Duhamel pull-through procedure in childhood. *Surgical Laparoscopy, Endoscopy and Percutaneous Techniques*. **8(1)**: 55–7.

Delanty S (1997) Neonatal necrotizing enterocolitis. *World Council of Enterostomal Therapists Journal*. **17(3)**: 26–9.

Fitzpatrick G (1996) The child with a stoma. In: Myers C (ed) *Stoma Care Nursing. A Patient-centred Approach*. London: Arnold.

Goyal A, Williams JM, Kenny SE, Lwin R, Baillie CT *et al.* (2006) Functional outcome and quality of life in anorectal malformations. *Journal of Pediatric Surgery.* **41:** 318–22.

Hanneman MJG, Sprangers MAG & De Mik EL (2001) Quality of life in patients with anorectal malformations or Hirschsprung's disease: development of a disease-specific questionnaire. *Diseases of the Colon and Rectum.* **44(11):** 1650–60.

Hartman EE, Oort FJ, Aronson DC, Hanneman MJG, van Heurn E *et al.* (2007) Explaining change in quality of life of children and adolescents with anorectal malformations or Hirschsprung disease. *Pediatrics.* **119(2):** e374–e383.

Huddart SN (1998) Hirschsprung's disease: present UK practice. *Annals of the Royal College of Surgeons of England.* **80(1):** 46–8.

Hyde C (2003) Diverticular disease. *Gastrointestinal nursing.* **1(5):** 34–9.

Ingram V, McKenzie F, Winslow F & Finlayson A (2004) Patient literature and diverticular disease. *Gastrointestinal Nursing.* **2(4):** 25–9.

Jallali N (2003) Necrotising fasciitis: its aetiology, diagnosis and management. *J Wound Care.* **12(8):** 297–300.

Jeter KF (1982) The pediatric patient: ostomy surgery in growing children. In: Broadwell DC & Jackson BS (eds) *Principles of Ostomy Care.* London: Mosby.

Johnson H (1992) Stoma care for infants, children and young people. *Paediatric Nursing.* **4(4):** 8–11

Kirkwood L (2006) An introduction to stomas. *Journal of Community Nursing.* **19(7):** 20–5.

Klostermann AR (1982) Congenital anomalies of the gastrointestinal tract. In: Broadwell DC & Jackson BS (eds) *Principles of Ostomy Care.* London: Mosby.

Lindley RM, Shawis RN & Roberts JP (2006) Delays in the diagnosis of anorectal malformations are common and significantly increase serious early complications. *Acta Pædiatrica.* **95:** 364–8.

Ludman L, Spitz L, Tsuji H & Pierro A (2002) Hirschsprung's disease: functional and psychological follow-up comparing total colonic and rectosigmoid aganglionosis. *Archives of Disease in Childhood.* **86(5):** 348–51.

McHoney M, Ransley PG, Duffy P, Wilcox DT & Spitz L (2004) Cloacal exstrophy: morbidity associated with abnormalities of the gastrointestinal tract and spine. *Journal of Pediatric Surgery.* **39(8):** 1209–13.

Mimura T, Nicholls T, Storrie JB & Kamm MA (2002) Treatment of constipation in adults associated with idiopathic megarectum by behavioural retraining including biofeedback. *Colorectal Diseases.* **4:** 477–82.

Mitchell ME (2005) Bladder exstrophy repair: complete primary repair of exstrophy. *Urology.* **65:** 5–8.

Nicholls RJ (1996) Surgical procedure. In: Myers C (ed) *Stoma Care Nursing. A Patient-centred Approach.* London: Arnold.

Nightingale JM (2003) The medical management of intestinal failure: methods to reduce the severity. *Proceedings of the Nutrition Society.* **62(3):** 703.

Pena A, Migotto-Krieger M & Levitt MA (2006) Colostomy in anorectal malformations: a procedure with serious but preventable complications. *Journal of Pediatric Surgery.* **41:** 748–56.

Pepin M, Schwarze U, Superti-Furga A & Byers PH (2000) Clinical and genetic features of Ehlers-Danlos syndrome type IV: the vascular type. *New England Journal of Medicine.* **342(10):** 673–80.

Sitzler PJ, Kamm MA, Nicholls RJ & McKee RF (1998) Long-term clinical outcome of surgery for solitary rectal ulcer syndrome. *British Journal of Surgery.* **85(9):** 1246–50.

Steele SE (2006) When trauma means a stoma. *Journal of Wound, Ostomy and Continence Nursing.* **33(5):** 491–500.

Telander RL & Brennom WS (1997) Congenital anomalies. In: Nicholls RJ & Dozois RR (eds) *Surgery of the Colon and Rectum.* London: Churchill Livingstone.

Vaizey CJ, Roy AJ & Kamm MA (1997) Prospective evaluation of the treatment of solitary rectal ulcer syndrome with biofeedback. *Gut.* **41**: 817–20.

Vaizey CJ, van den Bogaerde JB, Emmanuel AV, Talbot IC, Nicholls RJ *et al.* (1998) Solitary rectal ulcer syndrome. *British Journal of Surgery.* **85(12)**: 1617–23.

Ward J & Stanford E (2003) Conditions that may require surgery involving a stoma. In: Elcoat C (ed) *Stoma Care Nursing.* London: Hollister.

Williams J & Ebanks A (2003) Types of stoma and associated surgical procedures. In: Elcoat C (ed) *Stoma Care Nursing.* London: Hollister.

Chapter 8

Surgery

Alistair Windsor and Gemma Conn

Introduction

There are approximately 100 000 people in the UK with a stoma. Cancer operations remain the most common cause of stoma formation; however, there are a variety of other conditions which can result in the need for a stoma. These include inflammatory bowel disease, diverticular disease, familial adenomatous polyposis (FAP), Hirschsprung's disease, neurological conditions and trauma, to name a few.

Stomas can be broadly classified into temporary – those that there is an intention to reverse – and permanent. Ileostomies are the most common temporary stomas, while colostomies remain the most common permanent stomas. Permanent stomas are necessary when there is no distal bowel segment left to rejoin or the bowel cannot be rejoined for other reasons. This could be following, for example, an abdominoperineal resection for a low rectal tumour or a panproctocolectomy (usually for ulcerative colitis or FAP) unless an ileoanal pouch is constructed.

Temporary stomas

Temporary stomas are used to divert the faecal stream from the distal bowel. There are numerous indications for this including:

- to rest a distal segment of bowel which may be involved in a disease process such as an intestinal fistula or acute Crohn's disease;
- to protect an anastomosis which may have:
  - been technically difficult;
  - been compromised by sepsis;
  - poor blood supply;
  - other factors predisposing to post-operative leak;
- an emergency setting:
  - to relieve distal bowel obstruction;
  - to defunction distal trauma.

Stomas can also be classified by which part of the bowel is involved; for example, an ileostomy (small bowel), colostomy (colon), caecostomy (caecum) etc. Finally they can be classified according to their method of formation, whether one bowel lumen is diverted (end) or whether two lumens are used, giving an afferent and efferent lumen (loop or double barrelled).

Common operations resulting in a temporary stoma formation are anterior resection and a Hartman's procedure. This would be a temporary ileostomy and a colostomy respectively.

Anterior resection +/− a temporary ileostomy

An anterior resection involves resecting a rectal tumour while preserving the anal sphincters to allow anastomosis and faecal continence. A temporary ileostomy may be required and this would be formed in the right iliac fossa. The ileostomy may be required while the anastomosis is healing to prevent leakage occurring. If the join is low or if there are other reasons that the healing of the anastomosis will be delayed then a temporary ileostomy is performed. The ileostomy will usually be reversed after three to six months.

A clear margin of two centimetres is required from the distal end of the tumour, to minimise local recurrence rates. An anterior resection generally involves a midline incision to allow visualisation of the bowel. Then part of the rectum and sigmoid colon is removed and the bowel ends are anastomosed. This procedure is being increasingly performed by minimally invasive techniques. If adequate distal clearance cannot be achieved or the patient's pre-operative sphincter function is inadequate to provide continence then an abdominoperineal resection would be required, resulting in a permanent colostomy.

Hartmann's procedure and colostomy formation

Another common operation resulting in stoma formation is Hartmann's procedure. A Hartmann's procedure is also performed via a midline incision. Following a rectal or sigmoid resection the rectal stump is sutured closed and an end colostomy is formed in the left iliac fossa, from the proximal colon. This may be a temporary or permanent stoma depending on the indications for the operation and patient's condition. Rarely the rectum is brought to the midline incision and formed into a mucous fistula. In many situations the colostomy is never reversed.

Permanent stomas

A permanent stoma will result following an abdominoperineal resection of the rectum and a panproctocolectomy. The stomas formed would be a permanent colostomy and an ileostomy respectively.

Abdominoperineal resection of the rectum

An abdominoperineal resection of the rectum (APER) is performed via a midline and perineal incision. The rectum, anal canal and anal sphincter are removed and also some of the sigmoid colon. An APER is performed for low tumours or perineal Crohn's disease that has failed medical therapy for example. A permanent colostomy is formed in the left iliac fossa. The two surgical incisions are sutured. However, occasionally the perineal wound may have delayed healing, particularly if steroids were used pre-operatively in the treatment of Crohn's disease for example.

Panproctocolectomy

Another permanent stoma would result from a panproctocolectomy. This operation is also performed via a midline and perineal incision. In this procedure the colon, rectum, anus and sphincters are removed. A permanent ileostomy is formed in the right iliac fossa. This surgical procedure also produces two surgical wounds. Additionally there may be delayed healing of the perineal wound if pre-operative steroids are used.

Stoma formation

Siting

The stoma specialist nurse usually carries out siting of the stoma pre-operatively. It is a vital part of stoma surgery as correct siting of the stoma allows the patient to wear their normal clothes, helps with the appliance fit, the appliance change and greatly aids patient comfort. The stoma must be sited in an area away from skin creases, scars and bony prominences, thus reducing the risk of appliance leakage. The stoma must be in a position that is easily accessible to the patient so that they can change the appliance. The position should be checked in the lying, sitting and standing positions prior to marking with indelible ink. It is possible that siting the stoma so that it comes through the rectus muscle results in fewer post-operative complications such as parastomal herniae.

Surgical approach

To a certain extent the surgical approach depends on the indication for the operation and the stoma formation. For example, if the patient is undergoing a laparotomy for an obstructing bowel tumour then the decision may have already been made. The aim may be to perform a stoma to relieve the obstructing symptoms, prior to oncological therapy for instance. After chemo/radiotherapy further surgery can be planned to resect the tumour. In this situation a less invasive approach such as laparoscopy or trephining may be required when forming the defunctioning stoma.

With all approaches it is necessary to bring the stoma through peritoneum, muscle, fat and skin of the anterior abdominal wall.

Laparotomy

Laparotomy is the traditional approach. Its benefits are that it enables the surgeon good access, good visualisation of the bowel and the anatomy thus allowing excellent mobilisation. However it is major surgery with a prolonged recovery time so may not be the approach of choice in a patient who requires defunctioning prior to chemoradiation of a rectal tumour.

Since the development of laparoscopic techniques stomas are usually only formed during laparotomy if there is another reason to perform the laparotomy. For example, if the patient is undergoing an open anterior resection and a defunctioning ileostomy is formed then it is sensible to form the ileostomy at the same time via the laparotomy wound. It is best to bring the stoma out through a separate incision to the laparotomy wound. The formation of a stoma during laparotomy is a quick and relatively simple process, adding about 20 minutes to the operative time.

Trephine

Trephining is basically tunnelling through the abdominal wall. It results in a small wound with a good recovery time. However, it does not provide good access or views and thus there is a risk of damage to surrounding intra-abdominal structures. Adequate bowel mobilisation may be more difficult resulting in tension on the bowel and its associated complications, such as retraction. It may also be difficult to distinguish between the efferent and afferent loops of bowel, therefore creating an end stoma must be done with great care. It has been largely superseded by laparoscopic techniques and now is only used if laparoscopy is contraindicated or the surgeon is unfamiliar with laparoscopic techniques. It takes approximately 30 minutes.

Laparoscopy

Laparoscopy or keyhole surgery allows good views not only of the bowel, but also the rest of the abdomen and can provide valuable information about disease stage. If the patient does not require a laparotomy for other reasons and there is no contraindication to laparoscopy and the surgeon is trained in the technique then this is a good option. Laparoscopy is well tolerated with a good recovery time. There is an accepted risk of the need to convert to an open procedure that may be associated with slightly higher complication rates. However, all the limitations of a laparotomy approach are overcome by laparoscopy. During ileostomy formation for example, the camera port (10 mm) is usually inserted via the umbilicus. This can be achieved via an open, Hassan approach or a closed approach using a Verress needle. Two smaller (5 mm) ports are placed in the left and right iliac fossas, forming a triangle. Instruments can be inserted via these ports to manipulate the bowel. An incision is made through skin, muscle and peritoneum in the previously marked stoma site and the bowel is fashioned as described below. Operation time as always is influenced by the operator's experience and complexity of the case but on average takes 30–45 minutes.

Surgical technique

Ileostomy

An ileostomy is a stoma made from small bowel. The effluent is usually of a porridge like consistency, although it may be fluid. The bag normally needs to be emptied approximately four to six times per day, although there can be great individual variation. An ileostomy forms a spout of approximately 2–3 cm from the skin.

End/terminal ileostomy

A terminal or end ileostomy is a common permanent stoma. A 3 cm circular disc of skin is excised from the pre-chosen site. A cruciate (crucifix shape) incision is made in the anterior rectus sheath to expose the rectus muscle. The muscle fibres are split to expose the posterior rectus sheath that is then opened. The peritoneum is picked up and incised to reveal the intra-abdominal contents. The resulting defect should be able to accommodate two fingers. Six to eight centimetres of previously divided ileum are exteriorised through the defect. Care is taken not to twist or damage the mesentery and therefore compromise the blood supply. The bowel is everted and sutured to the skin with interrupted 2/0 vicryl. A spout of 2–3 cm is formed as the bowel is everted. This is also called the '554' stoma due to the lengths of bowel required for formation of the ileostomy spout.

Loop ileostomy

A loop ileostomy is usually formed as a temporary stoma. The initial steps are as for an end ileostomy. A loop of ileum is delivered through the resultant defect and then opened close to the skin level. A plastic rod is generally inserted to prevent the bowel slipping back into the abdominal cavity. The stoma should be positioned so that the proximal limb lies superiorly, with the potential risk of overflow of faeces into the distal limb of the bowel. As above the stoma is sutured to the skin using 2/0 vicryl, which dissolves in two to eight weeks.

Colostomy

A colostomy is a stoma involving the large bowel. It lies flush with the skin or is minimally raised. It usually produces formed stool although this varies according to which part of the large bowel is utilised. It is possible to irrigate the colostomy to gain control over passage of stool. This avoids the need to wear a permanent bag.

Transverse colostomy

Transverse colostomy is rarely used as a permanent stoma as it is associated with a high risk of complications, especially prolapse due to the mobility of the transverse colon within the abdomen. However, it is of use in the emergency setting when a temporary stoma may be required. It can be performed under local anaesthesia in a patient who needs urgent decompression of a distal obstruction and who is too unwell to withstand general anaesthesia. A loop or double-barrelled colostomy is usually formed although it is possible to fashion an end colostomy.

A 5 cm transverse incision is made in the right upper quadrant, between the umbilicus and the costal margin. The rectus sheath is divided and the rectus muscle split. After incising the peritoneum the transverse colon is identified by its omentum and the presence of taeniae. The right side of the transverse colon is used to reduce the risk of prolapse. The omentum is trimmed from the anterior surface to make a gap. A window is carefully made in the mesentery at the loop apex, without compromising the blood supply. A rubber catheter is passed through the window and used to deliver the loop of bowel into the wound. The loop is positioned so that the proximal opening lies to the right and the distal to the left. The apex of the loop is opened across half of the circumference. The colon edges are everted and full thickness, interrupted sutures using 2/0 vicryl are used to attach the colon to skin. A finger is inserted into each loop to ensure the lumen is patent and of adequate size. A stoma rod is left in situ; this is removed after 7–10 days.

Sigmoid colostomy

An end sigmoid colostomy is the stoma of choice when a permanent colostomy is required. The stoma is sited in the left iliac fossa. The sigmoid colon is identified by the presence of appendices epiploicae. Once again care is taken not to twist the mesentery and damage the blood supply. A loop of colon is delivered into the defect and divided. The distal end is closed and returned to the peritoneal cavity. The proximal loop ends are everted and sutured to the skin with full thickness interrupted 2/0 vicryl sutures. It is vital to ensure the correct (proximal) end of bowel is brought out as a stoma. Direct vision via laparotomy or laparoscopy should prevent any mistakes. If there is any doubt it is possible to inflate air per rectum resulting in the inflation and identification of the distal loop. If there is still doubt a loop colostomy could be performed.

Mucous fistula

A mucous fistula is formed at the same time as an ileostomy or colostomy. It is usually formed during emergency surgery, for example in acute colitis where primary anastomosis is unsafe. In this situation there are two options, to close the distal stump and return it to the abdomen or to bring out the distal end as a mucous fistula (non-functioning colostomy). The use of a mucous fistula reduces the risk of stump dehiscence that occurs in up to 10% of colostomies for acute colitis. The high risk of stump dehiscence in these cases is due to active rectal disease and pre-operative steroid use. Mucous fistulae do not produce faeces but may discharge small amounts of mucus. It is not always possible to form a mucous fistula as there may not be sufficient bowel length to bring the distal end to the abdominal wall and there may be no option but to return the distal end to the abdomen. The presence of a mucous fistula may make subsequent reversal an easier procedure. Most frequently the mucous fistula is formed at the base of the surgical wound, which often causes problems in the immediate post-operative period due to the wound oozing or difficulty in securing the stoma appliance.

Reversal/stoma closure

Reversal of an ileostomy or colostomy involves restoring continuity of the bowel. It should not be attempted before eight weeks after the original operation when bowel oedema has had chance to subside, to reduce the risk of complications (Perez *et al.* 2006). If a loop or a double barrel ostomy has been used then it may be possible to restore continuity without opening the abdomen. This is achieved by dissecting around the stoma to free it from the abdominal wall. In some cases this may not be possible and the case may have to be converted to a laparotomy. Techniques for closing the bowel are varied, but broadly speaking can be done with sutures or staples and can be performed as an end-to-end, or side-to-side anastomosis. The merits of each technique are in the main dictated by individual surgeon preference. Studies have shown no difference in leak rates, disease recurrence, morbidity or mortality with the use of stapled or hand sewn anastomosis.

Surgical alternatives

Restorative proctocolectomy

Restorative proctocolectomy is often used in ulcerative colitis patients as it avoids the need for a permanent stoma. It is also used in patients who have had a colectomy for FAP. In brief, the colon and the rectum are removed, leaving an intact anal sphincter. The terminal ileum is then fashioned into a reservoir and joined to the anal sphincter to restore bowel continuity. The small bowel can be fashioned in different ways to form a 'J', 'S' or 'W' pouch. A 'J' pouch is created from two side-by-side limbs that are stapled together to form a 'J' shape. A 'W' pouch is formed from four side-by-side limbs and so looks like two 'J' pouches stapled together. An 'S' pouch is created from three limbs. A temporary ileostomy may be required to protect the anastomosis, especially if the patient has been on high-dose steroids pre-operatively. A restorative proctocolectomy is not suitable for Crohn's patients, those who have a lax anal sphincter, patients who have had anal sphincter surgery or patients who have had significant small bowel resections. Patients are at risk of developing inflammation in the pouch, named pouchitis, which results in pain, diarrhoea, blood/mucus in the stool and urgency. Pouchitis may resolve with medications but in severe cases formation of an ileostomy may be required. This may be temporary to rest the bowel or permanent in intractable cases. Pouchitis is more common in patients who have undergone surgery for ulcerative colitis with 30% of patients experiencing at least one episode.

Kock's continent pouch

A Kock's continent pouch is another alternative to a permanent ileostomy. As above a reservoir is formed from small bowel and joined via a one-way valve to the abdominal wall. The valve is made by exteriorising a section of the wall of the small bowel reservoir to form a very small stoma at skin level. The valve is periodically accessed to drain the pouch contents to provide continence. This method may be of use in patients whose lax sphincter tone makes them unsuitable for a restorative proctocolectomy. As with a restorative proctocolectomy, it is not suitable for Crohn's patients. Complications include valve slippage, preventing access of the valve or inopportune stool leakage. Treatment may require corrective surgery. As above pouchitis may be a problem.

Complications

There are a number of complications associated with stomas. Arumugam *et al.* (2003) suggested that 50% of patients with stomas would experience complications within the first year of surgery. Complications can be broadly classified into early, those occurring within a few months of surgery and late. Complication rate is directly related to body mass index, nutritional status, presence of diabetes and emergency surgery.

Ischaemia

Ischaemia results from inadequate blood supply to the bowel brought out as a stoma. It can be recognised in the post-operative period by a dusky coloured, oedematous bowel.

Ischaemia can be caused by damage to the vascular supply during mobilisation, too much tension on the bowel, a tight fascial defect through which the stoma is brought out and sometimes secondary to the use of vasoconstricting inotropes such as noradrenalin in the septic patient. Patient factors such as smoking, diabetes and peripheral vascular disease may also impair blood supply.

Ischaemia often results in necrosis or tissue death. If superficial, this may result in the sloughing off of the necrotic tissue or the separation of the non-viable stoma from the surrounding skin. Long-term sequelae are stenosis and stricture formation that can cause practical problems, pain and carry a risk of bowel obstruction. At its worst ischaemia can result in infarction and necrosis of the stoma that can then retract causing peritonitis.

Conservative management includes good stoma care, well-chosen appliances and the use of barrier sprays and powders until the dead tissue has separated. However, surgical intervention and further mobilisation of well vascularised bowel may be required.

Obstruction

Obstruction is the prevention of passage of effluent along the bowel lumen and may be partial or complete. It may occur as an early or late complication.

Early obstruction is usually due to oedematous bowel or technical failure. Food bolus obstruction may also occur and the introduction of certain foods into the diet must be undertaken gradually. Late obstruction may be caused by adhesions, recurrent disease and secondary to other stomal complications such as parastomal hernia or bolus obstruction.

Initial management is conservative with surgery required if conservative management fails.

Parastomal herniation

A parastomal hernia is the bulging of peritoneum and abdominal contents through weakened abdominal musculature around the stoma. The hernial sac often contains omentum and small bowel but may contain any intra-abdominal viscera.

Herniation is generally a late complication and incidence increases with time. It occurs in approximately 30% of end colostomies and up to 30% of ileostomies. It may be predisposed to by technical or patient factors.

Too wide a fascial opening during formation of the stoma predisposes to this condition. It occurs more commonly if an end colostomy is brought out lateral to the rectus muscle rather than through a split in the rectus. It is also directly related to nutritional deficiency, raised intra-abdominal pressure and weight gain.

Complications of parastomal hernia are those of any hernia and include incarceration, obstruction and strangulation. They also cause practical difficulties with the fitting of appliances and clothing.

Although it may be possible to relieve discomfort via the use of a support belt, surgical correction is often required. Local repair may be attempted, either by mesh repair or suturing and it is now possible to do this laparo-scopically, or it may be necessary to resite the stoma. Resiting involves the need for relaparotomy with its attendant problems and there is limited space on the abdomen for resiting. Furthermore if the underlying problem, such as weak collagen, persists then the problem of herniation will inevi-tably recur.

Recent trial data from Scandinavia suggest that the use of mesh to support the stoma at the time of formation may reduce the incidence of parastomal hernia. Long-term data confirming this are not yet available.

Prolapse

Prolapse is the lengthening of the stoma due to bowel telescoping out (see Figure 8.1). Loop stomas tend to have higher rates of prolapse than end colostomies and ileostomies. Prolapse can occur as an early or late complication.

Prolapse can be related to a large redundant loop of bowel or too large a fascial opening. This may be related to a raised intra-abdominal pressure caused by chronic cough, chronic obstructive pulmonary disease, ascites and obesity.

If the prolapsed bowel is very oedematous there is a risk of necrosis and ischaemia as the blood supply becomes impaired. Reduction of oedema-tous bowel may also result in ischaemia.

Prolapses can usually be manually reduced; sometimes this may require sedation or general anaesthesia. If prolapse is recurrent following reduc-tion then surgical repair and/or resiting is required.

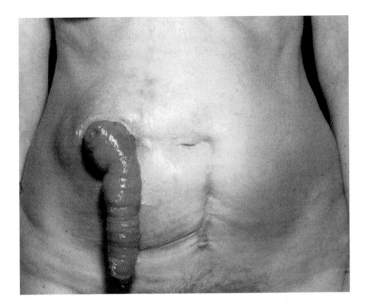

Figure 8.1 Prolapse of ileostomy.

Retraction

Retraction is defined as the stoma slipping back into the abdominal cavity. Retraction may occur due to technical failure related to inadequate mobilisation of the bowel, thus resulting in tension on the bowel, or due to mucocutaneous separation. It may also be due to premature removal of the plastic rod. Changes in the patient's weight post-operatively may predispose to retraction. It may be fixed or intermittent.

Retraction causes problems with the fitting of stoma appliances and may result in effluent leakage under the appliance. The use of specialist stoma appliances to ensure a good seal may avoid the need for surgery. However if conservative measures fail then surgical refashioning is required.

Stenosis

Stenosis is the narrowing of the stomal lumen. Stenosis is often related to ischaemia, ongoing underlying disease such as carcinoma or inflammatory bowel disease or technical failure.

Dilatation can be tried but is often unsuccessful. Surgical resiting or local revision whereby the bowel is literally advanced so the stenosed segment can be resected and discarded may be required.

Dehiscence/mucocutaneous separation

Dehiscence is the separation of the bowel mucosa from the skin. It may occur in a small area or the entire mucosal surface can be separated. It may be due to technical failure, where there is too much tension on the bowel, or secondary to ischaemia, necrosis or infection.

Dehiscence may result in a cavity that makes stoma care more difficult. This wound cavity is usually included in the appliance and barrier creams may need to be used. Surgical repair of the dehisced wound is uncommon.

Recurrent disease

Inflammatory bowel disease and carcinoma can both recur in a stoma. Crohn's disease may also recur proximally causing stenosis or fissuring lesions.

Pyoderma gangrenosum, peristomal fistulae and ulceration can also be seen around stomas in relation to inflammatory bowel disease. Medical therapy is the first line of treatment in inflammatory bowel disease. It may be necessary to resect more bowel. However, if the patient has already had a significant amount resected there is a risk of short bowel syndrome and nutritional problems must be considered. For recurrent carcinoma, if the disease is resectable and the patient fit for surgery then the disease should be resected and an oncological opinion sought regarding adjuvant therapy.

Bleeding

Bleeding from within or around a stoma can be due to a number of causes. Bleeding from within the stoma should be treated as for bleeding per rectum and an urgent referral for investigation should be made. Bleeding from the stoma itself may be caused by trauma from the appliance or cleaning, or by disease processes such as granuloma, ulceration or carcinoma. Most bleeding resolves spontaneously with time and supportive treatment such as correcting coagulation abnormalities, stopping antiplatelet/anticoagulation medications and transfusing as necessary. If there is bleeding due to recurrent disease then this may require resection as described above. Excess granulation tissue that bleeds easily can be cauterised with silver nitrate sticks and very infrequently surgery will be necessary.

Enhanced recovery after surgery (ERAS)

The ERAS protocol is basically aiming to reduce the stress response to surgery enabling faster recovery with a safe and early discharge. It differs from traditional post-operative care where prolonged immobility and bowel rest were standard, by promoting early mobility and gut function.

It begins with pre-operative patient counselling as it has been shown that patient understanding facilitates post-operative recovery and aids compliance with the care pathway. The role of the specialist colorectal nurse is vital.

Bowel preparation has traditionally been used prior to bowel resection and results in electrolyte disturbances and dehydration as well as being unpleasant for the patient. A recent Cochrane review has shown that there is no benefit in the use of bowel prep in most colorectal surgery.

Traditionally patients were fasted for six hours prior to surgery. The ERAS protocol recommends nil by mouth for six hours for solids and two hours for liquids. The patient is also given a clear, high carbohydrate drink prior to surgery (800 ml at midnight and 200 ml two hours before the operation). This reduces anxiety and decreases post-operative insulin resistance. Pre-operative malnutrition should be corrected prior to operation by enteral or parenteral routes.

Traditional fluid management results in overloading the patient. The ERAS protocol concentrates on prevention of pre-operative dehydration, IV fluid administration to maintain the patient's weight and to start oral fluids immediately (Fearon & Luff 2003) with the aim of discontinuing IV fluids quickly.

The ERAS protocol encourages early mobilisation. Prolonged bed rest increases risk of DVT, reduces lung function resulting in more chest infections, decreases muscle mass and increases insulin resistance.

The use of epidurals peri-operatively results in improved pain control, reducing the stress response and allowing earlier mobilisation. Following discontinuation of the epidural, adequate analgesia is vital and the pain team may be involved. Regular paracetamol should be prescribed. If there are no contraindications this should be supplemented with NSAIDs as they have been shown to decrease post-operative nausea and vomiting. The avoidance of pro-emetic drugs and the use of prophylactic anti-emetics also decrease problems of nausea and vomiting.

Urinary catheters, nasogastric tubes and drains contribute to decreased mobility and decreased comfort. Urinary catheters should be removed as quickly as possible, as they promote urosepsis and decrease mobility, or converted to leg bags to aid mobility. A Cochrane review showed that routine drainage of the abdominal cavity confers no benefit.

One article suggests that stoma forming surgery is possible as a day case for laparoscopic ileostomy formation and stoma reversal, suggesting that 11 out of 12 patients went home within 23 hours and four of these were discharged the same day (Gatt *et al.* 2007).

Conclusion

Informed consent and an adequate explanation of why a stoma is necessary are extremely important. Coupled with this, correct siting and good surgical technique should ensure a successful stoma. An understanding of the possible complications and their early recognition will also ensure good quality of life for the patient.

References and further reading

Arumugam PJ, Bevan L, Macdonald L, Watkins AJ, Morgan AR *et al.* (2003) A prospective audit of stomas – analysis of risk factors and complications and their management. *Colorectal Diseases.* **5(1)**: 49–52.

Bach SP & Mortensen NJ (2006) Revolution and evolution: 30 years of ileoanal pouch surgery. *Inflammatory Bowel Diseases*. **12(2)**: 131–45.

Barr JE (2004) Assessment and management of stomal complications: a framework for clinical decision making. *Ostomy Wound Management*. **50(9)**: 50–2.

Basse L, Hjort Jackobsen D, Billesbolle P, Werner M & Kehlet H (2000) A clinical pathway to accelerate recovery after colonic resection. *Annals of Surgery*. **232(1)**: 51–7.

Burch J (2005) The pre- and postoperative nursing care for patients with a stoma. *British Journal of Nursing*. **14(6)**: 310–18.

Burch J (2005) Exploring the conditions leading to stoma-forming surgery. *British Journal of Nursing*. **14(2)**: 94–8.

Carne PW, Robertson GM & Frizelle FA (2003) Parastomal hernia. *British Journal of Surgery*. **90(7)**: 784–93.

Chung CC, Tsang WW, Kwok SY & Li MK (2003) Laparoscopy and its current role in the management of colorectal disease. *Colorectal Diseases*. **5(6)**: 528–43.

Collett K (2002) Practical aspects of stoma management. *Nursing Standard*. **17(8)**: 45–52.

Fearon KCH & Luff R (2003) The nutritional management of surgical patients: enhanced recovery after surgery. *Proceedings of the Nutrition Society*. **6**: 807–11.

Gatt M, Reddy BS & Mainprize KS (2007) Day-case stoma surgery: is it feasible? *The Surgeon*. **5(3)**: 143–7.

Kirk RM (2006) *General Surgical Operations*. 5th edn. London: Churchill Livingstone Elsevier.

Lassen K, Hannemann P, Ljungqvist O, Fearon K, Dejong CH *et al.* (2005) Patterns in current perioperative practice; survey of colorectal surgeons in 5 European countries. *British Medical Journal*. **330(7505)**: 1420–1.

Oliveira L (2003) Laparoscopic stoma creation and closure. *Seminars in Laparoscopic Surgery*. **10(4)**: 191–6.

Onaitis MW & Mantyh C (2003) Ileal pouch-anal anastomosis for ulcerative colitis and familial adenomatous polyposis: historical development and current status. *Annals of Surgery*. **23(8)(6 Suppl)**: S42–8.

Perez RO, Habr-Gama A, Seid VE, Proscurshim I, Sousa AH *et al.* (2006) Loop ileostomy morbidity: timing of closure matters. *Diseases of the Colon & Rectum*. **49(10)**: 1539–45.

Rolstad BS & Erwin-Toth PL (2004) Peristomal skin complications: prevention and management. *Ostomy Wound Management*. **50(9)**: 68–77.

Taylor P (2001) Care of patients with complications following formation of a stoma. *Professional Nurse*. **17(4)**: 252–4.

Turina M, Pennington CJ, Kimberling J, Stromberg AJ, Petras RE & Galandiuk S (2006) Chronic pouchitis after ileal pouch-anal anastomosis for ulcerative colitis: effect on quality of life. *Journal of Gastrointestinal Surgery*. **10(4)**: 600–6.

Chapter 9

Pre- and Post-operative Care

Steve Wright and Jennie Burch

Introduction

This chapter covers issues related to the pre- and post-operative care of patients undergoing stoma-forming surgery. Informed consent following appropriate accurate information giving is essential. The need for bowel clearance prior to surgery will also be reviewed. After the decision to undertake stoma-forming surgery is made it is important to refer to the appropriate members of the multidisciplinary team, including the stoma specialist nurse. The principles of effective stoma siting are discussed. The post-operative needs of the new ostomate are examined, such as teaching stoma care, becoming independent and appliance choice.

Referral to health care professionals

To ensure the care of ostomates is holistic it is essential to involve all relevant health care professionals. The stoma specialist nurse should assess the patient either with the surgeons or soon after. The patient may be incapable of retaining all the necessary information so giving contact details and literature to take home is essential. Ideally the next appointment should be in the patient's home (Black 2000), but this is not always possible or appropriate. The rationale for meeting at the patient's home is to meet other family members and enables the patient to be relaxed so they can express their fears about the surgery. The Macmillan nurse should also see the patient if the reason for the stoma formation is cancer.

Pre-operative assessment and investigations

The aims of pre-operative assessment are to reduce the risks associated with surgery and anaesthesia, to increase the quality of peri-operative care and to restore the patient to a desired level of function (Garcia-Miguel *et al.* 2003). Patients undertaking elective stoma-forming surgery generally have a laparotomy and remain anaesthetised for a considerable period of time. Therefore, it is important that patients are adequately assessed and prepared for their procedure, in pre-operative assessment clinics within the outpatient department.

Historically, junior doctors undertook these clinics, but following change to postgraduate medical training and the UK junior doctors working hours initiative this has significantly reduced junior doctors' working time (UK General Medical Council 1995). Subsequently nurses in many hospitals offer nurse-led pre-operative assessment clinics (Kinley *et al.* 2002).

Before attending pre-operative assessment clinics patients are usually sent a pre-operative questionnaire to complete. The form requests information on pre-existing medical problems, past surgical history and smoking for example. In the clinic, patients have an assessment, a physical examination and routine tests, where individual assessment and formulation of an effective care plan are carried out.

Assessment

The assessment is undertaken in conjunction with the pre-operative questionnaire completed by the patient, reducing time spent asking the basic questions. Janke *et al.* (2002) advocate that the pre-operative interview includes the following aspects:

- a brief introduction;
- general and social history;
- medical, surgical and anaesthetic history;
- the presenting condition;
- medication;
- allergies.

Physical examination

The patient is made comfortable for the physical examination and vital signs are measured:

- temperature;
- blood pressure;
- pulse (rate and regularity);
- respiratory rate;
- weight;
- height.

The patient's airway and cardiopulmonary system are also assessed. The anaesthetist must be informed of abnormalities to initiate further appropriate investigation. Examination of the airway should include checking teeth for bridges, caps and crowns (Janke *et al.* 2002); also tongue size as a large tongue in a small mouth may impede laryngoscopy (Bellhouse & Dore 1988). A modified Mallampati test (Samson & Young 1987) is often used and documented on the patient's anaesthetic chart, determining how difficult laryngoscopy and intubation will be.

Auscultation of the heart is undertaken using a stethoscope, examining each component of the cardiac system. On examination normal heart sounds should be audible, added sounds or murmurs may be present. The patient should be asked if these were noted previously.

The lung fields are auscultated and percussed for abnormality. Munro and Campbell (2002) suggest abnormal findings may include bronchial breathing, rhonchi, crepitations and pleural sounds.

Patients undergoing elective stoma forming surgery require an abdominal and rectal examination. In the emergency situation a useful scoring system to predict post-operative outcome is the American Society of Anesthesiologists (ASA) score. This categorises patients into five subgroups by pre-operative fitness (Walker 2002). ASA scores are:

Class I   A completely healthy patient
      II   A patient with a mild systemic disease
      III   Severe systemic disease that is not incapacitating
      IV   An incapacitating disease that is a constant threat to life
      V   A moribund patient not expected to live 24 hours with or without surgery

At the pre-operative assessment patients have the surgical procedure explained often using diagrams. The patient's level of comprehension should be ascertained and questions actively sought from the patient to ensure understanding.

Investigations

The purpose of routine pre-operative testing is to assess pre-existing health problems, identify unsuspected medical conditions and predict potential complications. This establishes a baseline for future reference and screens patients. Indiscriminate pre-operative investigations are unnecessary and wasteful (Roizen 1989), therefore resources must be used appropriately.

Guidelines on routine pre-operative testing from the National Institute for Clinical Excellence (NICE 2003) use a traffic light system for investigations:

* red – not recommended;
* amber – consider testing;
* green – recommended.

During the pre-operative interview and clinical examination the routine tests required should be apparent. The main pre-operative investigations are an electrocardiogram (ECG), chest x-ray and blood tests. An ECG is appropriate if the patient has a history, suspicion or risk factors for cardiac disease (Janke *et al.* 2002). Patients with a cardiac history have a high incidence of new ECG abnormalities even in the absence of symptoms (Power & Thackary 1999). Any suspicions that are raised by the medical history, clinical examination or ECG may warrant further investigation with an echocardiogram or a cardiology referral.

Routine pre-operative chest x-rays are not indicated in patients below 60 years old undergoing non-cardiothoracic surgery (Royal College of Radiologists 2003). However, chest x-ray may be desirable in patients undertaking major colorectal surgery (Janke *et al.* 2002). Any abnormalities detected may necessitate the patient undergoing further pulmonary function testing.

Routine blood tests are normally:

- full blood count (FBC);
- urea and electrolytes (U&Es);
- clotting screen;
- group and save sample.

Patients undergoing stoma-forming surgery are usually venesected for routine blood tests. Colorectal cancer patients may be anaemic and require a pre-operative blood transfusion to optimise them prior to theatre. IBD patients must have their renal function and electrolytes checked, as profuse diarrhoea may lead to dehydration and imbalances in sodium, potassium and magnesium, and rectal bleeding might cause anaemia that may require pre-operative correction. All patients undergoing laparotomy with stoma formation should have a group and save sample, as blood may be required intra-operatively.

Pre-operative information

During the assessment the patient's understanding about their condition, the need and the implications of the stoma-forming surgery should be reviewed. It is also important to discuss post-operative expectations, which need to be realistic. The patient needs to understand the gastrointestinal tract and/or the urinary system to be able to understand what alters when the stoma is formed (McGrath & Black 2005).

If a patient has a new diagnosis, such as cancer, the stoma may be accepted in a different way to a chronically ill patient. For chronic diseases, such as Crohn's disease, a stoma may relieve symptoms and sometimes surgery has been discussed previously. In this case it may be easier to cope with a stoma or it may be something the patient has dreaded for years. Other factors that affect how a person copes with their stoma are whether it is temporary, permanent (Black 2000), elective or emergency surgery.

Information giving has been shown for many years to reduce anxiety (Hayward 1975), enabling patients to:

- make informed decisions about their surgery;
- have pre-operative counselling;
- ask questions;
- discuss feelings of anxiety;
- discuss any potential problems.

Oral and written information should be provided (Skene & Smallwood 2002). This has been recognised as important for over 40 years with the publication of patient information in a medical journal (Lenneberg & Mendelssohn 1969). Written information allows patients to revisit areas of interest or concern and additionally the patient's significant others can read them. There are many leaflets produced on stoma care by the appliance manufacturers, voluntary agencies and/or hospitals. It is also good practice to show an appropriate stoma appliance to the patient prior to surgery, as appliances are often not what patients expect and seeing one may reduce anxiety (Davenport 2003b).

Health care professionals should reinforce positive thoughts about stomas to help patients cope better after the stoma formation. However, it is essential to discuss the risks and potential complications (Quallich 2005). Clear information and explanations about stomas, how they work and potential lifestyle changes is beneficial to aid recovery and compliance (Skene & Smallwood 2002).

Patients have various concerns about stoma formation. The following list includes the more common issues that should be discussed prior to surgery:

- the stoma's appearance;
- smell;
- stoma size;
- will the stoma show under clothes;
- the stoma position on the abdomen;
- information on stoma appliances;
- expectations of the patient;
- expectations of and from the health care professional;
- the stoma function.

(Readding 2003)

Bowel preparation

Patients undergoing colonic surgery are usually given bowel preparation to rid the colon of solid stool, reducing bacterial load and minimising the risk of infection (Allen 2005). Bowel preparation has only been in use for 30 years, prior to this post-operative infectious complication occurred in 30–50% of all operations (Nichols *et al.* 2005). Oral sodium phosphate and sodium picosulfates/magnesium citrate are commonly used to evacuate the colon and rectum before colorectal surgery. These products are potent medications and have been associated with side effects such as electrolyte abnormalities, nausea, bloating, abdominal cramps and vomiting (BNF 2007). It may be necessary to commence intravenous fluid and electrolyte replacement prior to surgery to achieve optimum levels pre-operatively, particularly for the elderly. Additionally patients receiving intravenous fluids should be regularly venesected to check their renal function and electrolytes and any abnormalities corrected.

Contraindications to bowel preparation include cardiopulmonary disease, renal disease, hepatic disease and bowel obstruction (Frizelle & Colls 2005). Nichols *et al.* (2005) describe two approaches to bowel preparation. The first is whole gut lavage with a suitable agent on the day before the operation and the second option is dietary restrictions and cathartics for a two-day period. Patients undergoing stoma-forming surgery are routinely given bowel preparation to cleanse the gut the day before surgery and then take fluids only (Steele 1997). However, elderly patients are particularly vulnerable to becoming dehydrated and confused (Jester & Williams 1999). In the authors' clinical area surgical patients are brought into hospital the day prior to surgery for bowel preparation, with one dose given in the afternoon and a further dose in the evening. Patients then remain on clear fluids, for example tea and coffee without milk, after the first dose of bowel preparation. Patients prescribed bowel preparation will need to be situated close to a lavatory. Elderly patients and those with mobility problems may require a commode particularly at night. Frequent defaecation may cause sore peri-anal skin and a barrier cream can be useful.

Some authors doubt the efficacy of bowel preparation in routine pre-operative colorectal surgical patients and consider effective prophylactic antibiotics preferable (Mahajna *et al.* 2005; Ram *et al.* 2005; Santos *et al.* 1994). They consider the risk of the liquid bowel contents spilling, following bowel preparation, which may potentially increase wound infection and anastomotic dehiscence. Alternatively there is a three-tiered regimen (Nichols *et al.* 2005) of pre-operative bowel preparation, pre-operative antibiotic therapy and peri-operative intravenous antimicrobial therapy. This regime has shown to be efficacious in multiple reports from the last three decades but there are recent contrary reports.

Meeting another ostomate

It can be useful for the patient to meet another ostomate before or after surgery, to promote a positive attitude and to help them to realise that a normal life is possible with a stoma. The stoma specialist nurse may know of ostomates willing to speak to new ostomates. Stoma support groups also have trained visitors to provide support. Additionally joining a national or local support group can also help a new or established ostomate cope.

Informed consent

The patient must be able to comprehend the information given to provide informed consent (Quallich 2005). It is essential that prior to their operation patients understand:

- the implications of surgery;
- why surgery is required;
- risks and potential complications;
- diagnosis;
- alternatives;
- probability of success;
- the expected length of stay in hospital;
- the bowel preparation to clear the bowel – if any;
- expectations after surgery;
- equipment that may be required after surgery:
    - urinary catheter;
    - intravenous fluids;

- o   pain relief;
- o   post-operative observations, including blood pressure and stoma checks.

(Garretson 2004; Quallich 2005; Skene & Smallwood 2002)

It is well known that pre-operative information giving assists post-operative recovery (Salter 1997). Consent forms are increasingly complicated and cover more potential complications than before. This reflects patients wanting and expecting high standards of care from health care professionals, and more litigation. It is important to document questions or concerns raised by patients and the responses given (Skene & Smallwood 2002). The patient also needs to give verbal consent to have their stoma sited.

Stoma siting assessment

The term 'siting' means to mark the skin for the ideal stoma position. Stoma siting is required when a surgical procedure will potentially or definitely result in stoma formation. The stoma specialist nurse usually sites the patient the day before surgery (Readding 2003). The stoma specialist nurse has gained theoretical knowledge from a training course and then experience through supervised practice. In emergency situations, patients with pain and/or a distended abdomen siting can be difficult. The consensus is the patient should be sited (Rutledge *et al.* 2003); however, the site may not be in an ideal position and this should be explained to the patient.

Before stoma-forming surgery the stoma specialist nurse discusses with the patient the potential stoma site. Involving the patient can assist them to become independent with their stoma after surgery. Choosing a suitable stoma site helps to ensure the patient has an optimum quality of life as a poorly sited stoma may result in both management (Banks & Razor 2003) and psychological problems. Generally the stoma is sited over the outer third of the rectus abdominus muscle, below a line that joins the umbilicus (Erwin-Toth 2003) and in the left (see Figure 9.1) or right iliac fossa (see Figure 9.2). The stoma should be on the upper curve of the abdomen and not near the umbilicus or groin (Readding 2003). A colostomy is usually sited on the left and an ileostomy or urostomy on the right side (Davenport 2003a).

When siting a patient there are many aspects to consider. The nurse will need to assess:

- physical shape;
- obesity – site higher than usual;
- lifestyle;
- clothing – ideally site below the waistband, consider using high waisted trousers or braces;
- mobility;
- disabilities;
- level of independence with daily activities;
- hobbies;

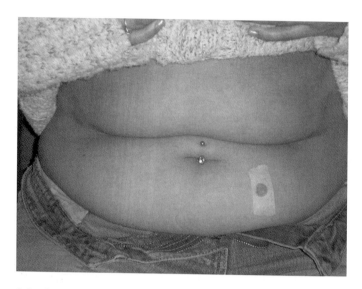

Figure 9.1   Colostomy site.

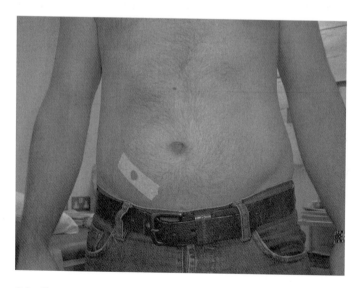

Figure 9.2   Ileostomy or urostomy site.

- dexterity;
- eyesight;
- leisure activities;
- prosthetics – should be worn when siting;
- sports;
- employment;
- cultural influences.

(Hunter 2004)

Cultural/religious issues related to siting

Some cultures or religions such as people from South Asian or Muslim faiths traditionally use one hand for eating and the other for cleaning and hygiene activities (Black 2000). Not all people from these groups will follow the traditions strictly, but for those that do it may be difficult to cope with a stoma. Pre-operative explanations can assist in planning care for the patient (Black 2004). A potential way around this issue is to place the stoma above the umbilicus (Pinches 1999); the output from the stoma is then considered to be food content and may be more acceptable.

Stoma siting

The stoma should be placed in a position that the patient can see, that allows freedom of movement and that their clothing can disguise. The appliance needs to be in a secure and comfortable position. The site should be agreed with the patient, stoma specialist nurse and surgeon, although sometimes a compromise has to be made. If the patient is usually in a wheelchair the stoma should be sited with them in the chair to help maintain independence with the stoma after surgery (Rutledge *et al.* 2003). If the patient is to have two stomas, it is better to have one site slightly above the other in case a stoma belt is required (Readding 2003).

The stoma specialist nurse should ensure the patient is fully informed, agrees to the surgery and has no further questions before siting begins. The process of siting is written below as a guideline, although practice varies.

- Explain the procedure.
- Obtain consent and co-operation from the patient.
- Assemble equipment, tape and pen.
- Clothes are loosened to reveal the abdomen from chest to groin.
- Ask the patient to lie on the bed, in the supine position, with a pillow under their head.
- Identify:
  - rectus abdominus muscle – to locate ask the patient to lift their head from the pillow;
  - umbilicus;
  - previous scars;
  - skin creases/folds;
  - bony prominences;
  - pendulous breasts.
- Draw an imaginary line between the umbilicus and the iliac crest.
- Place marked tape at the midpoint.
- Assess the patient:
  - lying;
  - sitting;
  - standing.
- The site marked should be:
  - on flat skin;
  - on healthy skin tissue;

  o   visible to the patient;
  o   in reach of the patient's hands;
  o   agreed by the patient.
- Mark the skin directly with a permanent marker pen.
- Cover the mark with a film dressing (this is not always required).
- Document in the notes and discuss any issues related to siting with the surgeons.

(Hunter 2004; Readding 2003)

Pre-operative fasting

Within the medical profession there is debate as to the amount of time a patient needs to remain nil by mouth pre-operatively. Bothamley and Mardell (2005) demonstrate patients continue to have excessive fasting times. Janke *et al.* (2002) suggest that not fasting increases the risk of regurgitation of stomach contents and pulmonary aspiration while under general anaesthetic. The rationale for ensuring that surgical patients remain nil by mouth is to facilitate a safe intubation by the anaesthetist.

Guidelines from the Royal College of Nursing (2005) suggest that nurses remember 'The two and six rule', that is intake of water two hours before surgery and a minimum of six hours fasting for solid food.

Complications of prolonged fasting before surgery include:

- headache
- irritability
- dehydration
- confusion
- electrolyte imbalance
- hypoglycaemia
- nausea and vomiting.
  (Jester & Williams 1999)

When caring for patients who are undergoing stoma-forming surgery it is important to be aware of research findings and to ensure surgical patients' oral intake, particularly of fluids is maintained pre-operatively. Patients at risk, such as the elderly, may benefit from intravenous fluids prior to surgery.

Post-operative aims

The importance of discharge planning has been recognised for over ten years. However, earlier discharges reduce the time for teaching stoma care (Mead 1994) and it is ideal for the ostomate to be independent with their appliance change prior to discharge (Thompson 2000). Therefore this time needs to be used effectively to optimise the teaching opportunities (O'Connor 2005).

Post-operative care

The aim of post-operative care for ostomates is to ensure a safe recovery. The patient requires observing for complications including nausea, vomiting and pain. Additionally vital signs include:

- temperature
- pulse
- respiration rate
- blood pressure
- oxygen saturation levels.
  (Butler-Williams 2005)

Zeitz (2005) showed that almost 50% of nursing interventions in the first 24 hours post-operatively involved a post-operative observation and almost 25% a set of vital signs. During the first four post-operative hours the intensity of the monitoring occurs, this is imperative as research demonstrates that five per cent of patients develop an early post-operative complication (Gamil & Fanning 1991).

Nurses caring for colorectal surgical patients must be aware of subtle changes in vital signs, indicating the patient's condition is deteriorating. An increasing temperature is primarily an indicator of infection (Wipke-Tevis 1999). The source of infection could be related to the wound, urinary tract or respiratory function; however, these usually occur several days post-operatively. A 'swinging' pyrexia over several days can indicate an abdominal collection.

Hypotension is defined as a systolic blood pressure of less than 90 mmHg or a reduction in a patient's systolic pressure of more than 40 mm Hg from their normal measurement (Robson & Newell 2005). Hypotension can be related to administration of analgesics, particularly epidural analgesia. Tachycardia is defined as a pulse rate above 100 beats per minute (Tortora & Grabowski 2003). Hypotension in conjunction with a tachycardia is normally indicative of shock.

McLuckie (2003) describes hypovolaemic shock as an inadequate intravascular volume caused by the loss of blood or other body fluids. This can be observed by a low urine output of less than 0.5 ml per kg an hour (about 30 ml an hour), which generally requires intervention to prevent the patient's condition deteriorating further. A fluid challenge is commonly administered to reverse the effects of hypovolaemia, usually in the form of a crystalloid or colloid solution given intravenously with much debate recently as to which of these is preferable (Rizoli 2003). A bolus of fluid is given over a short period of time to elicit an improvement in the patient's condition, although this practice has been questioned recently. Some patients may have a central venous catheter (CVC) for venous access and by using a manometer attached to the CVC the effectiveness of the fluid bolus can be assessed, by taking several measurements and observing the trend.

Normal respiratory rate is defined as nine to 14 breaths per minute (Butler-Williams 2005). Research suggests that an abnormal respiratory rate is a significant predictor of deterioration, cardiac arrest and/or the need for admission to the intensive care unit (Hodgetts *et al.* 2002). Surgical nurses need to be diligent and report an increasing respiratory rate; however, this vital observation is frequently not recorded (Chellel *et al.* 2002). To assist nurses in highlighting patients that are at risk many Trusts have instigated Early Warning Scoring on their observation charts (Stenhouse *et al.* 2000). Each vital sign is given a score (Allen 2004) which when added together gives a total. A total score of greater than four suggests that the patient's condition is deteriorating and will need medical intervention.

Blood tests

During their hospitalisation patients having undergone stoma-forming surgery will benefit from regular blood tests, usually haematology and biochemistry. The results of these investigations can be analysed and appropriate action taken. A full blood count will show anaemia following colorectal surgery; often if the haemoglobin is below 8 g/dl a blood transfusion is contemplated and a further cross-match sample may be required. Another useful indicator is the white cell count (WCC) and C-reactive protein (CRP) levels. These parameters are normally raised initially after surgery but as the patient's post-operative recovery continues these tests are useful for suspected infections. If either or both of the WCC and CRP increase then an infection may be present. If obvious causes, e.g. wound or chest infections, have been eliminated then investigation may be necessary to rule out an anastomotic leak or pelvic collection. The final aspects of blood testing to consider are the urea and electrolytes, giving an indication of renal function and therefore fluid requirement. Patients undergoing stoma formation usually have intravenous fluids until gut motility returns post-operatively. Electrolytes such as sodium, potassium and magnesium need to be monitored closely as levels can deplete especially if the patient has a prolonged ileus or is vomiting.

Nausea and vomiting

Zeitz (2004) showed that nausea and vomiting were the most frequent complications recorded in the first 24 hours post-operatively and continue to impact adversely on length of hospital stay (Fleisler *et al.* 1999). Colorectal surgical patients are susceptible to nausea and vomiting, as manipulation of the gut results in a paralytic ileus. Following stoma-forming surgery patients may return from theatre with a naso-gastric (NG) tube in situ, although this practice is declining. Regular aspiration of the NG tube and checking that tubing is not kinked will facilitate free drainage, reducing nausea and vomiting. If despite regular aspiration of the NG tube, nausea and vomiting still occurs an anti-emetic could be useful.

A number of anti-emetics are available, with differing modes of action: colorectal surgical patients will benefit from intramuscular or intravenous administration of these drugs. However, it is recommended that no more than two anti-emetics be administered concurrently. If nausea and vomiting continue for a prolonged period of time further investigation may be warranted to rule out bowel obstruction.

Nutrition

It is important that patients receive quality nutritional support to recover (Fulham 2004). Various aspects of nutrition are discussed in Chapter 14.

Post-operative analgesia

Patients undergoing stoma-forming surgery will be reviewed pre-operatively by an anaesthetist; during this consultation the patient's preferred method of pain relief is discussed. Svensson *et al.* (2001) showed that after undergoing elective abdominal surgery 76% of patients reported moderate to severe post-operative pain and of this group 5% reported unbearable pain. Therefore, ensuring surgical patients have adequate analgesia post-operatively is of paramount importance. Gan *et al.* (2004) state that pain after surgery can impede recovery and interfere with returning to normal activities. The most common pain relief strategies after major abdominal surgery are epidural analgesia and/or-patient controlled analgesia (PCA) (Bartha *et al.* 2006).

Epidural analgesia is highly effective for controlling acute pain following surgery to the abdomen and pelvis (Royal College of Anaesthetists 2004) and is common practice in acute care environments (Higgins 2006). Colorectal surgical patients usually have an epidural catheter inserted aseptically whilst in theatres, placed in the epidural space at the following level:

- upper abdomen T7 ~ T10
- lower abdomen T9 ~ L1
  (Dougherty & Lister 2004)

The synergistic combination of a local anaesthetic (such as bupivacaine) and a strong opioid (such as fentaynl) in low doses infused directly into the epidural space has the potential to provide analgesia (Melzack & Wall 2003) and benefits have been well established (Sakaguchi *et al.* 2000). As lower doses of opioids are needed to achieve effective analgesia a lower incidence of opioid related side effects such as sedation and prolonged ileus may occur. The epidural can run as a continuous infusion or as a patient-controlled system that allows the patient to administer small bolus doses in addition to a background continuous infusion (Higgins 2006).

Rigg *et al.* (2002) demonstrated that post-operative epidural analgesia was associated with lower pain scores during the first three post-operative days. When caring for patients with an epidural infusion it is essential to observe for potential complications:

- dural puncture causing headache;
- catheter migration;
- epidural haematoma and abscess.
  (Dougherty & Lister 2004)

An anaesthetist should be contacted immediately if complications with an epidural infusion are suspected including:

- respiratory depression
- hypotension
- sedation
- nausea and vomiting
- pruritis
- motor blockade.
  (Dougherty & Lister 2004)

Sugden and Cox (2006) state that the level of motor block should be checked regularly to ensure it is:

- covering the area and/or site of pain;
- not too high;
- not too dense, causing unnecessary motor blockade.

The epidural catheter site should be checked regularly for leakage, which will necessitate urgent discontinuation and a suitable alternative method of pain relief. The epidural infusion is generally discontinued on the third post-operative day and the epidural catheter removed. The administration of subcutaneous anticoagulant therapy should be organised around planned catheter removal to minimise the risk of haematoma formation (Higgins 2006).

PCA is widely used (Jeffs *et al.* 2002) enabling the patient to administer a bolus of opioid, usually morphine or a suitable alternative if the patient is allergic to morphine. This method may be viewed as inferior to epidural infusion because when the patient falls asleep the analgesic effects diminish and the patient awakes in pain. PCA also relies on intravenous opiates to relieve pain and therefore patients may experience more severe side effects compared to epidurals including:

- cough suppression
- nausea and vomiting
- respiratory depression
- sedation
- urinary retention
- constipation.
  (Unlugenc *et al.* 2003)

Regular paracetamol can be administered concurrently with the epidural or PCA to enhance pain relief, either intravenously or orally if tolerated. Other drugs that can be given in conjunction with a PCA are non-steroidal anti-inflammatory drugs, e.g. diclofenac sodium, and a limited number of intramuscular injections can also be used as adjuvant therapy. Once the epidural or PCA has been discontinued, the patient's pain needs reassessing and suitable oral analgesia administered. The timing of commencing oral analgesia is crucial when discontinuing other methods to ensure efficient pain relief (Brown *et al.* 2007). Synthetic opiates such as tramadol or compound analgesics, for example cocodamol or codydramol, can be useful. Sometimes a combination of analgesics is necessary to alleviate pain.

Acute pain is still a common occurrence after surgery despite improvements in treatment (Gan *et al.* 2004). Regular use of analgesia is usually warranted but assessment to ensure efficacy is essential and to monitor for side effects.

Post-operative exercises

Post-operative exercises should ideally be taught to the patient in the pre-operative phase. These exercises usually consist of leg and deep breathing exercises, which are taught by the physiotherapist and reinforced by the nursing staff. Patients undergoing stoma-forming surgery will benefit from such exercises to aid their recovery. In addition it can be useful to also perform pelvic floor exercises, arm raises, pelvic tilts, leg lifts, knee rolls, kneeling, calf raises and relaxation techniques.

Immobile colorectal surgical patients not able to mobilise due to pain, nausea and vomiting for example should be encouraged to participate in leg exercises. By plantar and dorsal flexion of the feet the circulation of the lower limbs will be enhanced, minimising the risk of blood stasis in the legs and reducing the risk of deep vein thrombosis.

During abdominal surgery patients are invariably anaesthetised for a prolonged period of time: this causes basal collapse of the lungs known as atelectasis. Post-operatively if patients are not encouraged to undertake deep breathing exercises and expand their lungs a chest infection may occur. Preferably, patients should be nursed sat upright in a chair at the earliest opportunity to facilitate lung inflation. As the post-operative recovery continues patients have to be encouraged to mobilise even if only for a short distance.

Post-operative appliances

Appliances used in the post-operative period are clear, drainable bags (Lee 2001). A clear appliance enables the stoma to be checked regularly for healthy bowel mucosa. The output can also be checked and emptied if required (Kirkwood 2006).

Post-operative stoma assessment

The stoma requires regular post-operative checks for any problems. The assessment should be done with each general observation and frequency of checks reduced as the patient's general condition stabilises.

Normal stomas

The bowel mucosa should be for all stoma types:

- red or pink – due to profuse blood supply; dark stomas can indicate poor blood supply; pale stomas may indicate a low haemoglobin;
- warm – the same temperature as the rest of the abdomen and can be felt through the plastic appliance;
- moist – due to the bowel secretions.

(McCahon 1999)

Colostomies are flush or minimally raised, whereas ileostomies and urostomies should have a 2.5 cm spout. Any abnormalities should be reported to the surgeon or the stoma specialist nurse, although intervention is not always required.

Initially following surgery the stoma may be oedematous. The oedema is usually minimal but in rare cases can almost double the size of the stoma. The oedema will reduce in up to eight weeks.

Normal stoma outputs

The long-term stoma outputs for each stoma are:

- colostomies – generally pass soft to formed stool, usually once or twice daily;
- ileostomies – usually pass semi-formed to loose stool; appliances should be emptied four to six times daily when a third to half full;
- urostomies – continually pass urine, with minimal mucus present; appliances are usually emptied four to six times daily when a third to half full.

(Fillingham & Douglas 2004; Trainor *et al.* 2003)

Post-operative urostomies

In the initial post-operative period the output from a urostomy should be immediate. The volume of urine should be about 30 ml an hour, depending on the patient's age, weight and size. There may be blood in the urine, but this should quickly cease. There may be mucus passed from the bowel used as the conduit: this reduces in volume but may always occur.

Urostomy stents

Post-operative urostomies may have stents (fine-bore catheters) to prevent stenosis of the anastomosis between the ureter and the bowel. The stents may be left in situ for 7–14 days. Stents should be checked regularly as occasionally they become blocked. If a blockage occurs a very gentle flush with saline may be required (Fillingham & Douglas 2004). If the stents are expelled unexpectedly, they should not be re-inserted. The patient, however, should be observed for pain, tenderness and urine volume. When the stents are due to be removed a gentle turn or pull can loosen them. If they do not easily drop out then a daily gentle turn is required until the stents fall out.

Post-operative faecal stomas

Faecal stomas will often pass nothing for a period of time; this may be hours to days, followed by haemoserous fluid, then flatus and faecal fluid. The faeces then gradually thicken as diet is increased. Uncommonly there may be a high faecal output of over one litre daily from the stoma. Outputs should be monitored and fluid losses replaced and resolution is generally spontaneously.

Rods/bridges

A loop stoma may have a rod/bridge under the stoma to prevent the bowel from pulling back into the abdomen. The rod is generally left in position for three to ten days and then removed, which is simple and painless. The rod has one end that is moveable and when the rod is removed the wing is turned to be in line with the rest of the rod. Finally the rod is gently removed from the stoma. The stoma should then be reviewed, as there may be damage to the stoma where the rod touched it. After removal there may be slightly sloughy edges to the bowel mucosa at the exit sites of the rod. This requires no treatment and the small openings quickly close over. The stoma should be observed for retraction after the rod is removed, particularly if there was tension on the rod.

Wound care

The mucocutaneous junction of the stoma and skin needs to heal after surgery. The dissolvable sutures are usually adequate to secure the wound edges, but if the wound breaks down action may be required.

The midline surgical incision is usually superficially healed within ten days when the clips/stitches are removed. However, care should be taken to protect the wound from contamination from the stoma output for several weeks or longer.

Post-operative stoma care teaching

A practical guide to stoma teaching promotes the patient's independence. The patient should be instructed so that they are aware what is normal for their stoma, in relation to appearance, size, output and function. It is important to also be aware of potential complications and the appropriate action to take if they occur.

The basic teaching schedule for new ostomates will need to be individualised. For example, a patient with poor balance should change their appliance sitting or lying down (Readding 2003). The nurse should demonstrate an appropriate appliance change and the patient should take over increasingly until they are confident and able to continue changing alone: the time to independence varies between patients. Nurses should wear gloves when participating in an appliance change but patients do not (Breckman 2005). When dealing with the ostomate there should be no signs of distaste or rejection to help the patient to cope with their stoma (Hunter 2004).

Teaching plan

The basic components of a teaching plan are as follows.

- Explain the procedure to the patient.
- Ensure privacy.
- Collect all the necessary equipment:
  - new appliance;
  - measuring guide (and pen);
  - scissors;
  - cleaning/drying cloths (or kitchen roll);
  - warm tap water (no soap);
  - disposal bag.
- Empty drainable appliances – to reduce risk of spillage.
- Gently remove the soiled appliance, use one hand to support the skin.
- Join together the edges of the used appliance flange, to avoid leakage of any contents and place in the disposal bag.
- Clean the peristomal skin thoroughly but gently – tiny spots of bleeding may be seen from the stoma surface if touched.
- *Note*: the stoma may move as part of peristalsis.
- Dry the skin well.
- Inspect the skin and stoma for any changes.
- Measure the stoma with the guide – the size will reduce for the first eight weeks after formation.
- Cut the appliance to the same shape as and 2–3 mm larger than the stoma – to give a small margin for error in appliance placement.
- Remove the backing from the pouch.
- Apply the flange to the skin around the stoma.
- Secure the adhesive to the skin by pressing firmly: start directly around the stoma and work outwards.
- If a two-piece appliance is used attach the bag, then hold the appliance on to the abdomen for 30 to 60 seconds to aid adhesion.
- Ensure that the fastening is closed (if appropriate).
- Seal the rubbish bag and dispose of it.
- Wash hands.
- Avoid bending the abdomen for ten minutes after application to help adhesion.

(Breckman 2005; Rust 2007; Trainor *et al.* 2003)

Stoma closure

A temporary loop ileostomy or loop colostomy is often constructed to protect a distal anastomosis (Rolandelli & Roslyn 2001), as an anastomotic leakage is a serious post-operative complication following colorectal surgery (Law *et al.* 2002). A loop ileostomy may be easier for patients to manage and cause fewer complications than a loop transverse colostomy (Haagmans *et al.* 2004). Ostomates normally return to hospital within three to six months following their initial procedure for closure of their temporary stoma (Black 2000). An early ileostomy closure reduces stoma-related complications and improves quality of life (Bakx *et al.* 2004). Prior to their stoma reversal, ostomates are generally admitted to the ward on the day before surgery. Typically in patients who have undergone a restorative proctocolectomy, a pouchogram may be performed to verify the integrity of the pouch and the pouch–anal anastomosis prior to the ileostomy closure.

Loop stomas often negate the need for laparotomy as a circumferential incision can be made around the stoma to mobilise the loop of bowel. Once the stoma has been taken down the anastomosis can either be hand sewn (Garcia-Botello *et al.* 2004) or stapled (Lane *et al.* 1998). On return to the ward the patient will need to have their observations maintained regularly as previously discussed until suitably recovered. Nurses must also be assiduous in checking the closure site regularly for signs of excessive bleeding and report any disproportionate swelling around the site.

Intravenous fluids will normally be required post-operatively to combat dehydration, until the surgeon feels it is appropriate to commence oral fluids and subsequent diet, which in some cases may be immediately post-operatively (Haagmans *et al.* 2004).

Overall complication rates from ileostomy closure have been reported to range between 10% and 30% (Wong *et al.* 2005). Therefore nurses should be aware of the potential problems that may occur following the closure of a loop ileostomy:

- small bowel obstruction
- wound infection
- abdominal sepsis.

Small bowel obstruction

The presence of a loop ileostomy may increase the chance of the small bowel twisting and the formation of adhesions adjacent to the stoma (Law *et al.* 2002). Metcalf *et al.* (1986) describe the incidence of intestinal obstruction as 14.8% after the closure of a loop ileostomy in patients with an ileoanal pouch anastomosis. Small bowel obstruction is normally managed conservatively with intravenous fluids and the patient is kept nil by mouth. However, surgery is sometimes required to relieve the obstruction that invariably is due to adhesions (Wong *et al.* 2005).

Wound infection

Treatment of minor wound infections is generally to make a small opening in the wound (Garcia-Botello *et al.* 2004) and possibly oral antibiotics (Wong *et al.* 2005). Using this technique, hospital stays did not increase but a better cosmetic result was achieved.

Abdominal sepsis

Post-operative leak rates following ileostomy closure are reported as up to 7% (Garcia-Botello *et al.* 2004). Post-operative leak management is dictated by the patient's condition and imaging. A localised leak causing abscess formation can be managed using percutaneous drainage. However, if the patient's condition deteriorates, a further laparotomy may be required as well as subsequent repair of the leak with a covering loop ileostomy.

Nurses caring for patients undergoing closure of a loop stoma should be attentive to the post-operative care of this patient group. Closure of a stoma may be regarded as a 'minor' operation; however, as discussed there are a number of serious complications that should be observed for.

References

Allen G (2005) Bowel preparation. *Association of Operating Room Nurses Journal.* **82(3)**: 489–92.

Allen K (2004) Recognising and managing adult patients who are critically sick. *Nursing Times.* **100(35)**: 34–7.

Bakx R, Busch ORC, Bemelman WA, Veldink GJ, Slors JFM *et al.* (2004) Morbidity of temporary loop ileostomy. *Digestive Surgery.* **21**: 277–81.

Banks N & Razor B (2003) Preoperative stoma site assessment and marking: trained RN's can improve ostomy outcomes. *American Journal of Nursing.* **103(3)**: 64A–E.

Bartha E, Carlsson P & Kalman S (2006) Evaluation of costs of epidural analgesia and patient-controlled intravenous analgesia after major abdominal surgery. *British Journal of Anaesthesia.* **96(1)**: 111–17.

Bellhouse CP & Dore C (1988) Criteria for estimating likelihood of difficulty of endotracheal intubation with the macintosh laryngoscope. *Anaesthesia and Intensive Care.* **16**: 329–37.

Black P (2000) *Holistic Stoma Care.* London: Baillière Tindall.

Black P (2004) Psychological, sexual and cultural issues for patients with a stoma. *British Journal of Nursing.* **13(12)**: 692–7.

BNF (2007) *British National Formulary. Number 53.* London: BMJ Publishing Group Ltd.

Bothamley J & Mardell A (2005) Pre-operative fasting revisited. *British Journal of Peri-operative Nursing.* **15(9)**: 370–5.

Breckman B (2005) *Stoma Care and Rehabilitation.* London: Elsevier Churchill Livingstone.

Brown D, O'Neill O & Beck A (2007) Post-operative pain management: transition from epidural to oral analgesia. *Nursing Standard.* **21(21)**: 35–40.

Butler-Williams C (2005) Increasing awareness of respiratory rate significance. *Nursing Times.* **101(27)**: 35–7.

Chellel A, Fraser J, Fender V, Higgs D, Buras-Rees S *et al.* (2002) Nursing observations on ward patients at risk of critical illness. *Nursing Times.* **98(46)**: 36–9.

Davenport R (2003a) Choosing the site for the stoma. In: Elcoat C (ed) *Stoma Care Nursing*. London: Hollister.

Davenport R (2003b) Pre-operative stoma care. In: Elcoat C (ed) *Stoma Care Nursing*. London: Hollister.

Dougherty L & Lister S (2004) *The Royal Marsden Hospital Manual of Clinical Procedures*. 6th edn. Royal Marsden Hospital. Oxford: Blackwell.

Erwin-Toth P (2003) Ostomy pearls: a concise guide to stoma siting, pouching systems, patient education, and more. *Advances in Skin and Wound Care*. **16(3)**: 146–52.

Fillingham S & Douglas J (2004) *Urological Nursing*. 3rd edn. London: Baillière Tindall.

Fleisler L, Yee K, Lillemore K, Talamini M, Yeo C et al. (1999) Is outpatient laparoscopic cholecystectomy safe and cost-effective? A model to study transition care. *Anaesthesiology*. **90(6)**: 1746–55.

Frizelle FA & Colls BM (2005) Hyponatremia and seizures after bowel preparation: Report of three cases. *Diseases of the Colon and Rectum*. **48(2)**: 393–6.

Fulham J (2004) Improving the nutritional status of colorectal surgical and stoma patients. *British Journal of Nursing*. **13(12)**: 702–8.

Gamil M & Fanning A (1991) The first 24 hours after surgery. A study of complications after 2153 consecutive operations. *Anaesthesia*. **46(9)**: 712–15.

Gan TJ, Lubarsky DA, Flood EM, Thanh T, Mauskopf J et al. (2004) Patient preferences for acute pain treatment. *British Journal of Anaesthesia*. **92(5)**: 681–8.

Garcia-Botello SA, Garcia-Armengol J, Garcia-Granero E, Espi A, López-Mozos CJF et al. (2004) A prospective audit of the complications of loop ileostomy construction and takedown. *Digestive Surgery*. **21**: 440–6.

Garcia-Miguel FJ, Serrano-Aguilar PG & Lopez-Bastida J (2003) Pre-operative assessment. *The Lancet*. **362(9397)**: 1749–57.

Garretson S (2004) Benefits of pre-operative programmes. *Nursing Standard*. **18(47)**: 33–7.

Haagmans MJ, Brinkert W, Bleichrodt RP, van Goor H & Bremers AJ (2004) Short-term outcome of loop ileostomy closure under local anaesthesia: results of a feasibility study. *Diseases of the Colon and Rectum*. **47(11)**: 1930–3.

Hayward J (1975) *Information: A Prescription Against Pain*. London: RCN.

Higgins D (2006) Practical procedures: how to remove epidural catheters. *Nursing Times*. **102(12)**: 28–9.

Hodgetts T, Kenward G, Vlachonikolis IG, Payne S & Castle N (2002) The identification of risk factors for cardiac arrest and formulation of activation criteria to alert a medical emergency team. *Resuscitation*. **54(2)**: 125–31.

Hunter H (2004) Case study: managing and caring for a patient undergoing stoma formation. *British Journal of Nursing*. **13(12)**: 698–700.

Janke E, Chalk V & Kinley H (2002) *Pre-operative Assessment: Setting a Standard through Learning*. Southampton: University of Southampton.

Jeffs SA, Hall JE & Morris S (2002) Comparison of morphine alone with morphine plus clonidine for post-operative patient-controlled analgesia. *British Journal of Anaesthesia*. **89(3)**: 424–7.

Jester R & Williams R (1999) Pre-operative fasting: putting research into practice. *Nursing Standard*. **13(39)**: 33–5.

Kinley H, Czoki-Murray C, George S, McCabe C, Primrose J et al. (2002) Effectiveness of appropriately trained nurses in pre-operative assessment: randomised controlled equivalence/non-inferiority trial. *British Medical Journal*. **325**: 1323–6.

Kirkwood L (2006) Postoperative stoma care and the selection of appliances. *Journal of Community Nursing*. **20(3)** (March): 12–18.

Lane JS, Kwan D, Chandler CF & Alexander P (1998) Diverting loop versus end ileostomy during ileoanal pull through procedure for ulcerative colitis. *The American Surgeon*. **64(10)**: 979–82.

Law WL, Chu KW & Choi HK (2002) Randomized clinical trial comparing loop ileostomy and loop transverse colostomy for faecal diversion following total mesorectal excision. *British Journal of Surgery.* **89(6)**: 704–8.

Lee J (2001) Nurse prescribing in practice: patient choice in stoma care. *British Journal of Community Nursing.* **6(1)**: 33–7.

Lenneberg E & Mendelssohn AN (1969) Colostomies: a guide for the patient. *Diseases of the Colon and Rectum.* **12(3)**: 201–17.

McCahon S (1999) Faecal stomas. In: Porrett T (ed) *Essential Coloproctology for Nurses.* London: Whurr.

McGrath A & Black P (2005) Stoma siting and the role of the clinical nurse specialist. In: Porrett T & McGrath A (eds) *Stoma Care.* Oxford: Blackwell.

McLuckie A (2003) Shock: an overview In: Oh TE, Bersten AD & Soni N (eds) *Oh's Intensive Care Manual.* 5th edn. Oxford: Butterworth Heinemann.

Mahajna A, Krausz M, Rosin D & Shabti M (2005) Bowel preparation is associated with spillage of bowel contents in colorectal surgery. *Diseases of the Colon and Rectum.* **48(8)**: 1626–31.

Mead J (1994) An emphasis on practical management – discharge planning in stoma care. *Professional Nurse.* **9(6)**: 405–10.

Melzack R & Wall PD (2003) *Handbook of Pain Management.* London: Churchill Livingstone.

Metcalf AM, Dozois RR, Beart RW, Kelly KA & Wolff BG (1986) Temporary ileostomy for ileal pouch-anal anastomosis. Functions and complications. *Diseases of Colon and Rectum.* **29**: 300–3.

Munro JF & Campbell IW (2002) *Macleod's Clinical Examination.* 10th edn. Edinburgh: Churchill Livingstone.

National Institute for Clinical Excellence (2003) *Pre-operative Tests. The Use of Routine Pre-operative Tests for Elective Surgery. Clinical Guideline 3.* London: NICE.

Nichols RL, Choe EU & Weldon CB (2005) Mechanical and antibacterial bowel preparation in colon and rectal surgery. *Chemotherapy.* **51**(supplement 1): 115–21.

O'Connor G (2005) Teaching stoma-management skills: the importance of self-care. *British Journal of Nursing.* **14(5)**: 320–4.

Pinches F (1999) Cultural issues. In: Taylor P (ed) *Stoma Care in the Community.* London: Emap Healthcare.

Power LM & Thackary NM (1999) Reduction of pre-operative investigations with the introduction of an anaesthetist-led pre-operative assessment clinic. *Anaesthesia and Intensive Care.* **27**: 481–8.

Quallich SA (2005) The practice of informed consent. *Dermatology Nursing.* London. **17(1)**: 49–51.

Ram E, Sherman Y, Weil R, Vishne T, Kravarusic D *et al.* (2005) Is mechanical bowel preparation mandatory for elective colon surgery? A prospective randomized study. *Archives of Surgery.* **140(3)**: 285–8.

Readding LA (2003) Stoma siting: what the community nurse needs to know. *British Journal of Community Nursing.* **8(11)**: 502–11.

Rigg JRA, Jamrozik K, Myles PS, Silbert BS, Peyton PJ *et al.* (2002) Epidural anaesthesia and analgesia and outcome of major surgery: a randomised trial. *The Lancet.* **359(9134)**: 1276–82.

Rizoli S (2003) Crystalloids and colloids in trauma resuscitation: a brief overview of the current debate. *Journal of Trauma.* **54** (supplement 5): S82–S88.

Robson W & Newell J (2005) Assessing, treating and managing patients with sepsis. *Nursing Standard.* **19(50)**: 56–64.

Roizen MF (1989) Pre-operative patient evaluation. *Canadian Journal of Anaesthesia.* **36**: 13–19.

Rolandelli RH & Roslyn JJ (2001) Colon and rectum. In: Townsend CM (ed) *Sabiston Textbook of Surgery.* Philadelphia: W.B. Saunders.

Royal College of Anaesthetists (2004) *Good Practice in the Management of Continuous Epidural Analgesia in the Hospital Setting.* London: Royal College of Anaesthetists.

Royal College of Nursing (2005) *Peri-operative Fasting in Adults and Children. An RCN Guideline for the Multidisciplinary Team.* London: RCN Publications.

Royal College of Radiologists (2003) *Making the Best Use of a Department of Clinical Radiology Guidelines for Doctors.* 5th edn. London: Royal College of Radiologists.

Rust J (2007) Care of patients with stomas: the pouch change procedure. *Nursing Standard.* **22(6)**: 43–7.

Rutledge M, Thompson MJ & Boyd-Carson W (2003) Effective stoma siting. *Nursing Standard.* **18(12)**: 43–4.

Sakaguchi Y, Sakura S, Shinzawa M & Saitos Y (2000) Does adrenaline improve epidural bupivacaine and fentanyl analgesia after abdominal surgery? *Anaesthesia and Intensive Care.* **28(5)**: 522–6.

Salter M (1997) *Altered Body Image, the Nurse's Role.* 2nd edn. London: Baillière Tindall.

Samson GLT & Young JRB (1987) Difficult tracheal intubation: a retrospective study. *Anaesthesia.* **42**: 487–90.

Santos JCM, Batista J, Sirimarco MT, Guimaracs AS & Levy CE (1994) Prospective randomization trial of mechanical bowel preparation in patients undergoing elective colorectal surgery. *British Journal of Surgery.* **81**: 1673–6.

Skene L & Smallwood R (2002) Informed consent: lessons from Australia. *British Medical Journal.* **324(7328)**: 39–41.

Steele RJC (1997) Colonic cancer. In: Phillips RKS (ed) *Colorectal Surgery.* 2nd edn. London: W.B Saunders.

Stenhouse C, Coates S, Tivey M, Allsop P & Parker T (2000) Prospective evaluation of a modified early warning score to aid earlier detection of patients developing critical illness on a general surgical ward. *British Journal of Anaesthesia.* **84(5)**: 663.

Sugden A & Cox F (2006) Practical procedures: how to assess epidural blockade. *Nursing Times.* **102(11)**: 26–7.

Svensson I, Sjostrom B & Haljamae H (2001) Influence of expectations and actual pain experiences on satisfaction with post-operative pain management. *European Journal of Pain.* **5**: 125–33.

Thompson J (2000) Part One: A practical ostomy guide. *RN.* **63(11)**: 61–8.

Tortora G & Grabowski S (2003) *Principles of Anatomy and Physiology.* 10th edn. New York: John Wiley & Sons, Inc.

Trainor B, Thompson MJ, Boyd-Carson W & Boyd K (2003) Changing an appliance. *Nursing Standard.* **18(13)**: 41–2.

UK General Medical Council (1995) *The New Doctor.* London: GMC.

Unlugenc H, Ozalevli M, Gunes Y, Guler T & Isik G (2003) Pre-emptive analgesic efficiency of tramadol compared with morphine after major abdominal surgery. *British Journal of Anaesthesia.* **91(2)**: 209–15.

Walker R (2002) ASA and CEPOD scoring. *World Anaesthesia.* **14**: Article 5.

Wipke-Tevis DD (1999) Vascular infections: medical and surgical therapies. *Journal of Cardiovascular Nursing.* **13(2)**: 70–81.

Wong KT, Remzi FH, Gorgun E, Arrigain MA, Church JM *et al.* (2005) Loop ileostomy closure after restorative proctocolectomy: outcome in 1,504 patients. *Diseases of the Colon and Rectum.* **48(2)**: 243–50.

Zeitz K (2004) Post-operative complications in the first 24 hours: a general surgery audit. *Journal of Advanced Nursing.* **46(6)**: 633–40.

Zeitz K (2005) Nursing observations during the first 24 hours after a surgical procedure: what do we do? *Journal of Clinical Nursing.* **14(3)**: 334–43.

Chapter 10

Intestinal Pouches

Zarah Perry-Woodford

Introduction

This chapter will discuss the three main types of intestinal pouches.

- the ileoanal pouch;
- the coloanal or colonic 'J' pouch;
- the Kock pouch.

In the last 30 years, the ileoanal pouch has become the standard procedure for patients requiring surgery for ulcerative colitis (UC) and some patients with familial adenomatous polyposis (FAP). This 'procedure of choice' is based largely on a perceived improved quality of life (Jimmo & Hyman 1998). The aim of pouch surgery is to restore intestinal continuity and hopefully continence, therefore avoiding the need for a permanent ileostomy.

This chapter will explore the benefits and complications associated with an intestinal pouch with the main focus on the ileoanal pouch. Issues surrounding patient suitability and selection for surgery will be discussed along with the advantages and drawbacks of the 'J', 'W' and 'S' shaped pouches. Pre-operative counselling, early post-operative and long-term care issues will be considered from a nursing perspective. The common problems associated with pouches such as frequency, sore perianal skin and defaecation difficulties will be explored and suggestions made to resolve or manage these issues. Finally this chapter will reflect on the recent changes and research-based evidence involved with the continued development and modernisation of the intestinal pouch.

The coloanal or colonic 'J' pouch

In some situations, such as cancer of the rectum, where the entire rectum is removed, a coloanal pouch can be formed from the distal colon and offers an alternative to simply joining the end of the colon on to the anus. This neo-rectum restores function of the intestine and provides bowel continence and control to the patient. Overall the function is better than with a straightforward coloanal anastomosis. The colonic pouch is usually protected with a loop ileostomy, while it heals. Patients can usually manage to eat a normal diet a few weeks post closure of the ileostomy and do not appear to encounter dietary difficulties. Faecal evacuation can be a problem. Some patients report faecal frequency and urgency in the immediate postoperative period and may experience nocturnal leakage or soiling. This can be managed with sphincter exercises, anal skin care advice and allowing time for the pouch to become adapted to its new role. The colonic pouch appears to be the superior choice for patients compared to the straight coloanal anastomosis (Furst *et al.* 2002; Remzi *et al.* 2005). However, for those unsuitable or for whom function is poor, a permanent colostomy is an option.

The Kock pouch/reservoir

A Kock pouch is formed from ileum following a colectomy. This differs from an ileoanal pouch as the faeces pass from the abdomen. The Kock pouch is different to an ileostomy as it has a valve that gives faecal continence, which requires emptying via the abdominal stoma. The Kock pouch is not a common continent internal pouch in the present surgical climate and most surgeons would be reluctant to form one as a first option. The reasons for this are the high risk of malfunction and complications of the Kock reservoir and the success of the ileoanal pouch. The continent ileostomy may be offered at specialist gastrointestinal centres as an attractive long-term option to select patients whose only alternative is a permanent ileostomy (Nassar *et al.* 2006).

A medina catheter (see Figure 10.1) is inserted into the pouch in theatre and sutured to the skin. The medina is allowed to drain freely for three to six weeks depending on the surgeon's preference and the patient's recovery. This will allow the internal anastomosis time to heal, prevent overfilling of the pouch and irrigation can occur if necessary. Blackley (1998) suggests that the pouch be irrigated if necessary to gently wash out accumulating mucus. Once the patient starts eating the Kock pouch may become blocked and drainage impaired. To remove a blockage 500–1000 ml

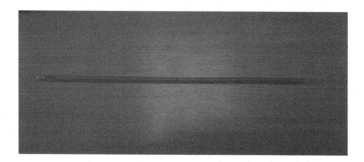

Figure 10.1 A medina catheter.

of tepid tap water can be inserted and drained via a bladder syringe, in divided doses of 30–40 ml, to improve flow (Williams 2002). A Kock pouch cannot hold large volumes and the irrigation fluid needs to be drained before inserting more fluid and careful observation for abdominal pain should be made. Patients should be encouraged to eat a light, soft, low fibre diet. When the catheter is removed patients are taught by the stoma or pouch specialist nurse how to insert the catheter themselves and empty their pouch.

The procedure may have to be practised, as the patient can be reluctant to attempt catheterisation when there is resistance between the catheter and the valve into the pouch. This stress can cause tensing of the abdominal muscles, which in turn hinders catheterisation. Water-based lubricants can also be used to ease the process. Patients should be reassured and encouraged to relax during the procedure. When the pouch is empty a flush can be used to ensure complete emptying and also ease the medina's eyelets from the pouch. The flush is approximately 30–40 ml of tepid tap water. Once the pouch is empty and the medina removed, a stoma cap, dressing or small stoma appliance can be worn. The pouch is emptied approximately every three to four hours. Berndtsson *et al.* (2005) in their study of people with a long-term continent ileostomy found them to have good self-care and quality of life.

The ileoanal pouch

An ileoanal pouch is an internal pouch made from the ileum and attached to the anal canal after a colectomy. There is no documented evidence of the exact number of ileoanal pouches in the UK; however, this figure is ever increasing as centres in the UK submit data on to a national database and more surgeons elect to perform the operation. Most patients requiring pouch surgery are elective patients who opt for either a two- or three-stage operation, commonly referred to as restorative proctocolectomy (RPC). Rarely, some patients opt for a one-stage operation but this carries considerably more risk and is reserved for patients with a complete repulsion towards a temporary ileostomy and who are medically stable.

The two-stage operation involves a total colectomy with the formation of the ileoanal pouch and a defunctioning ileostomy. The patient then returns in approximately three months for a closure of the ileostomy. The three-stage operation differs as a total colectomy, end ileostomy and/or mucous fistula are performed first therefore preserving the rectal stump. The bowel is allowed to rest for a period of two to three months before the rectum is removed and the pouch formed and then the ileostomy closed (either at the second or more often as a separate third procedure). The three-stage pouch procedure is usually performed as an emergency option, for example in near bowel perforation as a result of toxic megacolon or if the patient presents with severe, non-resolving active disease.

Technical improvements allow colectomy for benign disease, for example, to be increasingly performed by minimally invasive techniques (Larson *et al.* 2006). The ongoing debate about the advantage of laparoscopic RPC over conventional methods appears to be the goal of future work.

Patient suitability and selection

Elective patients must have a diagnosis of UC, indeterminate UC or FAP. Crohn's disease is a contraindication for an RPC because of the unacceptably high pouch failure rate of 40–60% (Lovegrove *et al.* 2006). A successful patient for an RPC requires adequate anal sphincter muscle squeeze and control in order to hold large volumes of semi-formed faeces, which will be present in the pouch. The viability of the sphincter muscles can be assessed using a combination of clinical examination, manometry and anorectal physiology. It must be clear that there is an absence of low rectal cancer, especially in the FAP patient group. However, if a patient presents with an established carcinoma that can be excised with good clearance margins and it has not extended into the surrounding tissues an RPC can be performed. As far as possible, patients are weaned off steroid and immunosuppressant therapy prior to surgery. The nutritional status of the patient is assessed and improved with supplements to enhance surgical results. There appears no absolute contraindication for pouch surgery on the grounds of age. According to Nicholls *et al.* (1993) patients as young as three years of age and those in their early 80s have had a successful RPC. There are studies that suggest patients over the age of 55 may have increased problems with continence following pouch surgery. Deterioration of the sphincter muscle is more common in women than in men. Children are usually considered for RPC when there is failure of growth and normal development.

Blood tests are performed to ensure safe biochemistry levels and may identify conditions such as primary sclerosing cholangitis (PSC). PSC is inflammation of the bile ducts and liver associated with extra-intestinal manifestations of UC. The prevalence of PSC in patients with inflammatory bowel disease (IBD) is more common with UC patients than those with Crohn's disease. The characteristics of UC in patients with PSC differ from those without PSC. The colitis is usually substantial; the clinical course quiescent and rectal sparing is common. However, patients with UC and PSC have a higher risk of developing colorectal dysplasia/carcinoma than UC patients without PSC (Broome & Bergquist 2006). PSC is a relative contraindication to RPC in patients with UC as it is also a risk factor for the development of pouchitis. Lohmuller *et al.* (1990) found pouchitis in 39% of RPC patients with extra-intestinal manifestations of UC compared to 26% of those who had not. The same study reported that patients who develop extra intestinal manifestations post-operatively had an incidence of pouchitis of 53% compared to 25% in the group of patients without extra-intestinal manifestations.

The 'S', 'J' or 'W' pouch

Pouch configuration depends highly upon the surgeon's preference and the patient's pelvis. The 'S' shaped pouch is more difficult to construct and was one of the first designs. It has been suggested that it reaches the perineum more easily and has a lower stricture rate with a higher volume than the 'J' shaped pouch. However, the elongated limb to the ileoanal anastomosis was responsible for a failure of spontaneous evacuation in some patients and the technique is now rarely used. The 'J' pouch is easily constructed with the conventional stapling device and fits well into the pelvis. It empties easily as it lacks the efferent limb of some other pouch types. The 'W' shaped pouch is noted for the highest volumes but may not fit into a smaller pelvis. Each of the pouch designs tends to have similar functional results for the patient; however, satisfaction and quality of life studies rate the 'J' shaped pouch as more effective. In some studies adaptation to normal life was comparable for patients with or without a pelvic pouch (Tiainen & Matikainen 1999).

Pre-operative counselling (surgical vs. medical approach)

The intestinal pouch operation does not result in a return to normal bowel function and great care must be taken to explain the advantages and drawbacks to potential patients. Informed patients are likely to be more cooperative and compliant and therefore recover quicker (Skene & Smallwood 2002). Patients for an RPC should be given as much information and preoperative counselling as possible. Most patients are provided with their surgeon's statistics to their success rates for the operation. In order to obtain informed consent patients must be aware of the failure rate of the pouch, which is documented as between 5% and 10% in the first year, increasing with time, up to 10–15% by ten years (Nicholls *et al.* 1993). Most patients experience some form of complication with rates ranging from 20 to 60%.

Patients are primarily under the care of the gastroenterology team and are known to their IBD specialist nurse who manages their medication, provides practical advice and overall support. Together the gastroenterology team decide when the patient is no longer suitable for medical intervention and may benefit from surgery. The common reasons for surgery are failure of medical treatment and the risk of associated drug side effects, for example the prolonged use of steroid therapy, failure of growth in a child, an increased risk of colorectal cancer or high density of polyps, i.e. over 1000 in the FAP patient, or conversion of an ileorectal anastomosis to an internal pouch. The overall aim of pouch surgery is a satisfactory functional outcome, good quality of life and excellent patient satisfaction.

Patients should be made aware that even though surgery for UC is considered curative for the disease manifestations within the bowel, it might not resolve extra-intestinal manifestations, which can develop over time (Rayhorn & Rayhorn 2002). Extra-intestinal manifestations that may occur in the UC patient after RPC fall into three main groups:

- Arthropathy – includes conditions such as peripheral arthritis with active disease and ankylosing spondylitis and sacroilietus, which occur independently of active disease. Ankylosing spondylitis and sacroilietus are arthritis of the spine, sacroilietus affecting the lower regions of the spine. Stiffness, pain and possible mobility limitations may occur if untreated (Feldman *et al.* 1998). Osteoporosis is common in patients with UC due to reduced bone density; however, it is difficult to separate the effect of long-term steroid use. Pouch patients may complain of joint pain especially in the knees or ankles.

- Skin conditions – pyoderma gangrenosum and erythema nodosum tend to occur with active intestinal disease. These skin conditions are usually associated with underlying disease such as IBD. Pyoderma gangrenosum is a rare ulcerative cutaneous disorder commonly occurring on the lower extremities but may present in the peristomal area (Bull 1997). Erythema nodosum are painful, tender, red circular nodules that usually present on the outside of the lower leg but can be found on the calf, ankle and sometimes arms. Steroid treatment may aid the conditions, however treatment of the underlying condition is the long-term option (Lichtman & Sartor 1994).

- Ophthalmic conditions – iritis, uveitis, episcleritis and conjunctivitis. These eye conditions relate to the specific part of the eye which becomes inflamed. Uveitis affects the coloured part of the eye. Symptoms may include sensitivity to light, blurred vision and eye pain. Headaches are also associated. If left untreated it may lead to damage of the optic nerve, which in turn can cause blindness (Levene 2000). Episcleritis is inflammation of the coating of the white part of the eye. Associated burning and redness may occur but vision is not usually affected (Lichtman & Sartor 1994). Most of these conditions can be treated by an ophthalmologist prescribing steroid eye drops.

It is important that pouch patients are made aware that even though the colon and rectum have been removed by RPC, routine checks are required to observe skin and eye conditions. Blood tests or DEXA scans are used to monitor calcium and bone density levels. The British Society for Gastroenterology (BSG 2004) suggests that patients requiring surgery for IBD are best managed under the joint care of a colorectal surgeon and gastroenterology team. Only when the two specialist areas combine can the patient attempt to view surgery as an extension of their medical management and not as a last resort or medical failure. Patients that undergo RPC for UC with a long-standing history of relapses may accept surgery better than those who have had a diagnosis of UC for over ten years but experience no associated inflammatory problems or those who are well preoperatively, such as the FAP patient. The latter patient group may be shocked by the need for surgery and may need extra care and convincing about the requirement for invasive surgery. The FAP patient may also have issues of grief or guilt as they usually have experienced a parent or sibling contemplating or dealing with surgery.

Some pre-operative assessments may be invasive and result in embarrassing or uncomfortable situations for the patients. The patient with the introduction of anal examination, rigid or flexible scopes and x-rays may experience feelings of indignity and repulsion. Every effort must be made to protect the patient's dignity and keep them informed of the routine pre-operative requirements, for example restricting diet before examinations and effective emptying of the bowel.

Post-operative care

Patients with an ileoanal pouch performed either in two or three stages initially post-operatively require stoma care. This involves regular observation of the stoma colour, output and temperature. Patients need to be reminded that if the rectal stump is left in situ that they may feel the need to empty their bowels rectally. This is quite normal as the rectal mucosa will still produce mucus and may also contain old blood-stained fluid or fresh if there is still active rectal disease. If the pouch has been formed at the same time some patients can pass old blood, mucus and may even pass small amounts of faeces or wind if it bypasses the loop ileostomy. Patients need to be reassured that this is normal. It is also helpful to provide advice on follow-up procedures so that they can prepare for the last stage when the ileostomy is closed and the pouch is active. Follow-up usually takes place six to eight weeks after RPC when the doctors feel that the ileoanal anastomosis is fully healed. If there is doubt an examination under anaesthetic may be performed prior to closing the ileostomy.

When the ileostomy is closed the pouch will usually start to work in a couple of days. The patient may experience faecal urgency and frequency and this is again normal. The pouch needs to adapt to hold the faeces and gently expand into its new role. Patients can encourage this by extending the time when they get the urge to use the toilet to the time they empty the pouch. The increasing 'holding' time can start at just a few minutes and be increased within reasonable measures and within personal pain tolerance. The sphincter muscles that were defunctioned by the ileostomy will need to regain strength and may occasionally leak at night when the patient relaxes. This is normal and reassurance can be provided that these nocturnal episodes will get less frequent or stop over time. Some patients use pads at night for peace of mind. Small panty liners or sanitary pads can be used by both sexes as these are discrete and seepage is usually minimal. Pouch frequency can be as often as every couple of hours during the day so barrier creams and good quality anal hygiene should be introduced as soon as the ileostomy is reversed and the pouch is active. Follow-up in the community can be provided by the GP, practice nurse and/or pouch or stoma specialist nurse.

Anal skin care

Anyone who has frequent bowel motions, such as someone with an ileoanal pouch, may get sore perianal skin from time to time. Faecal frequency and leakage are the commonest cause of perianal soreness. Taking good care of the skin around the anus can help stop these problems occurring (see Box 10.1). A good barrier cream or wipe is recommended and these can be acquired through the GP or chemist. With the absence of the large bowel the faeces still contain the digestive acids and enzymes that can very easily damage healthy skin. If the pouch output is high (eight times or more in 24 hours) sore skin is likely as the perianal area is not ideally suited to this new situation. Sometimes patients may also complain of an associated rectal burning or an anal itch. This could arise from the faeces being

Box 10.1 Hints and tips to avoid anal soreness and itching

- Keep the area clean by washing and drying after every motion
- Have regular baths or use a bidet. Portable bidets are available from chemists.
- Use a mirror to assist cleaning and application of barrier creams
- Use moist toilet paper or wipes
- Keep the anal area dry
- Avoid rubbing
- Avoid perfumed talc or soap
- Wear loose cotton underwear and avoid tight fitting trousers
- Avoid excessive use of creams and make sure these are completely washed away before reapplication
- Consider thickening the bowel output by use of drugs such as loperamide or codeine phosphate
- Some foods can increase itching or burning, e.g. coconut and citrus fruit

in contact with the pouch–anal anastomosis. Anecdotally a haemorrhoid preparation or aloe vera gel can be helpful. However it is important to confirm that an anal fissure is not present. An anal fissure can be treated topically with either a steroid based cream or glyceryl trinitrate ointment but this will need to be prescribed. In more complex cases where anal pain persists, it is worth considering possible nerve damage, infection such as cuffitis, ulceration, abscess or collection and in very rare situations, a carcinoma.

Fertility, pregnancy and childbirth

Young women with UC who are considering becoming pregnant were generally advised to complete their family before an RPC. There is now good evidence to show that fertility is approximately halved in women who have had an ileoanal pouch (Cornish *et al.* 2007). However, with the improved success of the pouch operation, the increased knowledge of first-time mothers, advances in research and the growing confidence of surgeons, it is viewed safe for mothers with an ileoanal pouch to carry a baby to full term with little or no problems. The rate of spontaneous abortion may be higher than in the normal population but this is controversial due to the lack of comparable studies (Tiainen *et al.* 1999). During gestation the mother may suffer with pouch disruptions such as frequency, urgency, perianal irritation or nocturnal incontinence as the foetus develops. This is worst in the third trimester when there is greater pressure on the small bowel, but function returns to normal after delivery. Advice on anal skin care, diet and general management can be helpful. Some women find it useful to speak to others who have experienced pregnancy and childbirth with a pouch.

The main controversy lies in the chosen method of delivery. Polle *et al.* (2006) suggest that little is known about the long-term function of the pouch in women who have had vaginal deliveries, especially when child-birth occurred before RPC. In the study 60% of the 86 women who attempted vaginal delivery had an increased risk of obstetric injury and impaired continence according to predefined obstetric risk factors. It is advised that patients with an ileoanal pouch be informed of the considerable risks of a vaginal delivery on long-term pouch function with ageing. Elective caesar-ean sections are generally advised in order to avoid straining and tearing of the anal sphincter muscle in the case of traumatic or prolonged deliver-ies. Women with a Kock pouch, however, favour a vaginal delivery. The chosen method of delivery wholly depends on the size of the baby and obstetrician decision.

Before considering RPC men must be made aware of the potential risk of ejaculatory and erectile dysfunction following surgery deep within the pelvis. Surgeons take utmost care to avoid pelvic nerve damage; however, studies predict approximately 5% nerve damage in men (Gorgun *et al.* 2005). There are also hypothetical dangers to the foetus from the precon-ception exposure of the father to immunosuppressive drugs such as aza-thioprine. It is advisable that steroid use is monitored if planning a family, however drug therapy must never be stopped without medical advice. Sperm banking is not usually necessary as RPC does not affect the manu-facture of sperm but may reduce the effectiveness of the delivery method. If erectile dysfunction occurs sperm can be removed from the testis after RPC and stored or inseminated successfully.

Sexuality and sexual counselling is a vital part of pre- and post-operative information. It is not usually the easiest of subjects to approach by health care professionals; however it is one of the most vital to the patient. Sexual questioning should be direct but considerate and professional. This support is essential in helping patients to deal effectively with adverse conse-quences should they occur. The RPC patient group is more commonly young adults who are still developing their own sexuality or personal relationships. A continent procedure is seen to improve the quality of sexual life in approximately 85% of both men and women (Nicholls *et al.* 1993). It is important to note that if a patient has unresolved problems with their pouch then their perception of a good quality of life is greatly reduced. After abdominal surgery patients may complain of lack of libido, fear of incontinence or discomfort when having intercourse. Women may com-plain of vaginal dryness, which can be relieved with the use of water-based lubrication.

It is documented that following RPC dyspareunia increased after the operation but sexual satisfaction was enhanced, as the fear of leakage during coitus was reduced and general health following surgery improved (Tiainen *et al.* 1999). It appears that patients who have had a continent Kock pouch have a greater incidence of dyspareunia than those who underwent RPC (Metcalf *et al.* 1986). Coitus should be resumed when the patient has recovered from the effects of surgery and feels ready to resume a sexual relationship. Gay male patients should be informed pre-operatively that they should refrain from anal sex as this could damage the sphincter muscles leading to incontinence and faecal leakage. Curran & Hill (1990) suggest that 67% of males and 78% of females in their study reported unchanged or increased sexual activity following pouch surgery.

Pouch absorption and diet

The RPC patient who has experienced life with an ileostomy usually adapts well with the dietary requirements of the internal pouch. It is important to understand the effect of pouch formation on water, sodium and nutrient absorption in order to detect potential problems and provide dietary advice. Removal of the colon in an RPC results in reduced ability to absorb water and sodium. People with an ileoanal pouch open their bowels approximately three to eight times a day and those with a Kock reservoir intubate the pouch on average two to four times in 24 hours passing on average 600–800 g of faeces (Williams 2002). The ileoanal pouch is formed from 30–60 cm of terminal ileum, which is vital for the absorption of bile acids and vitamin B_{12}. Supplementary therapy with vitamin B_{12} is necessary in about one-third of patients, dependent on the time duration since RPC. Bile acid malabsorption appears to be related to villous atrophy of the pouch mucosa and therefore differs considerably in patients following RPC and/or ileostomy formation when compared with UC patients who have not had an operation.

Patients who have bile acid complications may be offered a ^{75}Se-homo-taurocholate (SeHCAT) investigation (Santavirta *et al.* 1990). Unabsorbed bile salts can cause liquid faeces and therefore bowel frequency for the pouch patient. It appears that intestinal adaptation as far as absorption is concerned is minimal within the first three months after RPC (Hylander *et al.* 1991). Patients need to be aware that pouch function may take anywhere between six months to a year to settle into a routine where the patient is comfortable with the frequency and consistency of the faeces. The ileal mucosa must also adapt to its new role as a faeces reservoir. The ileum of the pouch after an RPC is no longer required solely for absorption of nutrients. Additionally the micro flora of the pouch changes to become intermediate between that of an ileostomy and of normal faeces.

In the early days post-operation a soft, light and low fibre diet is required. This will reduce the risk of problems with the newly formed pouch. Food and drink can usually be increased to whatever the patient can tolerate or chooses within two to three weeks. Most patients enjoy a healthy well balanced diet. High protein, high energy diets will help the patient recover from surgery preventing weight loss and lethargy. Carbohydrates and starches found in rice, potatoes and pasta can help to thicken the pouch output. Some patients are able to tolerate spicy food such as curries, but they can lead to anal irritation and burning. Over time most patients realise the effects of certain foods on their pouch function.

However, from the literature it appears that pouch function and predictability is not solely based on dietary intake. Fruit, vegetables and high fibre may cause blockages within the pouch or pre-pouch ileum or increase bowel frequency. It is important to make vegetarians aware of the risk of taking too much fibre prematurely. Fruit and vegetables should be peeled, cooked and chewed well. A dietary obstruction is usually resolved by avoiding food for 24 hours and only drinking fluids. Mobilising activities such as walking or massaging the abdomen may shift a blockage. Some patients have a warm bath, which can relax muscles and therefore disperse a blockage relieving the associated pain and bloating. If the pouch fails to work, the patient starts vomiting or function is severely disabled from an intestinal blockage, the patient is advised to seek medical advice.

Problems following RPC

Poor function can be caused by four major factors:

- Mechanical – examples are pouch outflow obstruction or strictures within the pouch or in the pre-pouch ileum, a small reservoir or weak sphincter muscles.
- Functional – examples are evacuation disorders, a motility disorder (a slow or sluggish transit) or psychological disorders (anxiety or stress).
- Inflammation – for example, pouchitis, retained rectal mucosa or bacterial overgrowth/disturbance.
- Sepsis – a collection within the pelvis which can lead to the breakdown of the ileoanal anastomosis.

Pouch failure

Pouch failure resulting in the formation of a temporary defunctioning ileostomy or even the excision of the pouch and the creation of a permanent end ileostomy is a multi-factorial event. The main causes of pouch failure are anastomotic leaks causing pelvic sepsis, recurring abscesses and fistulae. The prevalence of these conditions varies between 6% and 37% (Reissman *et al.* 1996). Other factors include poor pouch function, outlet obstruction and sphincter dysfunction. The diagnosis of Crohn's disease, fistula or fissure in ano pre-operatively, significant haemorrhoids or skin tags, extra-intestinal inflammatory bowel disease, patient co-morbidity (cardiac, respiratory, renal impairment or obesity), previous abdominal surgery or the female gender are all increased risk factors for pouch failure. A less common cause is chronic pouchitis (Fazio *et al.* 2003). Lifetime analysis studies show the incidence of pouch failure as 5% in the first five years and increasing over time to 10% at ten years. Pouch failure in some studies is as low as 3%; however, this figure is likely to increase with longer follow-up periods (Michelassi *et al.* 2003).

Pouchitis

Pouchitis is an inflammatory response to changes of the bowel mucosa within the pouch (see Figure 10.2). Pouchitis presents with varying degrees of severity but is associated with bowel frequency, urgency and in most cases bloody diarrhoea. Although the aetiology of pouchitis after RPC is unknown its manifestations resemble those of non-specific IBD including the ability to provoke extra-intestinal manifestations of IBD (Lohmuller *et al.* 1990). Pouchitis is more commonly seen in patients with UC than FAP. It is also likely that, due to the positive response of most patients with pouchitis to antibiotics, changes in the intraluminal bacteria also play a role. The research on pouchitis varies and statistics range from 20% to

undertaken by a specialist nurse and 96% were happy to discuss their concerns or related issues without a doctor present. It has generally been acknowledged that nurse-led services offer patients a service that had previously been reduced following an over-stretched NHS. The specialist nurse is able to reduce clinic waiting times by adding patients to their own list and assess the patient's problems without necessarily requiring a doctor. The nurse specialist is well supported by the medical team in clinic should they need advice or assistance.

Nurse-led initiatives continue to identify areas of independent practice where they are able to initiate and deliver care to patients and incorporate certain aspects of clinical work previously carried out by medical staff (NMC 2006). Many centres have now moved towards telephone clinics run by specialist nurses in order to combat the problems associated with long waiting lists, wasted clinic appointments and cost restraints (Hennell *et al.* 2006). Consultants now view nurse specialists as a vital asset to the clinic and acknowledge the nurses' diverse knowledge and skills in other areas such as providing psychological and practical support, referring to other members of the multidisciplinary team and continuation of patient care. Nurses view this extended role as resulting in an increase in job satisfaction, confidence and the ability to be responsible for assessing patient needs, developing and managing areas of research to improve the quality of care and outcomes of their patients (Campbell *et al.* 1999).

In conclusion, the RPC with ileoanal pouch anastomosis confers good long-term functional results to patients with UC in need of surgical treatment. After an initial period of adjustment lasting 12–18 months, bowel frequency stabilises at six motions per day with the majority of patients fully continent and able to postpone a bowel motion until convenient. Subjective assessments of quality of life, overall satisfaction and adjustment are high (Michelassi *et al.* 2003).

References

Alves A & Panis Y (2005) Laparoscopic ileal pouch anal anastomosis. *Annales de Chirurgie.* **130(6–7)**: 421–5. Full text [online]. PubMed-indexed for Medline (accessed 21.06.06).

Berndtsson I, Lindholm E & Ekman I (2005) Thirty years of experience living with a continent ileostomy. *Journal of Wound, Ostomy and Continence Nursing.* **32(5)**: 321–6.

Blackley P (1998) *Practical Wound and Continence Management.* Victoria, Australia: Australia Research Publications Pty Ltd.

British Society of Gastroenterology (BSG) (2004) *Guidelines for the Management of Inflammatory Bowel Disease in Adults* [online]. Available: http://www.bsg.org.uk (accessed 14.03.06).

Broome U & Bergquist A (2006) Primary sclerosing cholangitis, inflammatory bowel disease and colon cancer. *Seminars in Liver Disease.* **26(1)**: 31–41.

Bull RH (1997) Pyoderma gangrenosum: a diagnosis not to be missed. *Journal of Tissue Viability.* **7**: 107–13.

Camilleri-Brennan J, Munro A & Steele-Robert J (2003) Does an ileoanal pouch offer a better quality of life than a permanent ileostomy for patients with ulcerative colitis? *Journal of Gastrointestinal Surgery.* **7(6)**: 814–19.

Campbell J, German L & Lane C (1999) Radiotherapy outpatient review: a nurse led clinic. *Nursing Standard.* **13(22)**: 39–44.

Cornish JA, Tan E, Teare J, Teoh TG, Rai R *et al.* (2007) The effect of restorative proctocolectomy on sexual function, urinary function, fertility, pregnancy and delivery – a systematic review. *Diseases of the Colon and Rectum.* **50(8)**: 1128–38.

Curran FT & Hill GL (1990) Results of 50 ileo-anal J pouch operations. *Australian and New Zealand Journal of Surgery.* **60(8)**: 579–83.

Das P, Johnson MW, Tekkis PP & Nicholls RJ (2007) Risk of dysplasia and adeno-carcinoma following restorative proctocolectomy for ulcerative colitis. *Colorectal Disease.* **9**: 15–27.

Delaney CP, Remzi FH, Gramlich T, Dabak D & Fazio VW (2002) Equivalent function, quality of life and pouch survival rates after ileo pouch anal anastomosis for indeterminate and ulcerative colitis. *Annals of Surgery.* **236(1)**: 43–8.

Duff SE, O'Dwyer ST, Hulten L, Willen R & Haboubi NY (2002) Dysplasia in the ileoanal pouch. *Colorectal Disease.* **4(6)**: 420–9.

Fazio VW, Ziv Y, Church JM, Oakley JR, Lavery IC *et al.* (1995) Ileal pouch-anal anastomosis complications and function in 1005 patients. *Annals of Surgery.* **222**: 120–7.

Fazio VW, Tekkis PP, Remzi F, Manilich E, Connor J *et al.* (2003) Quantification of risk factors for pouch failure after ileo pouch anal anastomosis surgery. *Annals of Surgery.* **238(4)**: 605–17.

Fedorak RN (2007) Probiotics in the management of inflammatory bowel disease? *American Journal of Gastroenterology.* **102(S1)**: S22–S28.

Feldman M, Friedman LS & Brandt LJ (1998) *Gastrointestinal and Liver Disease.* Philadelphia: W.B. Saunders Co.

Furst A, Burghofer K, Hurzel L & Jauch KW (2002) Neo-rectal reservoir is not the functional principle of the colonic J pouch: the volume of a short colonic J pouch does not differ from a straight coloanal anastomosis. *Diseases of the Colon and Rectum.* **45(5)**: 660–7.

Gionchetti P, Rizzello F & Venturi A (2000) Oral bacteriotherapy as a maintenance treatment in patients with chronic pouchitis: a double blind placebo-controlled trial. *Gastroenterology.* **119**: 305–9.

Gorgun E, Remzi FH, Montague DK, Connor JT, O'Brian KO *et al.* (2005) Male sexual function improves after ileal pouch anal anastomosis. *International Journal of Colorectal Disease.* **7**: 545–50.

Hennell S, Spark, Wood B & George E (2006) An evaluation of nurse-led rheumatology telephone clinics. *Musculosketal Care.* **3(4)**: 233–40.

Hylander E, Rannem T, Hegnhoj J, Kirkegaard P, Thale M *et al.* (1991) Absorption studies after ileal J pouch anastomosis for ulcerative colitis. A prospective study. *Scandinavian Journal of Gastroenterology.* **26(1)**: 65–72.

Iwaya A, Liai T, Okamoto H, Ajioka Y, Yamamoto T *et al.* (2006) Change in bacterial flora of pouchitis. *Hepatogastroenterology.* **53(67)**: 55–9.

Jimmo B & Hyman NH (1998) Is ileo anal pouch anal anastomosis really the procedure of choice for patients with ulcerative colitis? *Diseases of Colon and Rectum.* **41(1)**: 41–5.

Larson DW, Cima RR & Dozios EJ (2006) Safety, feasibility and short term outcomes of laparoscopic ileal pouch anal anastomosis: a single institutional case matched experience. *Annals of Surgery.* **243**: 667–70.

Levene JB (2000) *Extra Intestinal Manifestations of Inflammatory Bowel Disease.* 5th edn. Philadelphia: W.B. Saunders Co.

Lichtman SN & Sartor RB (1994) *Extra Intestinal Manifestations of IBD, Clinical Aspects and Natural History. Inflammatory Bowel Disease from Bench to Bedside.* Baltimore: Williams & Wilkins.

Lohmuller JL, Pemberton JH, Dozois RR, Ilstrup D & Van Heerden J (1990) Pouchitis and extra intestinal manifestations of inflammatory bowel disease after ileal pouch anal anastomosis. *Annals of Surgery.* **211(5)**: 622–6.

Lovegrove RE, Tilney HS, Heriot AG, von Roon AC, Athanasiou T *et al.* (2006) A comparison of adverse events and functional outcomes after restorative proctocolectomy for familial adenomatous polyposis and ulcerative colitis. *Diseases of the Colon and Rectum.* **49(9)**: 1293–1306.

Metcalf AM, Dozois RR & Kelly KA (1986) Sexual function in women after proctocolectomy. *Annals of Surgery.* **204(6)**: 624–7.

Michelassi F, Lee J, Rubin M, Fichera A, Kasza K *et al.* (2003) Long term functional results after ileal pouch anal restorative proctocolectomy for ulcerative colitis. A prospective observational study. *Annals of Surgery.* **238(3)**: 433–45.

Mimura T, Rizzello F, Helwig U, Poggioli G, Schreiber S *et al.* (2002) Four-week open-label trial of metronidazole and ciprofloxacin for the treatment of recurrent or refractory pouchitis. *Aliment Pharmacological Therapy.* **16**: 909–17.

Moskowitz RL, Shepherd NA & Nicholls RJ (1986) An assessment of inflammation in the reservoir after restorative proctocolectomy with ileo-anal ileal reservoir. *International Journal of Colorectal Disease.* **1**: 167–74.

Nassar G, Fazio VW, Tekkis PP, Connor J, Wu J *et al.* (2006) Long term outcome and quality of life after continent ileostomy. *Disease of Colon and Rectum.* **49(3)**: 336–44.

Nicholls RJ, Bartolo D & Mortensen N (1993) *Restorative Proctocolectomy.* London: Blackwell Scientific Publications.

NMC – Nursing and Midwifery Council (2006) *Independent Practice* [online]. Available http://www.nmc-uk.org/ (accessed 12.06.06).

Oresland T, Fasth S, Nordgren S & Hulten L (1989) The clinical and functional outcome after restorative proctocolectomy. *International Journal of Colorectal Disease.* **4**: 50–6.

Perrin A (2005) Development of a nurse led ileo-anal pouch clinic. *British Journal of Nursing.* **14(16)**: S21–S24.

Perry-Woodford ZL & McLaughlin SD (2007) A guide to ileo-anal pouch surgery and related complications. *Gastrointestinal Nursing.* **5(4)**: 18–24.

Polle SW, Vlug MS, Slors JF, Zwinderman AH, Van Der Hoop AG *et al.* (2006) Effect of vaginal delivery on long term pouch function. *British Journal of Surgery.* **93(11)**: 1394–1401.

Rayhorn N & Rayhorn D (2002) An in-depth look at inflammatory bowel disease. *Nursing.* **32(7)**: 36–46.

Reissman P, Teoh TA & Weiss EG (1996) Functional outcome of the double stapled ileoanal pouch in patients more than 60 years of age. *American Surgical.* **62**: 178–83.

Remzi RH, Fazio VW, Gorgun E, Zutshi M, Church JM *et al.* (2005) Quality of life, functional outcome and complications of coloplasty pouch after low anterior resection. *Diseases of Colon and Rectum.* **48(4)**: 735–43.

Sandborn WJ, Tremaine WJ, Batts KP, Pemberton JH & Phillips SF (1994) Pouchitis after ileo pouch anal anastomosis: a pouchitis disease activity index. *Mayo Clinic Proceedings.* **69(5)**: 409–15.

Santavirta J, Mattila J, Kokki M, Poyhonen L & Matikainen M (1990) Absorption of bile acids after ileo anal anastomosis. *Annales Chirurgiae et Gynaocologiae.* **79(3)**: 134–8 full text [online] PubMed-indexed for Medline (accessed 19.07.06).

Setti-Carraro P, Talbot IC & Nicholls RJ (1998) Patterns of endoscopic and histological changes in the ileal reservoir after restorative proctocolectomy for ulcerative colitis. A long-term follow-up study. *International Journal of Colorectal Disease.* **13(2)**: 103–7.

Skene L & Smallwood R (2002) Informed consent: lessons from Australia. *British Medical Journal*. **324**: 39–41.

Tiainen J & Matikainen M (1999) Health related quality of life after ileal J pouch anal anastomosis for ulcerative colitis: long term results. *Scandinavian Journal of Gastroenterology*. **34(6)**: 601–5.

Tiainen J, Matikainen M & Hiltunen KM (1999) Ileal J pouch anal anastomosis, sexual dysfunction and fertility. *Scandinavian Journal of Gastroenterology*. **34(2)**: 185–8.

Tulchinsky H, Hawley PR & Nicholls RJ (2003) Long term failure after restorative proctocolectomy colitis. *Annals of Surgery*. **238(2)**: 229–34.

Ulisse S, Gionchetti P, D'Alo S, Russo FP, Pesce I *et al.* (2001) Expression of cytokines, inducible nitric oxide synthase and matrix metalloproteinases in pouchitis: effects of probiotic treatment. *American Journal of Gastroenterology*. **96(9)**: 2691–9.

Williams J (2002) *The Essentials of Pouch Care Nursing*. London: Whurr.

Chapter 11

Urinary Diversion

Sharon Fillingham

Introduction

In recent years patients undergoing surgery for diseased or malfunctional bladders have had a wider choice of potential procedures. Each of these operations requires the patient to adapt to an altered voiding pattern and often requires that they acquire a new skill.

Reasons for urinary diversion

The most common reasons for urinary diversion are:

- tumour – confined to bladder and radical pelvic clearance (Blackley 1998);
- tumour – obstructive (usually palliative);
- trauma – resulting in fistula formation;
- congenital abnormalities – bladder exstrophy, spina bifida;
- bladder failure – neuropathic, severe incontinence, interstitial cystitis;
- failure of previous reconstructive surgery.

Urinary diversion can be either incontinent or continent in nature. Urinary diversion and reconstruction can be classified broadly into four groups:

- the incontinent urinary diversion – the ileal conduit;
- the continent cutaneous urinary diversion – the Mitrofanoff (+/– enterocystoplasty);
- enterocystoplasties – neobladder, cystoplasty;
- rectal bladder – Mainz II sigma pouch.

Urostomy

An incontinent type of urinary diversion is the urostomy. All of the 'urinary stomas' require the patient to wear an external appliance to collect the urine (Fillingham & Fell 2004). There are various types of urostomy that have now become rather outdated but still present occasionally in the outpatient department. These include:

- cutaneous vesicostomy – where the bladder is brought through the abdominal wall;
- cutaneous pyelostomy – where the pelvis of the kidney is brought to the abdominal surface;
- cutaneous ureterostomy – in which the ureters are brought to the abdominal surface.

Currently the most usually formed urostomies are:

- colonic conduit
- ileal conduit.

Colonic conduit

A colonic conduit is a section of colon fashioned into a stoma and brought through the abdominal surface to form a spout. Colonic conduits are rarely formed unless it is impossible to find a sufficient length of ileum. It is more usual for the colonic conduits to be sited on the left side of the abdomen, to be larger in circumference and to produce greater amounts of mucus than an ileal conduit.

The ileal conduit

Described by Bricker (1950) the ileal conduit remains the most popular form of urinary diversion worldwide.

Specific pre-operative care and investigations

There are a number of pre-operative investigations that are required prior to the formation of an ileal conduit:

- blood – baseline urea and electrolytes, bicarbonate, chloride, vitamin B_{12} plus full blood count and group and save;
- intravenous urogram – to determine the anatomy of the renal tract;
- glomerular filtration rate (GFR) – isotope study to provide a quantitative measurement of the renal function;
- computed tomography (CT) – to assess the abdomen and renal system for tumour staging and evidence of metastatic spread.

Bowel preparation

The use of bowel preparation varies between centres and urologists. Today it rarely involves the use of purgative laxatives unless the patient has a history of constipation. A low residue diet and then clear fluids on the day before surgery with hydration maintained via an intravenous infusion are recommended.

All patients who are about to undergo potential stoma-forming surgery should be assessed by the stoma specialist nurse prior to surgery. The majority of urostomies are formed as an elective procedure and there is generally ample time for patients to be seen in an outpatient setting.

Written information in the form of booklets as well as videos and a CD-ROM can be shown to the patient. These can be invaluable when describing the surgical procedure that they are about to undergo as well as an aid in the understanding of the post-operative management.

Siting the stoma

The ileal conduit is normally sited on the right-hand side of the abdomen below the umbilicus. It is generally considered necessary to site the stoma within the rectus sheath to prevent parastomal hernia (Pearl 1989). However, most studies have been undertaken on patients with bowel stomas and there are an increasing number of surgeons who do not believe that siting within the rectus sheath will prevent hernia formation (Ortiz *et al.* 1994).

Formation of ileal conduit

During the formation of an ileal conduit a section of ileum is isolated, of approximately 15–25 cm in length. The mesentery remains intact and the section of bowel is chosen for its healthy appearance. The distal end is securely fixed to the peritoneum and the proximal end is closed and the ureters are implanted after surgical removal from the bladder (see Figure 11.1). The distal end is then brought through a pre-marked opening on the

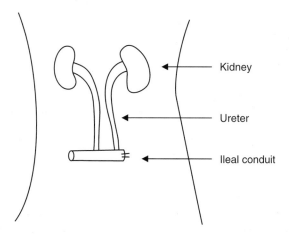

Figure 11.1   Urostomy formation.

abdominal wall and a spout is created in the form of a Brooke's ileostomy (Brooke 1952). The remaining ends of the ileum are re-anastomosed in order to maintain continuity.

Post-operative care

The general care of the patient with a urinary stoma is consistent with any patient who has undergone major abdominal surgery. It is essential that accurate fluid balance is recorded and any imbalance reported to the medical staff. Observations for the stoma are to check the stoma condition, urine output and the patency of the stents (see Table 11.1).

Stents

The purpose of the stents is to protect the anastomosis between the ureters and the newly formed conduit. Patency of the stents should be checked regularly. If blocked they should be very gently flushed with 5 ml of normal saline.

Stents may fall out spontaneously before they are due for removal at seven to ten days. No pressure should be required to remove the stents. If any resistance is felt they should be left in situ and the procedure attempted the next day.

Urostomy appliance selection

Immediately post-operatively, patients should be fitted with a two-piece appliance with 'floating flange'. This allows removal and reattachment of the pouch to be carried out without putting pressure on the patient's abdomen.

Urostomy pouches differ from appliances designed for bowel stomas by incorporating an inner pouch (see Chapter 12 on appliances). This is designed to prevent urine pooling around the stoma.

Urinary stomas are active as soon as they are formed. Patients are encouraged to maintain a two litre fluid intake and therefore the ideal time to change the appliance is first thing in the morning. All urostomy pouches have an integral drainage tap. These vary in shape and ease of use and selection should be made with regard to the patient's manual dexterity.

Table 11.1 Stoma observations

Stoma	Pink, warm, moist, soft
Urine	Fluid balance – equal Colour – clear or light haematuria
Urinary stents 1 stent for each ureter	Remains patent until removed

Source: Fillingham & Fell 2005.

Night drainage system

The capacity of most urostomy appliances is approximately 350 ml. To prevent the need for waking regularly at night urostomates will usually choose to attach a night drainage bag. These have a two litre capacity enabling the individual to have an uninterrupted night's sleep.

Ileal conduit complications

While the ileal conduit is regarded as the simplest form of urinary diversion to create, recent studies show that patients with urostomies have a significant complication rate (see Table 11.2). The most common problems encountered were deteriorating upper tracts 27%, stomal problems 24%, urinary tract infections 23% and parastomal hernias 19%. However, these results compare equally with studies undertaken of patients with other types of urinary diversion (Greenwell *et al.* 2001; Suzer *et al.* 1997).

Urinary tract infections

Symptoms of the presence of a urinary tract infection include loin pain, pyrexia, feeling 'feverish', rigors, vomiting, cloudy and offensive urine. The only absent symptom will be dysuria (pain on passing urine). The patient may experience some or all of the other symptoms.

Whenever gastrointestinal tissue is used to create a stoma or pouch a small amount of *Escherichia coli* (*E. coli*) will be found on urine testing. Dip stick analysis will be positive for leukocytes and nitrites in nearly all urinary stoma samples. Antibiotic therapy should not be instigated unless the patient is symptomatic. To avoid contamination the sample should be taken from the stoma via a single use catheter using an aseptic technique. Microscopy and culture will identify any organisms present and the antibiotic sensitivities.

Cranberry juice – hippuric acid

The build-up of mucus in the bowel segment used to form the ileal conduit can provide an ideal medium for the colonisation of *E. coli*. Cranberry is an excellent source of hippuric acid (Gray 2002). This has the effect of breaking down and flushing out the mucus and thus preventing further increase of any bacteria in the urinary system. Patients on warfarin must limit or avoid cranberry products because of a possible interaction affecting the INR (international normalisation ratio) values (Suvarna *et al.* 2003).

Table 11.2 Urostomy complication rates

Number of patients	Complication rate	Author(s)
60	42%	Allen & Greenwell (2003)
137	15%	Kouba *et al.* (2007)

Colour and odour changes

Several foods, drinks and medications can affect the colour and odour of urine. These changes are particularly noticeable when observed through a urostomy appliance. Offensive odours are often mistaken for urinary tract infections. Pharmacists are a good source of information (Watson 1987) and established urostomates provide anecdotal information regarding many food and medicine related changes.

Internal urinary pouches

The technique to create internal urinary diversions (continent diversions) varies throughout Europe (Busuttil-Leaver 2004). However, the operation most commonly performed in the UK is the Mitrofanoff with augmented bladder (see Figure 11.2). Continent urinary diversions consist of:

- reservoir
- tunnel or channel
- continence mechanism.

The reservoir/augmented bladder

This reservoir can be created from various tissue structures:

- The bladder – if the bladder is present and intact with a low pressure this is always regarded as the first choice.
- The augmented bladder. As stated, various organs can be used for creating the augmented bladder which include:
  - ileum – clam ileocystoplasty
  - colon – colocystoplasty
  - ileum and colon – ileocolocystoplasty   } enterocystoplasties
  - caecum – caecocystoplasty
  - patch or stomach – gastrocystoplasty

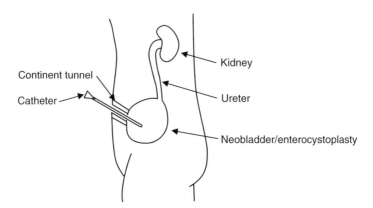

Figure 11.2   Mitrofanoff channel and neobladder.

The Mitrofanoff principle

This procedure was developed by a French surgeon called Paul Mitrofanoff. In this procedure urinary continence is achieved by creating a catheterisable channel into the reservoir by forming a tunnel from the internal reservoir to an abdominal opening which can be catheterised and the new bladder emptied. What makes this channel continent is the formation of a non-return valve formed from the tissues used to create the tunnel. Various types of tissue have been used for this procedure including the appendix, the ureter, Fallopian tubes, ileum or even a skin flap.

Individual assessment

Prior to being considered for this operation the patient needs to be assessed for their understanding of the necessity of intermittent clean self-catheterisation (ICSC). They need to have sufficient dexterity as it is necessary to catheterise this channel at least every four to six hours and, unless they have a 24-hour carer, this must be done by the individual. They must also be able to have sufficient understanding of the principles of intermittent self-catheterisation. It is also felt that they should be highly motivated as this particular operation carries with it a high re-operation rate.

Indications for continent urinary diversion

The most common reasons for this procedure in the younger person are for congenital abnormalities, including bladder exstrophy and spina bifida. Urological disorders affecting the bladder and severe incontinence are the second most common reasons. Now that this type of surgery is offered in an increasing number of centres, patients who have been diagnosed with bladder cancer are more likely to consider this operation over the ileal conduit as their first choice. However, many individuals with bladder cancer regard the complexity of Mitrofanoff and neobladder (complete refashioning of a bladder from bowel) formation as unsuitable for their personal circumstances.

Pre-operative investigations

In addition to the investigations required for urinary diversion the patient who is having an ileal conduit converted to any other form of urinary diversion will require a loopogram. This will identify the length and structure of the stoma and allow the surgeon to calculate how much viable tissue is available in the loop.

Surgical procedure – enterocystoplasty and Mitrofanoff formation

The enterocystoplasty involves replacing part of or the entire bladder with bowel. The abdomen is opened in the midline, adhesions are divided and the intra-peritoneal contents are mobilised. In the case of a bladder cancer a cystectomy (removal of bladder) will be performed and the bladder is entirely reconstructed using bowel. This is termed a neobladder (with Mitrofanoff access).

Tissue for the creation of the Mitrofanoff channel is identified, such as the appendix, and is mobilised on its mesentery. A segment of detubularised bowel is used to augment the bladder. This is known as clam cystoplasty, usually utilising the ileum or colon (see Figure 11.3). A substitution cystoplasty is a procedure where the bulk of the bladder is removed and refashioned using caecum (see Figure 11.4).

Specific post-operative care

The patient will return to the ward with:

- intravenous infusion – to maintain hydration in the early post-operative period;
- patient-controlled analgesia (PCA) – to maintain pain relief;
- nasogastric tube – paralytic ileus present in the early post-operative period, to remove stomach contents;
- wound drains – to prevent build-up of intra-abdominal fluids;
- ureteric stents – to protect the anastomosis between the ureters and the newly formed reservoir;
- supra-pubic catheter – to promote urinary drainage;
- Mitrofanoff catheter – to keep Mitrofanoff channel patent and allow healing to take place.

The care of catheters and stents is shown in Table 11.3.

Bladder washout

As bowel has been used to create the reservoir, mucus and debris will be produced. It is important that the catheters remain patent and that they are flushed regularly both in hospital and at home. It is essential that the reservoir is kept empty of urine to allow the pouch to heal, prior to expand-

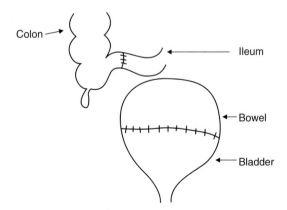

Figure 11.3 Clam cystoplasty.

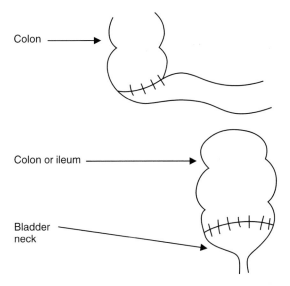

Colon

Colon or ileum

Bladder neck

Figure 11.4 Substitution cystoplasty.

Table 11.3 Care of catheters and stents

Stents	Function – to protect the anastomosis between the ureters and the newly formed reservoir. Ureteric stents are used if the ureters are implanted into a new segment of bowel Care – removed seven to ten days post-operatively
Supra-pubic catheter	Function – to promote urinary drainage Care – remains in situ for six weeks and is removed on the second admission to hospital
Mitrofanoff catheter	Function – to keep Mitrofanoff channel patent and allow healing to take place Care – remains in situ for six weeks and is removed on the second admission to hospital

ing and increasing the bladder capacity. This is achieved by flushing both catheters with 20 ml normal saline twice daily on days one, two and three. After day three until re-admission for a trial without catheter, the bladder washouts are commenced twice daily using 50 ml of saline until clear.

Discharge

The patient will be discharged home with both catheters in situ. The one which has consistently drained the least can be spigotted using a 'flip flo' device. This will allow the washouts to be carried out without the need for disconnection.

The following equipment should be provided and further supplies ordered:

- bladder syringes;
- sterile jug;
- saline;
- leg bag;
- night drainage bag;
- a single use catheter (size is dependent on the Mitrofanoff catheter already in situ; this is provided to replace the original catheter if it falls out; the patient is advised to contact the department immediately if this happens).

Both catheters need to be taped securely even if sutured. District nurse visits will be requested to support the patient and family in catheter care. One catheter should be on free drainage at all times either connected to a leg bag or two litre night drainage bag.

Readmission

Six weeks after the surgery the patient is readmitted for removal of catheters; and also to be taught intermittent self-catheterisation (ISC) via the Mitrofanoff channel.

The intermittent self-catheterisation procedure

- The supra-pubic catheter is clamped/spigotted.
- The catheter in the Mitrofanoff channel is removed and a single-use catheter is inserted (see Figure 11.5). This is a 'clean procedure'.
- This will be repeated every two to three hours initially until the pouch has expanded.
- A catheter will usually be left in situ overnight initially until expansion has occurred. There should be no longer than four to six hours between catheterisation (there should be a maximum volume of no more than 600 ml).
- Catheterisation should not be painful; however, it may take some time for the patient to become used to the sensation of the catheter pushing through the valve into the bladder.
- When the patient feels confident with catheterisation the supra-pubic catheter is removed under antibiotic cover.
- With a size 12–14 French gauge catheter it should only take three to five minutes to empty the bladder completely.
- When the patient feels confident and is competent in ISC they will be discharged home.
- The patient should be encouraged to drink at least 2.5 litres of fluid per day.

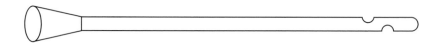

Figure 11.5 Single-use catheter.

Follow-up

This surgical procedure requires lifelong follow-up (Woodhouse 2002). The tests that are required to be regularly carried out are to measure the renal function, pouch pressure and check for the presence of stones and debris:

- Bloods
  - full blood count
  - urea, electrolytes, creatinine
  - bicarbonate
  - chloride
  - vitamin B_{12}
- Scans
  - intravenous urogram
  - bladder and renal ultrasound
  - glomerular filtration rate (GFR)
  - pouch pressure studies.

Complications

Complications are common with this surgery and the patient should be advised when and where to get help:

- Urinary tract infections – *E. coli* will be present in small amounts in all urine samples. Samples should be sent for culture and sensitivity and any appropriate antibiotic prescribed, but only if the patient is symptomatic.
- Stenosis of the channel – if catheterisation becomes increasingly difficult, advice will be given to leave the catheter in situ for a few days and then reattempt ISC. A further surgical procedure may be required if the situation does not resolve.
- Leaking – further surgery may be required to 'tighten' the valve.
- Stone formation – the build-up of mucus and repeated infections are precursors to stone formation. Bladder washouts are encouraged to decrease mucus build-up. Drinking cranberry juice containing hippuric acid may help (caution should be taken with patients who take warfarin). Larger stones will be removed surgically.
- Metabolic acidosis – patients with enterocystoplasties may require oral bicarbonate supplements.
- Malabsorption – vitamin B_{12} levels should be checked and supplements given intramuscularly if required.

Medic alert identification

The medic alert identification should read – no urethral access.

Neobladder

Following cystectomy the patient may be given the choice of having a neobladder created. This type of bladder reconstruction is also called an orthotopic reconstruction. The advantage of the neobladder is that it alleviates the need to wear an external appliance or to catheterise abdominally. However, the patient's suitability for this procedure must be carefully assessed prior to offering it as an option. Co-morbidity including a history of bowel disease, radiotherapy or an invasive tumour of the urethra would be unsuitable for a neobladder.

Pre-operative assessment

Prior to surgery it is important that the patient is given sufficient information about the reconstructive surgery to decide whether this would be their preferred option. The individual must also be willing and able to self-catheterise urethrally.

Intermittent self-catheterisation

It is essential that the patient is taught ISC prior to having the surgery. The male urethra is 15–20 cm long and broadly shaped like an 'S'. Therefore catheters used for male patients must be in excess of 40 cm long. The female urethra is approximately 4 cm long and catheters designed for female use vary from 6 cm to 23 cm.

Single-use catheters come in both coated and uncoated varieties. Uncoated varieties are generally used with lubricating gel. ISC is a clean procedure and the patient is taught to thoroughly clean their hands prior to use. The frequency of ISC is obviously dependent on whether the patient is able to void spontaneously or not. In those who rely on catheterisation to empty their bladder the procedure should be carried out every three to four hours during the day and often once at night. Advice will be given on how many catheters to order and their storage, volumes of fluid to be drunk in a 24-hour period and what adverse symptoms to look out for and who to contact if they occur. Excellent information booklets are prepared by all manufacturers of single-use catheters, along with DVDs to enhance the teaching provided by continence advisers and urology specialist nurses.

Pelvic floor exercises

The function of pelvic floor exercises both pre- and post-operatively is to increase the support of pelvic organs and thus help to prevent leakage of urine from the newly created neobladder. It is important that the pelvic floor muscles undergo regular exercise to retain good muscle tone. If muscles are not exercised they may become slackened, stretched, weak and no longer work effectively. Pelvic floor exercises have proved both to be useful in terms of continence and sexual function (Dorey 2005). The patient should be taught to identify their pelvic floor to ensure that they are exercising the right muscles:

- Women (vaginal examination):
  - This involves tightening the vagina round two inserted fingers. This can also be done using a vaginal probe.

- ○ Stop test – the patient should be advised to stop the flow of urine midstream.
- ○ The patient is asked to imagine they are trying to avoid passing wind/flatus.
- ○ The patient is asked to imagine themselves preventing a tampon from falling out of the vagina.
- Men:
  - ○ Asked to try and stop the flow of urine midstream.
  - ○ Imagine themselves trying to avoid passing wind/flatus.

The continence adviser or physiotherapist is the ideal person to advise the patient how to perform pelvic floor exercises. They generally advise that exercises should become a lifetime habit as part of a preventative programme.

Bowel preparation

Bowel preparation for this procedure will vary according to the consultant urologist. However this is less frequently requested when the ileum is used to create the pouch.

Formation of a neobladder

This procedure involves creating a pouch or reservoir using a section of small bowel approximately 45–60 cm long (see formation of enterocystoplasty). Various configurations have been used in constructing the pouches and are named after the urologists who developed them, i.e. Hautmann and Studer. The ureters are disconnected from the bladder and reimplanted into the new pouch. This new reservoir is then connected to the urethra and thus becomes one internal integral unit.

Post-operative care

Bladder reconstruction is major surgery and patients will need careful monitoring after the procedure. They will return to the ward with a nasogastric tube in situ, as a segment of bowel is used, and bowel peristalsis is often slow to return. At least one wound drain will be required and hydration via an intravenous infusion will remain until the patient is able to maintain their own oral intake. Adequate analgesia will be provided via PCA.

Urinary drainage

Ureteric stent care

Ureteric stents are placed into the ureters to maintain patency. These stents are left on free drainage and usually remain in situ for up to ten days postoperatively. It is important for the ureteric stents to remain patent in the early post-operative period. They will be individually attached to drainage bags. If the stents become blocked they should be gently flushed with normal saline. Stents are removed by daily gentle 'tweaking' until they can be easily removed.

Catheter care

Patients usually return from theatre with two catheters in situ, one urethrally and the other supra-pubically inserted. One or both of the catheters will remain in situ for at least four weeks, depending on the surgeon's preference. If the patient is to be discharged with only one catheter the second catheter will be removed at approximately seven days postoperatively. The catheter(s) remain on free drainage to allow the newly reconstructed bladder time to heal, to prevent any pressure being exerted on the pouch by overfilling.

Pouch care

The aim of pouch and catheter care is to ensure that the pouch does not stretch before adequate healing has taken place and to ensure that as much mucus as possible is removed from the bladder. The neobladder, being made entirely of bowel, will therefore produce a greater amount of mucus than that of a clam cystoplasty which contains more of the native bladder in its construction.

Discharge home

The patient will usually be discharged home with the supra-pubic catheter in situ. Urologists' preferences vary and occasionally patients are sent home with either both their urethral and supra-pubic catheters or their urethral catheter alone in situ. This is to allow sufficient time for the new bladder to heal. Bladder washouts will be carried out at least twice daily during this period and more frequently if mucus blockage occurs. Prior to discharge the patient will be taught to be self-caring in the management of their catheter(s) although the district or practice nurses should be informed of the operative details to provide support in the community.

Cystogram and catheter removal

Readmission is usually four weeks after surgery. A cystogram will usually be requested prior to removal of the catheter(s). This radiographic examination involves instilling a contrast medium via the catheter into the neobladder. Leaks or bladder reflux will be observed and if present removal of the catheters will be delayed.

Prior to readmission the patient may be asked to spigot their catheters on a clamp and release basis to increase bladder capacity. This should be commenced in week three.

Catheters are generally removed under antibiotic cover. It may take some time for the capacity of the new bladder to increase, approximately three to six months to hold 500 ml. The sensation described when the bladder is full is 'like having wind'. In the first few weeks the patient may need to empty their bladder every one to three hours. They should always be advised to get up at least once in the night and not leave voiding for more than six hours even when they have good capacity.

Bladder control may take some time to be achieved. Leakage is more common at night particularly in the male patient. Pelvic floor exercises are helpful to restore tone to the pelvic muscles.

Intermittent self-catheterisation

Approximately 10–30% of patients (Greenwell *et al.* 2001) will retain a sufficient amount of urine that they will need to catheterise. Retention of urine will cause problems such as:

- urinary tract infection
- leakage
- high pressure bladder
- hydronephrosis.

Complications

Complications for neobladder are similar to other forms of enterocysto-plasty but also include the risk of narrowing at the anastomosis between the ureter and the bladder. Stone formation can be reduced by encouraging the patient to maintain a high fluid intake and continue regular bladder washouts to reduce mucus.

Follow-up

The follow-up for orthotopic/neobladder will be similar to that of all other reconstructive procedures.

The Mainz Sigma II pouch (modified ureterosigmoidostomy)

The Mainz Sigma II pouch is a further type of urinary diversion where urine is passed via the anus. Rectal bladders have been around for many years and were first described in *The Lancet* in 1852 (Simon 1852). Many serious problems were encountered with this procedure which included pyelonephritis, anastomotic neoplasm, hyperchloraemic metabolic acidosis and renal function deterioration, and resulted in a higher mortality rate. Such complications led to the development of alternative types of urinary diversion. However, in recent years research has been driven by the concept of ridding the patient of the need to use an external appliance.

Patient selection

Patients suitable for a Mainz Sigma II pouch should be carefully selected. They need to be highly motivated and more importantly they need to be in possession of a competent anal sphincter. Anyone who leaks stool with or without sensation or is incontinent of faeces when they describe 'suffering from an upset stomach' or have diarrhoea for any other reason should consider other options.

Pre-operative preparation

It is very important that the patient understands the complexity of this surgery. Pre-operative counselling is essential. It is desirable that contact with another person who has had the surgery previously, either face to face or by phone, is offered prior to them making their final decision to have this surgery.

Pre-operative care

Patients undergoing this procedure will be assessed for the competency of their anal sphincter. Even for those patients with a highly competent anal sphincter regaining continence can take some months to achieve, particularly nocturnal continence. Patients must be aware of potential complications and have a high degree of motivation. Complications resulting from the formation of a Mainz II appear higher than in other reconstructive bladder surgery (Nitkunan *et al.* 2004). Despite this rectal bladders are becoming increasingly popular particularly in poorer countries where the cost of stoma appliances prohibits surgery requiring an external device.

Patients should be aware in pre-surgery that where there is a mixture of faeces and urine together, a strong odour is produced. Some people describe this as being extremely offensive and something they would find unacceptable. The potential embarrassment caused by this odour must be addressed pre-operatively, as an unprepared patient may suffer from social isolation.

Anal sphincters assessment

To ensure that the individual has the potential of being continent post-operatively it is important that the strength and control of the anal sphincters are assessed. A simple 'porridge test' can be done in outpatients. During this procedure 300–400 ml of water are mixed with a wheat-based cereal or porridge. This is instilled into the bowel with a large-size rectal catheter (20–22 French gauge) and a bladder syringe. The patient should be able to hold this for three to four hours without leaking. This simple test along with more refined recto-dynamic evaluation will ensure that the most appropriate patients are offered this surgery.

Bowel preparation

All patients undergoing this particular procedure will require bowel preparation. Prior to surgery it is essential to clear the bowel of as much faecal matter as possible. An effective diarrhoeal agent will be used in conjunction with clear fluids and an intravenous infusion to maintain hydration.

Urological surgeons differ in their protocol for pre-operative bowel clearance. Limited research has been carried out using this client group and with the absence of empirical evidence urologists remain divided in their approach. However for the Mainz II, a light, low residual diet is eaten on the second and third days prior to surgery and on the day preceding the operation supplementary drinks and clear fluids are taken. An intravenous infusion will be commenced in the evening prior to surgery to maintain good hydration.

Surgical procedure

Formation of the Mainz Sigma II pouch involves opening the bowel over a length of 12 cm both distal and proximal to the rectosigmoid junction (Fisch *et al.* 1996). The uninterrupted colon is detubularised to eliminate pressure thus reducing the problems encountered in the past with ureteric reflux and pyelonephritis because of the high pressure peristalsis in the bowel. During surgery a side to side anastomosis of the posterior wall is used to form a reservoir. The ureters are implanted and ureteric stents are inserted to maintain the anastomosis (see Figure 11.6). Finally the anterior wall is closed. Urine collects in the reservoir until the patient is ready to void. Faeces and urine will mix and the subsequent output will be usually diarrhoea like in nature.

Post-operative care

Routine monitoring will be consistent with protocols for major abdominal surgery. The patient will return with:

- intravenous infusion;
- naso-gastric tube;
- wound drains (one or two).

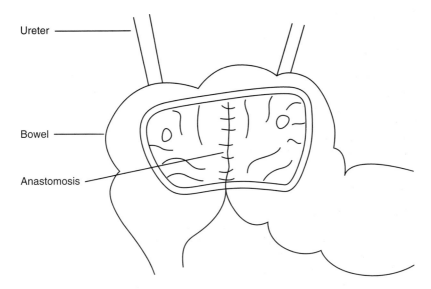

Figure 11.6 Formation of the Mainz Sigma II pouch.

Specific drains/urinary drainage

Both the stents and the rectal catheter need to remain patent and may require flushing with normal saline (see Table 11.4). These should be carefully secured to prevent movement which can cause discomfort.

Mucus

To prevent build-up and blockage from mucus the rectal catheter requires flushing. The flush is performed twice a day with saline via a bladder syringe.

Urinary continence

When the stents are removed the pouch begins to fill with urine which is then drained via the catheter until it is removed. If blocked the catheter may bypass and should be flushed until it is due for removal. After removal of the rectal catheter it may take some time for the voiding pattern to establish, the pouch to expand and continence to be achieved. Frequency may be experienced, especially in the early post-operative period, until the pouch expands.

Pelvic floor exercises

Prior to surgery the patient the patient will have been taught pelvic floor exercises. These are continued after their operation.

Complications

- Incontinence – less than 1% of patients continue to be incontinent after the first six months (Nitkunan *et al.* 2004).
- Pyelonephritis/urinary tract infections – repeated symptomatic infections may lead to stone formation and renal damage.
- Metabolic acidosis – 50% of patients develop hyperchloraemic acidosis and require oral sodium bicarbonate (600–2400 mg twice daily). Regular blood analysis is required (Woodhouse 2002).
- Anastomotic neoplasia – remains the most major of the long-term complications at 24% (Nitkunan *et al.* 2004). Yearly endoscopy is performed after ten years.

Table 11.4   Specific drains/urinary drainage

Ureteric stents	One into each re-implanted ureter. These will drain urine immediately	Removed 7–10 days post-operatively
Rectal catheter	Drains urine from the newly formed rectal pouch.	Removed 10–14 days post-operatively

Medic alert

It is advisable for all patients who have undergone surgery to reconstruct their bladder to wear some form of medic alert identification. For ileal conduit, Mitrofanoff and Mainz Sigma II details should include 'no urethral access'.

Support groups

The Urostomy Association is a self-help organisation which provides advice and support to all patients who have or are going to have any type of urinary diversion or reconstruction (see Chapter 1).

References

Allen S & Greenwell T (2003) Ileal conduit friend or foe? *Urology News*. **7(5)**: 6–8.

Blackley P (1998) *Practical Stoma Wound and Continence Management*. Victoria, Australia: Research Publications Pty Ltd.

Bricker EM (1950) Bladder substitution after pelvic evisceration. *Surgical Clinics of North America*. **30**: 1151.

Brooke BN (1952) The management of an ileostomy including its complications. *Lancet*. **ii**: 102–4.

Busuttil-Leaver R (2004) Reconstructive surgery for the promotion of continence. In: Fillingham S & Douglas J (eds) *Urological Nursing*. 3rd edn. Edinburgh: Churchill Livingstone.

Dorey G (2005) Restoring pelvic floor function in men: review of RCTs. *British Journal of Nursing*. **14(19)**: 1014–21.

Fillingham S (2005) Care of patients with urological stomas. In: Breckman B (ed) *Stoma Care and Rehabilitation*. Edinburgh: Elsevier Churchill Livingstone.

Fillingham S & Fell S (2004) Urological stomas. In: Fillingham S & Douglas J (ed) *Urological Nursing*. 3rd edn. Edinburgh: Churchill Livingstone.

Fisch M, Wammack R & Hohenfeller R (1996) The sigma rectum pouch (Mainz pouch II). *World Journal of Urology*. **14**: 68–72.

Gray M (2002) Are cranberry juice and cranberry products effective in the prevention or management of urinary tract infection? *Journal of Wound Ostomy Continence Nurse*. **29(3)**: 122–6.

Greenwell T & Venn SN (2002) Zen and the art of Mitrofanoff maintenance. *Urology News*. **6(2)**: 12–15.

Greenwell T, Venn SN & Mundy AR (2001) Review: augmentation cystoplasty. *British Journal of Urology International*. **88(6)**: 511–25.

Kouba E, Sands M, Lentz A, Wallen E & Pruthi RS (2007) A comparison of the Bricker versus Wallace ureteroileal anastomosis in patients undergoing urinary diversion for bladder cancer. *Journal of Urology*. **178(3)**: 945–9.

Nitkunan T, Leaver R, Patel HR & Woodhouse CR (2004) Modified ureterosigmoidostomy (Mainz II): a long-term follow-up. *British Journal of Urology International*. **93(7)**: 1043–7.

Ortiz H, Sara MJ, Armendariz P, de Miguel M, Marti J *et al.* (1994) Does the frequency of paracolostomy hernias depend on the position of the colostomy in the abdominal wall? *International Journal of Colorectal Disorders*. **9(2)**: 65–7.

Pearl RK (1989) Parastomal hernias. *World Journal of Surgery*. **13(5)**: 569–72.

Simon J (1852) Ectopia vesclicae (absence of the anterior walls of the bladder and pubic abdominal parieties): operation for directing the orifices of the ureters into the rectum: temporary success; subsequent death; autopsy. *Lancet*. **2**: 568–70.

Suvarna R, Pirmohamed M & Henderson L (2003) Possible interaction between warfarin and cranberry juice. *British Medical Journal.* **327(7429)**: 1454.

Suzer O, Vates TS, Freedman AL, Smith CA & Gonzales R (1997) Results of the Mitrofanoff procedure in urinary tract reconstruction in children. *British Journal of Urology International.* **79(2)**: 279–82.

Watson D (1987) Drug therapy – colour changes to faeces and urine. *Pharmaceutical Journal* **236**: 68.

Woodhouse CR (2002) British Society for Gastroenterology and Association of Colo-proctology for Great Britain and Ireland Guidelines for monitoring of patients with ureterosigmoidostomy. *Gut.* **51(suppl 5)**: V15–V16.

Chapter 12

Appliances

Jo Sica and Jennie Burch

Introduction

Stoma appliances are forever evolving to meet the needs of the ostomate. History of appliances used gives a background to methods in which patients had to cope with their stoma in the past. Appliances will never fulfil all patients' needs but skin reactions are much reduced and security is greatly improved. The different patient requirements are discussed in relation to stoma appliances to assist the reader.

History of stoma care products

Stoma surgery dates back as far as 400 BC and has a plotted history through to Leonardo da Vinci and his drawings made from dead bodies. Historically there were no stoma appliances available to the ostomate. A variety of devices were used to collect faeces, offering poor skin care and very little odour control. These included tins, cloths and leather bags during the seventeenth century (Lewis 1999). In 1944 the Koenig–Rutzen bag was introduced; this black rubber bag (see Figure 12.1) adhered to the skin with a latex solution. The bag incorporated a screw at the bottom that was used to empty the device (Black 2000). Most rubber bags required renewal after four to six months or longer (Brooke 1952). These bags solved many problems but were far from ideal. The black bags were large and the adhesives used with them led to severe skin irritation in many cases. The appliances were washed, dried, powdered and reused but however thorough the wash, the faecal smell would permeate the appliance and they soon become malodorous. A later option was a disposable bag that was held in place by a ring and belt. This was not snug fitting and led to leakage, odour and excoriated skin.

In the 1960s there were several revolutionary developments for ostomates with the use of karaya gum (see Figure 12.2) and hydrocolloid skin wafers. Karaya is produced from trees (Broadwell *et al.* 1982) and can be used to protect the peristomal skin. Karaya comes in a variety of configurations: powder, a ring/washer or as an integral part of the stoma appliance. The use of karaya greatly reduced excoriated skin. Although karaya-based products are still available it is not a part of modern appliances.

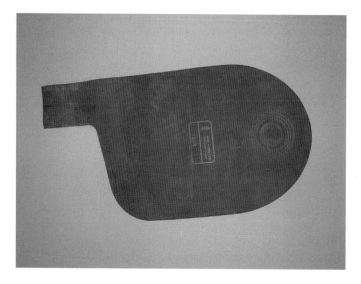

Figure 12.1   Koenig-Rutzen bag.

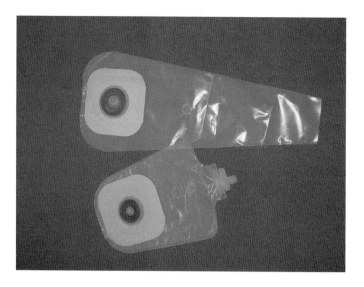

Figure 12.2   Karaya gum adhesive appliances.

A further advancement for ostomates was the use of hydrocolloid. Initially hydrocolloid wafers were used to reduce the incidence of excoriated skin and to provide security (Williams 2006a). The hydrocolloid adhesive is made from carboxymethylcellulose, polyisobutylene, pectin and gelatine (Lewis 1999). Hydrocolloid flanges hold moisture and are more skin friendly than the older acrylic adhesives (Black 2007). Variations of hydrocolloid are currently used, some in a more flexible and comfortable version.

Laminated plastic pouches also superseded the polythene pouches in the 1960s. These were more odour-proof, less noisy, more environmentally friendly and felt more comfortable for the patient.

Modern pouches

The aims of the modern appliance are to be leak-proof, odour-proof, easy to apply and remove, secure and skin friendly (Black & Stutchfield 2007). Appliances have evolved to offer ostomates more choice, comfort and discretion. This is important for the new ostomate to help them to adapt (Cottam & Porrett 2005). There are many variations of stoma products, attempting to suit different ostomates, as it has long been recognised that one bag will not suit all (Brooke 1952). Stoma appliances are designed to contain faeces or urine within them whilst not allowing odour to permeate through the appliance. Appliances are available in one and two pieces and with clear or opaque coverings. Clear appliances are used after surgery so that nurses and ostomates can observe the stoma without removing the appliance. Some ostomates choose to continue wearing clear appliances. Generally, however, in the United Kingdom (UK) most ostomates choose opaque appliances to disguise the faecal content, but clear urostomy appliances. Many manufacturers produce paediatric, small, medium and large size appliances to suit the different ostomates' needs.

Stoma appliances are available with cut to fit flanges. This is essential in the first eight weeks after surgery, when the stoma is changing shape and size. Companies also offer pre-cut sizes once the stoma size settles; however, these are only circular in shape and many stomas are not. It is imperative to ensure that the aperture size in the appliance flange is correct for the stoma. If the aperture is too large sore skin can occur, whereas if it is too small there may be leaks or constriction of the stoma. Pre-cut appliances are very beneficial for ostomates with manual dexterity or visual problems; however, it should be noted that delivery companies will hand cut unusual shaped apertures if that suits the ostomate.

The ostomate when using a two-piece appliance can leave the adhesive in place for up to five days (Lee 2001), although it is generally advisable to change every two to four days. The pouch can then be changed as required.

Colostomy appliances

Colostomy appliances are closed bags and used to collect soft to formed stool (see Figure 12.3). There is also flatus passed and modern appliances include a filter to release the air but not the odour (Plant 2001). The stool consistency depends upon the position of the colostomy in the colon, e.g. a transverse colostomy tends to produce a looser stool and may require use of a drainable bag. Colostomy appliances are replaced when dirty which can be up to three times daily. One study found the majority of

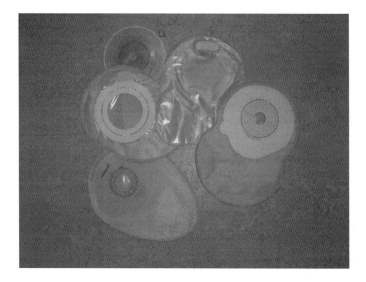

Figure 12.3   Closed one- and two-piece appliances.

colostomates change their appliance twice daily (Voergaard *et al.* 2007). The frequency of appliance change depends on the faecal consistency and the output volume. However, when there is nothing in the appliance it does not require changing.

Ileostomy appliances

Ileostomy appliances are drainable and collect loose to porridge-like faeces (see Figure 12.4). However, ileostomies fashioned in the upper ileum produce more liquid faeces. The drainable pouches historically fastened with either a hard plastic clip or a soft tie. However, clip-less fastenings such as Velcro have largely superseded this in the UK. Ileostomy appliances are replaced daily to every four days and appliances are emptied about four to six times daily when a third to half full.

Urostomy appliances

The urostomy appliance is used to collect urine (see Figure 12.5). The taps and bungs are simple to use to empty the urine into the toilet. However, some can be bulky and catch in the groin if not positioned well. Urostomy appliances are worn for one to three days and emptied about five or more times daily (Lee 2001), when a third to half full. Both urostomy and night bags have a non-return reflux valve. The valve helps prevent urine refluxing and is key in preventing urinary tract infections (Kirkwood 2006).

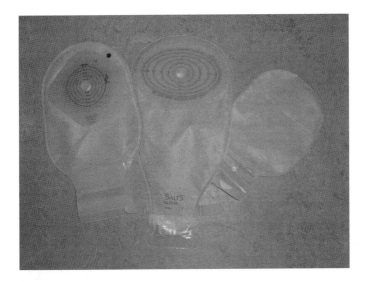

Figure 12.4   Drainable appliances.

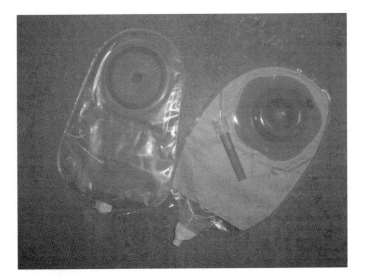

Figure 12.5   Urostomy appliances with adapter.

Additional drainage bags

Urostomates can have a larger storage capacity by attaching an extra drainage system to their urostomy bag, particularly helpful at night. The night drainage bag may require a connector to attach the urostomy bag tap to the night bag. Leg bags can also be used in the daytime, particularly when travelling.

Additional drainage bags are often used for one week and cleaned daily. However, some urostomates prefer to use a sealed or single-use disposable night drainage bag that is emptied in the morning, by tearing the end of the night bag off and draining the urine into the toilet. It is thought that by using a single-use night drainage bag, the risk of infection is reduced, although anecdotally if the drainage bag is cleaned thoroughly infections do not happen.

One- and two-piece appliances

Most manufacturers make ostomy products in both one- and two-piece appliances. One-piece appliances tend to be thinner, more flexible and more discreet, while two-piece appliances offer the ostomates the opportunity to keep the flange in situ and change the bag, useful to protect the skin from damage due to repeated appliance changes (McPhail 2003). Two-piece appliances historically join using plastic clicking ring type connectors. Many manufacturers now also produce two-piece appliances that join together with adhesive (White & Berg 2005).

One-piece colostomy appliances are generally suitable for colostomates with a faecal output that requires appliance changes of two or fewer daily. However, it may be more time-efficient, more skin-friendly and more cost-efficient to use a two-piece appliance if the colostomy is active two or more times daily. If the colostomy output is loose then a drainable appliance may be more suitable.

One-piece ileostomy appliances are popular in the UK. In other countries two-piece appliances can be more cost-effective and thus have greater usage where patients self-fund or have limited insurance cover. Two-piece appliances may be useful if the ileostomate wishes to change the bag daily or to wear a smaller appliance during the day and a larger one at night, for example.

Two-piece urostomy appliances are popular, allowing the angle of the appliance to be changed if necessary; for example at night when the night drainage bag is attached. Some urostomates also find that mucus can build up in the appliance lining and prefer to change the bag daily and leave the flange in situ.

Adhesive coupling system

Two-piece appliances have been developed to be less bulky. There are now appliances that come in two adhesive parts. This offers the ostomate all the benefits of the two-piece system but with a thin and discreet profile.

Toilet flushable colostomy appliances

Each year over 36.5 million used stoma pouches are disposed of, many to landfill sites (Black 2000). It is not just the environmental aspect that needs to be considered but also the psychological effect of pouch disposal on the individual. There are colostomy appliances available that can be flushed down the toilet and biodegrade as they go through the sewage system. Flushable appliances are useful when the ostomate is away from home and disposal of used colostomy appliances could prove difficult but they can also be used at any time. Despite worries about these appliances blocking the toilet, there have been no proven cases of this occurring (Buckland 2006a). Due to the impact on the environment stoma appliance manufacturers should be considering the disposal of all appliances as a real issue.

Stoma caps

For the colostomate there are small caps that are designed to cover the colostomy (see Figure 12.6) but have little more than a pad inside, so the absorption capacity is minimal. Caps can be used in a variety of situations:

- after irrigation (with no expected output for one to two days);
- for sexual activities (for a short period of time);
- for sport and hobbies (for a limited period).

Caps are available in both one and two pieces.

   A cap has also been designed for the urostomate, useful for a very limited amount of time, when discretion is required.

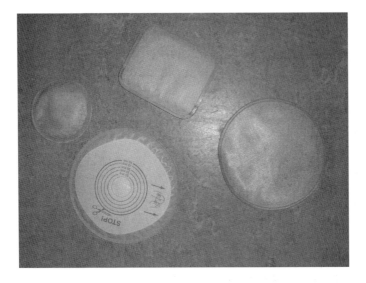

Figure 12.6   Stoma caps.

Stoma plug

The Conseal plug is available as a one- or two-piece system and allows the colostomate to be free from wearing a colostomy pouch. The plug itself looks like a mushroom with the stalk part being placed in the colon to stop faeces from leaving the colostomy for up to 12 hours. Plugs do need to be used in conjunction with an appliance or colostomy irrigation, to allow passage of faeces from the colostomy. It may take time for the colostomate to learn how to use the plug and a number of weeks for them to be able to wear it for extended periods of time.

Appliances for high-output stomas

There are a few very rare stomas, the jejunostomy or duodenostomy, that are made from the higher gastrointestinal tract. These ostomates pass high faecal outputs often in excess of one litre daily from their stoma. There is also a small group of ostomates that have a high output from their ileostomy or colostomy, passing up to several litres daily (Forbes 1997). Management of high faecal outputs can be difficult, the appliance fills quickly and the storage capacity of many appliances may be inadequate. Some manufacturers make a larger size bag in their range that can be useful in this situation (see Figure 12.7). However, there is also a limited choice of high-output bags, available only in two pieces. The appliances are large for extra storage and instead of the outlet being like an ileostomy appliance, the opening is round and about one centimetre in diameter. This allows the connection of a catheter night drainage bag or a specialised

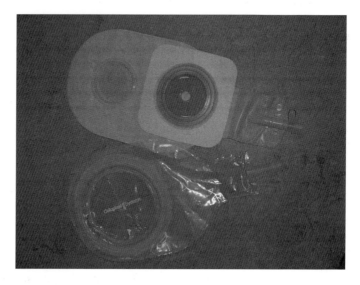

Figure 12.7   High output appliances.

drainage bag. Extra drainage is particularly useful overnight to reduce the frequency of appliance emptying. Many ostomates feel the need to apply extra adhesive around the stoma flange to help improve adherence or wear a stoma belt to help with the weight of the pouch when full.

Another method of caring for a high output stoma with a very liquid output is to use a urostomy pouch. This has the benefit of being able to be connected directly into a night drainage system. However, should the output become thicker, the non-return valve can block and the pouch will not function properly or the outlet may be too small to drain the faeces. Using a urostomy appliance can be a good short-term solution for ostomates with post-operative high outputs that resolve soon after surgery.

Fistula appliances

For a limited but complicated patient group the fistula appliance is required. There is a variety of manufacturers that make these appliances and in many different sizes to accommodate the largest fistula or wound. Appliances are clear, so that the fistula site and output can be observed. These products are expensive, but can potentially be left in situ for up to one week. Some appliances have an opening in the plastic surface of the bag for access to the fistula. This can be beneficial in the care of the fistula or for fistuloclysis (see Chapter 16 for more information). All fistula appliances have drainable ports, to attach to drainage bags, as the output is generally greater than one litre daily.

Fistula appliances adhere to the skin in the same way as a stoma bag, but are larger. These appliances are often used in conjunction with other ostomy products, such as skin protection wipes/sprays, paste and/or seals to aid adhesion. To apply a fistula bag is generally time consuming and can be difficult for the inexperienced (see Chapter 16).

Convex flanges

Convexity may be a solution to poorly spouted ileostomies or urostomies or a retracted colostomy to prevent leaks and/or skin excoriation (McKenzie & Ingram 2001). The construction of the convex shoulders of the appliance applies pressure on to the immediate peristomal skin, thus encouraging the stoma to protrude. A thorough assessment of the individual patient should be made before using a convex appliance due to the potential risks to the skin (Boyd *et al.* 2004).

Convex pouches are available in one and two pieces for the colostomate, ileostomate and urostomate. Generally the convexity of choice would be integral to the appliance, but convex inserts are available to make convex flanges from older type two-piece appliances. There has been a huge influx of convex systems into the stoma care market in recent years with companies striving to manufacture a pouch that is comfortable for the ostomate. Most convex pouches are rigid near the aperture due to the plastic insert that is used to create the dome. This can often make the pouch uncomfortable to wear. There has been a recent trend to move towards softer, cushioned convex pouches as they are less likely to cause skin damage and can be more comfortable for the ostomate.

Problems associated with convexity include peristomal skin bruising, ulceration and exacerbation of rare underlying conditions such as pyoderma gangrenosum (Lyon & Beck 2001). Convex appliances are contraindicated for ostomates with a parastomal hernia, as the skin can be friable due to its being stretched by the hernia putting the skin at high risk of breakdown. Several appliances are available with soft convexity or thick hydrocolloid around the aperture to provide pressure. The Curvex pouch from Welland Medical has a soft domed plateau that will anecdotally invert when used with a parastomal hernia. An international study showed a dramatic reduction in the incidence of leakages when using the Curvex pouch (Buckland 2006b).

Stoma accessories

For ostomates with 'normal' stomas the use of stoma accessories is not generally required (see Figure 12.8). However, for ostomates with problems, accessories can be invaluable. Stoma accessories can be expensive and should be regularly reviewed, but can actually reduce prescription costs if repeated leaks are prevented.

Protective wafers/sheets

Wafers are hydrocolloid squares that come in various sizes. They are flexible and applied directly to the peristomal area prior to the pouch being

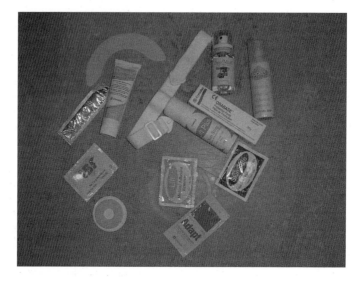

Figure 12.8 Stoma accessories.

applied. Protective wafers were historically useful to help treat large areas of sore skin, especially with some of the 'older' type pouches when skin reactions were more common. Wafers are still worn beneath old type appliances, e.g. karaya by ostomates to protect their peristomal skin from the appliance adhesive.

Skin cleansers

Some ostomates find that a skin cleanser is particularly useful when they are away from home. Skin cleansers can be applied to a dry wipe and used to cleanse the peristomal skin. They can also be used to cleanse hands after an appliance change if no water is available. However, skin cleansers should be used with caution as they may irritate sore or broken skin. Skin cleansers should not be used routinely and warm water is advised for general cleansing. There is an array of cleansers available and some are free with certain delivery companies.

Paste

If the peristomal skin is uneven, i.e. there is a small skin crease near the stoma, using a filling paste may be helpful. By levelling the skin there is less chance of a leaking appliance and thus skin integrity should be maintained. Paste can be applied directly on to the skin or around the flange aperture to aid adhesion for uneven skin, for example. It should be noted that paste takes time to 'dry' and should therefore be used sparingly for best effects.

Pastes are made from hydrocolloid and generally mixed with alcohol to aid squeezing the paste from the tube and moulding it. Paste with alcohol should be used with caution as it can sting broken skin. Using the paste on the appliance flange can be useful as this allows the alcohol to evaporate and thus reduces the pain if used on broken skin. Anecdotally some ostomates apply paste from a 10 ml syringe, which has several benefits: less paste is used and/or more accurate application of the paste is possible. Paste can be difficult to use when the tube becomes less full; this can be overcome by placing the tube (with the cap on) into some warm water as the warmth softens the paste. This method should be used with caution to ensure that ostomates do not burn themselves on the water.

Most ostomates do not need to use paste. Paste can be difficult to remove from the skin, although there are adhesive remover wipes and sprays that help. A simple method to remove the old paste is to leave the skin and paste open to the air for a few minutes to allow the paste to dry out and then the paste can be gently removed. However, picking at the paste can cause skin damage and should be avoided. If the paste is fresh, clean and secure on the skin it may be advantageous to simply leave the paste in situ, for example on a recently changed appliance that needs premature removal for a leak. Adhesive paste should not be confused with protective paste, which will actually hinder adhesive.

Seals and washers

If there are skin dips around the stoma a seal/washer can raise the skin to a smooth level. Another situation where seals are useful is for stomas with a corrosive output that has a tendency to break down the inner edge of the flange or the peristomal skin. Seals are moisture absorbing, securing, skin-friendly and contain no alcohol. Seals can be stretched and/or moulded to fit almost any stoma size.

Seals can also be cut or broken in half or into smaller pieces and applied to problematic peristomal skin, i.e. a half moon type dip in the skin at the base of the stoma.

Convex seals have been introduced that can be used alone or to increase convexity. They can be used with any system.

Seals can be useful in the care of enterocutaneous fistulae. For fistula management the seal can be placed directly around the wound edges to aid skin protection, to improve 'wear-time' of the fistula appliance and to build up any skin dips. To fill deeper skin creases the seal can be used by rolling it into a sausage shape. The shaped seal is then gently pushed into the skin crease with a small amount of paste below it to aid adhesion.

Flange securing tape

Securing strips can be used on the outer edges of the stoma bag flange or fistula appliance to aid appliance security. There can be many reasons that a ostomate may require extra flange security; for example with parastomal hernias, prolapsed stomas or badly sited stomas such as those in a crease or near a bony prominence. High-output stomas may require extra adhesion to help secure the pouch on to the body when full.

Ostomy belts

To add extra security a thin elastic belt can be attached to some appliances. The belt is often used with convex or two-piece products. Some appliances have small plastic loops on the flanges that are used to hold the belt. If the bag does not have these hooks there are belt plates available that can be placed around the bag, on top of the flange and will fit any standard bag. Belts need to be adjusted to fit the ostomate and should be worn level with the stoma – not on the waistline. Belts may be washed by hand or on a gentle machine wash when required.

Adhesive

There are adhesive sprays or glues used to increase the adhesive qualities of the flange. These should be used with caution, as they can be difficult to remove and thus increase the risk of peristomal skin damage. It should be noted that there are adhesive remover sprays/wipes available to help remove the appliance.

Adhesive removers

Some ostomates find removing their stoma appliance to be uncomfortable. Adhesive removers are available as sprays and wipes and are particularly useful for these ostomates. There has been a move by ostomy manufacturers to develop adhesive removers with no alcohol so they do not sting the patient when used on sore or broken skin. Adhesive removers are available as either oil or silicone based (Berry *et al.* 2007). Additionally the sticky residue from the hydrocolloid flange may be left on the peristomal skin and this can collect fluff from clothes and is difficult to remove with water alone. Although soap generally removes the residue it can also dry the skin. Adhesive removers can be useful in these situations; however, in general ostomates do not require an adhesive remover.

Odour treatment options

Some ostomates find the smell of their faeces, from either their ileostomy or colostomy, unacceptable. It is important to remember that odour should only occur when either changing or emptying the pouch. There are many options to reduce odour, including diet manipulation and generic air fresheners, but there are possible solutions on drug tariff. There is a range of drops or powders that can be put directly into the new appliance before use to eradicate the odour. There are also sprays that are specially formulated to eliminate odour rather than mask it, although their efficacy may be limited (Smith 2003). Sprays are best used just prior to emptying or changing rather than afterwards, as the faecal odour may cling to clothes.

Protective powder

A protective powder can be used on broken skin that is reddened, sore or irritated, to promote healing. Protective powder should be used sparingly and any excess needs to be removed to be effective, as excessive powder can reduce the adhesion of the flange (Williams 2006b). The correct amount of powder is achieved by gently 'dusting' the excess powder from the skin. The cause of the red skin should be investigated so that the powder is not used as a long-term solution. For a limited number of ostomates there is a slight discomfort when the powder is applied; this soon passes.

Protective film

Protective films come as wipes or sprays and are used on the skin prior to the appliance being adhered. There has been a recent move from skin protection films that contain alcohol to formulations without it. Alcohol is contraindicated for use on broken skin, due to the pain on application. Protective films can be used on red and broken skin, as well as skin at risk of excoriation. Films can act as a barrier against stoma effluent, maceration of the peristomal skin and repeated removal of a stoma pouch. Ostomates with sensitive skin may also find a film beneficial.

Another use of protective films is for those who have sweaty skin, as the film can add extra tackiness to the skin. The tackiness can aid adhesion and extends wear time of the appliance in hot weather. It should be noted that most ostomates do not generally require protective films.

Protective cream

Protective creams can be highly effective in the treatment of dry and flaky peristomal skin. Creams can also be beneficial on perianal skin after the reversal of a stoma or when the patient has had an ileoanal pouch formation. Creams are designed to soothe, condition and moisturise the skin but allow a stoma pouch to adhere, as they are not greasy. However, most ostomates do not need to use a protective cream. Those that are assessed to need cream should be educated to ensure that the cream is used sparingly or adhesion of the appliance can be compromised.

Pancaking prevention agents

Pancaking (see Chapter 15 on complications) can be a real issue to some colostomates and cause appliances to leak. There have been lots of accessories produced to help with pancaking. Several accessories are designed to keep apart the inside edges of the appliance. There are foam bricks available that are stuck to the top of the inside of the clean stoma appliance. This keeps the two plastic edges of the appliance apart and allows the faeces to drop to the bottom of the appliance. Plastic bridges can be placed on the outer surface of the appliance, at the top of the pouch so that it bends the top surface and stops the inside edges of the pouch from sticking together.

Lubricating gels and solutions can be used to make the inside of the pouch more slippery. The gel is applied inside the fresh bag and the plastic is rubbed together to distribute the gel. This helps encourage the faeces to travel down inside the pouch. Some of these lubricating products also act as a deodorant.

Ostomates also use their own homemade inventions. These include baby/olive oil, which is applied directly into the pouch to help the faeces to slide down inside the bag. A piece of crumpled tissue in the pouch can also be effective in keeping the inner surfaces apart.

Discharge solidifying agents

Thickening agents generally come in the form of sachets or tablets and are placed into the appliance and not taken orally. These are used to solidify the stoma output, help reduce pouch noise and reduce the chances of the appliance ballooning. Unfortunately there is nothing currently on the market that reduces the volume of the stomal output.

Whilst solidifying agents are extremely useful in the management of a loose faecal output, the reason behind the loose output should be investigated. Only after assessment should this type of treatment be used, as an infection may be present or loose stool may be diet related.

Pouch clips and soft ties

With the advent of the new clip-less ileostomy appliances there are few appliances that require additional clips or ties. Companies will generally supply, on prescription, extra fastenings.

Soft ties can also be applied to the base of a urostomy pouch to prevent it from twisting. This is particularly useful at night when attached to a night drainage bag, allowing the urine to flow freely into the night drainage bag.

Pouch covers

The newer stoma pouches have integral soft, non-woven coverings. Some people, however, choose to wear a separate cloth pouch cover, either to disguise their pouch or for enhanced comfort. Pouch covers are generally made from light cotton and slip over the pouch. Covers are available in both plain and patterned fabrics and some people choose to make their own pouch covers. However, it is important that the right pouch cover is ordered, as there are different codes for covers to fit one- and two-piece systems.

Flatus filters

Filters are integral in modern faecal stoma appliances to release flatus (Davenport & Sica 2003). However, the filters can become ineffectual if made wet, so covering the filter when bathing or swimming is advised (Skipper 2002). Filter covers are generally small stickers supplied in each box of appliances. Covers can also be useful if the ostomate needs to keep some flatus in their pouch to help prevent pancaking.

Filters need to be effective for the two different types of faecal odour; sulphorous and complex organic odours containing indoles and skatoles that are found in faeces. Each appliance manufacturer uses a different type of construction for their treated carbon filter so if a patient finds one filter ineffective trying a different appliance may be useful.

Hernia support garments

Parastomal hernias can be treated non-surgically with a hernia support garment. Unisex support garments can range from elasticated underwear to support belts and can provide light to firm support. There are mixed opinions as to whether there should be a hole in the belt to pass the stoma appliance through or not; general consensus is in favour of no opening. Undergarments are made by different companies in various forms to try and suit different tastes and requirements. However, many ostomates do not use support garments (see Chapter 15 on complications).

Protective shields

Plastic shields are made to protect the stoma from direct blows that may be sustained in sporting activities or occupations, for example. Shields are available on prescription and attached over the stoma appliance and under clothing and held in place with a thin elastic belt.

A stoma cup is also available, designed to hold absorbent material to catch any stomal output. The stoma cup is worn when the ostomate is in the shower and allows bag-free bathing. This is not available on drug tariff.

Clothing

Some companies produce underwear, swimwear or clothes that are especially designed for ostomates to make the stoma less visible, but none is available on drug tariff. Some specialist underwear is available with small pockets inside to hold and support the appliance. However, it should be remembered that most ostomates do not need to change their pre-surgery clothes. Male ostomates may feel more comfortable wearing high waisted trousers, which are available at a cost.

Stoma appliance costing

Stoma appliances are costly, at over £2 per bag. Although cost should not be an issue it is increasingly becoming so. For the average ostomate with an uncomplicated stoma the use of an appliance from any manufacturer would be suitable and provide a comfortable, odour-free system. However, patient choice remains crucial and each stoma pouch offers different benefits that may be suitable for one ostomate and not another. There has been some evidence that using a two-piece system can be marginally cheaper than a one-piece (Black 2000). However, no correlation was found between high morbidity and appliance costs of ostomates, which may be a reflection of the quality of stoma appliances, but colostomates' appliance usage was nearly twice as costly as ileostomates' (Hughes 2005).

The cost of accessories and appliances is increasing and their use should be reviewed to ensure products are appropriate. Even as far back as 1989 it was felt that stoma specialist nurses may be able to keep prescribing costs down (Elcoat 1989). Many stoma specialist nurses find an annual review beneficial (Jefferies *et al.* 1995), as they are able to reassess and advise the ostomate on practical stoma care. Stoma appliances are largely funded through the GP, and the PCTs (primary care trusts) are increasingly interested in the costs of stoma equipment and need to keep the ever-escalating costs down. Many GPs have set up audits with the help of the stoma specialist nurse to ensure ostomates use cost-effective and appropriate appliances.

Conclusion

With developing technology and research by the stoma care companies, new products are constantly being brought to the market place. Whilst this benefits the patient, it can also be daunting and confusing. Stoma specialist nurses are invaluable in the process of appliance choice to aid and guide the ostomate. For those ostomates with uncomplicated stomas the choice of appliances is extensive; however, an increasing number of ostomates develop peristomal and stoma problems that necessitate the need for specialist products. The stoma specialist nurse is instrumental in this situation to address and resolve any problems.

Having a stoma is not just a physical problem, but can also be a psychological one. Thus it is essential to ensure that the appliance is secure and discreet. This allows the ostomate to feel confident when performing their daily activities.

References

Berry J, Black P, Smith R & Stuchfield (2007) Assessing the value of silicone and hydrocolloid products in stoma care. *British Journal of Nursing.* **16(13)**: 778–88.

Black P (2000) *Holistic Stoma Care.* London: Baillière Tindall.

Black P (2007) Peristomal skin care: an overview of available products. *British Journal of Nursing.* **16(17)**: 1048–56.

Black P & Stutchfield B (2007) *Caring for Stoma Patients – Best Practice Guidelines.* CREST CliniMed Resource for Education and Specialist Training. High Wycombe CliniMed.

Boyd K, Thompson MJ, Boyd-Carson W & Trainor B (2004) Use of convex appliances. *Nursing Standard.* **18(20)**: 37–8.

Broadwell DC, Appleby CH, Bates MA & Jackson BS (1982) Principles and techniques of pouching. In: Broadwell DC & Jackson BS (eds) *Principles of Ostomy Care.* London: Mosby.

Brooke BN (1952) The management of an ileostomy including its complications. *The Lancet.* **2(3)**: 102–4.

Buckland SJ (2006a) Problems encountered when discarding stoma pouches. *The Journal of Stomal Therapy Australia.* **26(1)**: 16–20.

Buckland SJ (2006b) A global study to determine if soft convexity can be utilised in the management of parastomal hernias. Oral presentation. Hong Kong: WCET.

Burch J & Sica J (2005) Frequency, predisposing factors for and treatment of parastomal hernia. *Gastrointestinal Nursing.* **3(6)**: 29–32.

Cottam J & Porrett T (2005) Choosing the correct stoma appliance. In: Porrett T & McGrath A (eds) *Stoma Care – Essential Clinical Skills for Nurses.* Oxford: Blackwell.

Davenport R & Sica J (2003) A new modern drainable appliance for people with ileostomies. *British Journal of Nursing.* **12(9)**: 571–5.

Elcoat C (1989) Coping with stoma care in the community. *The Practitioner.* **233**: 776–9.

Forbes A (1997) *Clinicians' Guide to Inflammatory Bowel Disease.* London. Chapman & Hall.

Hughes D (2005) Ostomists – the real cost. *Gastrointestinal Nursing.* **3(2)**: 28–30.

Jefferies E, Joels J, Wood EJ, Butler M, Cullen R *et al.* (1995) A service evaluation of stoma care nurses' practice. *Journal of Clinical Nursing.* **4(4)**: 235–42.

Kirkwood L (2006) Postoperative stoma care and the selection of appliances. *Journal of Community Nursing.* **20(3)**: 12–18.

Lee J (2001) Nurse prescribing in practice: patient choice in stoma care. *British Journal of Community Nursing.* **6(1)**: 33–7.

Lewis L (1999) History and evolution of stomas and appliances. In: Taylor P (ed) *Stoma Care in the Community.* London: Nursing Times Books.

Lyon CC & Beck MH (2001) Dermatitis. In: Lyon C & Smith A (eds) *Abdominal Stomas and Their Skin Disorders. An Atlas of Diagnosis and Management.* London: Martin Dunitz.

McKenzie FD & Ingram VA (2001) Dansac Invent convex in the management of flush ileostomy. *British Journal of Nursing.* **10(15)**: 1005–9.

McPhail J (2003) Selection and use of stoma care appliances. In: Elcoat C (ed) *Stoma Care Nursing.* London: Hollister.

Plant C (2001) Coping with a colostomy. *Nursing and Residential Care.* **3(6)**: 260–4.

Skipper G (2002) Esteem® one-piece closed pouch in the management of stomas. *British Journal of Nursing.* **11(21)**: 1412–15.

Smith C (2003) Not to be sniffed at. *Gastrointestinal Nursing.* **1(6)**: 16–18.

Voergaard LL, Vendelbo G, Carlsen B, Jacobsen L, Nissen B *et al.* (2007) Ostomy bag management: comparative study of a new one-piece closed bag. *British Journal of Nursing.* **16(2)**: 95–101.

White M & Berg K (2005) A new flangeless adhesive coupling system for colostomy and ileostomy. *British Journal of Nursing.* **14(6)**: 325–8.

Williams J (2006a) Stoma care part 1: choosing the right appliance. *Gastrointestinal Nursing.* **4(6)**: 16–19.

Williams J (2006b) Stoma care part 2: choosing appliance accessories. *Gastrointestinal Nursing.* **4(7)**: 16–19.

Chapter 13

Discharge to the Community

Jennie Burch

Introduction

To plan an effective discharge starts at admission. There are many issues that need to be addressed for a new ostomate in addition to the usual discharge criteria of being sent to a safe environment. The stoma-specific issues include ensuring that the patient is proficient in their stoma care, knows how to dispose of used appliances and is able to obtain further stoma supplies. Other matters are also discussed.

Discharge criteria

The ideal plan for discharge home with a newly formed stoma is that the ostomate can independently perform their stoma care prior to discharge (Erwin-Toth & Doughty 1992). It is important to remember that early self-care with the stoma can enhance psychological adaptation but that does not mean that there will not be emotional difficulties (O'Connor 2005). Psychological issues are discussed in Chapter 18. If a patient is not able to perform their own stoma care when discharged from the hospital, community nurses or the family can assist (Pringle & Swan 2001). In most areas in the UK the community or district nurses do not routinely visit ostomates after their discharge home from hospital after their stoma-forming surgery. It has also been documented that some community nurses do not feel confident to care for ostomates and would welcome further training (Skingley 2004). This could be achieved possibly by undertaking a secondment (Adams *et al.* 2003) with the stoma specialist nurse. It can be important to establish goals so that the patient can see that they are meeting their targets and becoming ready for discharge home. It can also be important when planning for discharge home to consider any potential problems the ostomate may have and to discuss and try to resolve them.

Prior to discharge home the following are some of the criteria that need to be met:

- Can the ostomate/carer independently change their appliance?
- Does the ostomate understand how to dispose of used appliances?
- Has the ostomate received written and verbal advice to help them to care for their stoma?

- Can the ostomate identify normal and abnormal stomas and do they know what action to take if changes occur?
- Is the ostomate aware of the normal stoma function and when to gain advice?
- Can the ostomate recognise healthy peristomal skin and do they know what to do if changes occur?
- Does the ostomate have adequate stoma appliances and know how to obtain further stoma supplies?
- Is the ostomate aware of which activities they should undertake and when to further increase them?
- Does the ostomate know how to contact the stoma specialist nurse for help and advice at any time in the future?

(Allison 1996)

Other aspects to consider are: does the ostomate understand the changes that will occur with their stoma in the first few weeks after discharge? Generally there will be a reduction in the size of the stoma, as the swelling subsides for up to eight weeks (Readding 2005). The stoma may also slightly change shape and the stool will generally become thicker with the introduction of the ostomate's usual diet. The colour of the stoma should not change and it should remain moist. Diet needs to be discussed to prevent complications such as constipation for the colostomate, obstruction for the ileostomate or a urine infection for the urostomate (see Chapter 14 on nutrition). It can be useful when the ostomate is still learning about their stoma to place newspaper on the floor when changing the appliance in case of accidents, although care should be taken not to slip on this. Additionally when performing their stoma care some patients find it useful to use a peg or two to hold their clothes out of the way when changing or emptying their appliance.

Stoma supplies

It is essential to ensure that the new ostomate is discharged from the hospital with adequate supplies. Many stoma specialist nurses will provide one to two weeks' supply of stoma appliances and any accessories required. These discharge products are usually provided by the appliance manufacturing companies free of charge in most of the UK, saving the hospitals and primary care trusts money; however, this is frequently reviewed and questioned. The general practitioner or nurse prescriber will continue to prescribe appliances to the ostomate in the community.

Stoma appliances should be stored at room temperature. Care must be taken in hot climates and appliances should never be stored in a refrigerator, as both will cause problems with the adhesive. It is also not advisable to have large stocks of appliances, even though they do have a shelf life of several years, as the appliances take up space. Appliances are generally quick and easy to obtain and it is possible that the ostomate's needs may alter and that the current appliances become unusable and are wasted. Alternatively the appliances may not be used in the sequence obtained and then their sell by date may expire. Ordering a maximum of three months' supply of appliances means less potential wastage. The ostomate can be advised to ensure that they reorder when they have about two to three weeks of stock remaining to ensure they do not run out if a problem is encountered, such as a leaking appliance. If the stock is obtained from the chemist, supplies may take a little longer and therefore this advice will need to be individually adjusted.

Disposal of appliances

Stoma appliances are once-only use. However, there is debate about how dirty appliances should be disposed of as they are not generally biodegradable and therefore cannot be flushed into the sewage system (Black 2000). There are colostomy appliances available that can be disposed of in the toilet (see Chapter 12 on appliances). The Royal College of Nursing wrote in their guidelines that the contents of colostomy appliances should be flushed down the toilet prior to disposal of the appliances into the household waste (Mead 1994; RCN 1994). Many stoma specialist nurses advise the colostomate to empty their appliance into the toilet prior to sealing it in a disposable bag and discarding it in the household rubbish (Berry 2006). This can be achieved by cutting the top corner of the appliance off to dispose of the faeces in the toilet. Others advise that the appliance flange should be sealed prior to placing it in a disposable bag. Ultimately the used appliance should not pose a problem to others (Rust 2007) by potentially spilling from bin bags. A study that partially looked into the disposal of used colostomy appliances found that 42% emptied their stool into the toilet before disposal (McKenzie *et al.* 2006). For an ileostomate or urostomate it is advisable to always empty the appliance before changing it to reduce the risk of spillage.

Obtaining further supplies

Prescriptions and exemptions

Stoma appliances are free of charge to ostomates under the age of 16 or over the age of 60 years and to those with a permanent stoma and some other medical conditions, on production of an exemption certificate. Ostomates with a temporary stoma, who are not already exempt, will generally need to pay for their equipment or obtain a pre-payment certificate for their prescriptions. Stoma exemptions need to be considered on an individual basis, as not all potentially 'temporary' stomas are reversed or patients may prefer not to undergo any further surgery.

In the UK the prescription can be sent to the local chemist for collection or possibly delivery; alternatively the prescription can be given to a specialist stoma product delivery company (Pullen 2002). There are a number of benefits to having the appliances delivered. Elderly ostomates after surgery may find it difficult to travel for example. The delivery companies also offer many incentives that include free wipes and disposal bags. The delivery companies can obtain the prescription directly from the general practitioner (GP), which means that the ostomate does not need to visit the

GP for a repeat prescription. Delivery companies will also usually cut appliances. However, it should be noted that after eight weeks the stoma will usually have stopped changing size (unless the ostomate loses or gains weight) and many companies make a range of pre-made holes in their appliances that might suit the ostomate. There are currently a large number of delivery companies that may meet the needs of the ostomate.

Nurse prescribing

Nurses are now able to prescribe a variety of drugs and also stoma equipment. The choice and range of ostomy products is huge and may cause difficulty to the nurse and patient in choosing the most appropriate stoma products. There are over ten companies that manufacture stoma appliances each with its own unique product range (Lee 2001).

Appliances

Prior to discharge home the patients are required to choose a stoma appliance to wear when they have very little experience of what they need or want. In some cases it is more appropriate for the stoma specialist nurse to advise on the first appliance used. It can be necessary for some ostomates to try several different stoma appliances before selecting an appropriate one (Lee 2001). There are a number of considerations that can influence appliance choice, such as:

- the faecal consistency;
- the volume of the output;
- the stoma size;
- any problems with the stoma;
- manual dexterity;
- any problems with eyesight.

The various appliances are discussed in Chapter 12.

It can be useful for the ostomate to carry a small bag that contains an extra supply of stoma equipment for emergency situations if a leak occurs. This can be kept in the car or handbag. However, it is important to ensure periodically that the appliance is not creased or ageing and would therefore reduce the adhesive powers.

Follow-up visits

Home visits were in the past arranged for the first week following discharge home (Mead 1994). Unfortunately home visits are becoming more difficult to sustain, due to reduced nursing staff for example. A study found that, due to the number of complications and social adaptation required, home visits were still required and useful (Pringle & Swan 2001). Despite this, home visits are frequently being cut to an absolute minimum.

However, contact with the stoma specialist nurse is needed and the patient can attend stoma clinics for review. It is also considered important to have a yearly review to ensure that any issues are addressed.

Home visits are used to assess how patients are coping with their stoma after they are discharged home. They also allow the stoma specialist nurse to assess the family and home. Home visits can be essential to the housebound or very elderly who would have difficulty attending hospital clinics following discharge home. District nurses in some areas are able to perform home visits but this may not be possible due to staffing constraints.

Clinic visit frequency will vary between patients. Some ostomates require only one follow-up and know that more are possible if problems occur. Ostomates, particularly those with problematic stomas, may require more contact with the stoma specialist nurse. A clinic visit at three months is ideal to assess how the ostomate is coping physically and psychologically.

Post-operative psychological adjustment

There has been work undertaken on the coping mechanisms adopted by ostomates. White (1998) felt that to enhance the psychological adaptation to stoma-forming surgery, early learning of stoma skills was required. Gaining these skills promotes independence and is usually achieved prior to discharge home from the hospital. However, with the shorter hospital stays careful planning may be needed to achieve this, which may include pre-operative teaching.

It is unlikely that much adaptation to the stoma will have occurred in the hospital. However, by three months it is usual for many ostomates to have returned to their previous employment or activities. This can also be a stressful time for the new ostomate who will now be feeling stronger and the full impact of their situation may become evident. It is important for health care professionals to be aware of this and follow-up at this time can be beneficial.

It must be remembered that adjustment to a stoma is an ongoing process. The health care professional is ideally placed to ensure that adaptation occurs as smoothly as possible and to try to prevent the ostomate from worrying about stoma-related issues. Depression is also a potential problem after stoma-forming surgery and may be identified and addressed at a clinic visit. Pringle & Swan (2001) found that, in their study of patients with a stoma for colorectal cancer, depression was reported by more than a quarter one week after discharge home but this had reduced to ten per cent at one year. Thus it is essential for the health care professional to be aware of the risk of depression on discharge and that it can be a long-term problem.

Returning to work

It is generally possible for ostomates to return to work after their stoma-forming surgery. The length of time off work will depend upon general health, recovery and the type of work undertaken. Many ostomates find that six weeks to three months is adequate time to recover from surgery. This time may be reduced with laparoscopic surgery. It might be advisable to return to work on a part-time basis initially or to light duties. It may take several months to return to jobs that require heavy lifting (Kirkwood 2006). Toilet facilities at work need to be available but this should not pose a problem. There is usually no job that cannot be undertaken with a stoma.

Resuming social activities and hobbies

After returning home and following a period of recovery, it is important for the ostomate to recommence activities, such as hobbies and sports. For most patients the activities and employment undertaken prior to surgery can be resumed. Pringle and Swan (2001) found that one week after discharge home virtually no social activities were undertaken. However at one year only a third of their patients with a stoma formation for cancer had completely resumed their social lives. The high percentage of ostomates who did not return to their previous lifestyle after their stoma was formed mainly chose not to go out as much after their surgery. Anecdotally many patients do alter their life after surgery, which is not always necessary or beneficial.

It may be useful for the ostomate to join one of the support groups (see Chapter 1). These groups can provide a network of other ostomates to discuss coping mechanisms and many groups also arrange social activities (Williams 2007). Sport and hobbies can be recommenced gradually following surgery.

Exercises

After the surgical wound heals, the abdominal muscles are considerably weakened and need toning to regain their strength and support. Walking is encouraged while still in hospital and this can be increased to the patient's tolerance. Other activities should be gradually recommenced but individual assessment and advice should be provided. Chapter 18 provides further information.

Driving

There is no definitive recommendation when driving should be recommenced after stoma-forming surgery. Generally the advice is not to drive for a minimum of six weeks; however, each person is individual and some ostomates may be able to drive safely after only two weeks. It is recommended that the ostomate should be able to perform a safe emergency stop, if required while driving, without hurting themselves. It can also be advisable to seek guidance from the car insurance company.

Clothing

Ideally after a planned stoma is formed the same clothes can be worn after surgery as was possible before. However, siting is often not possible before emergency surgery and therefore the stoma may not be in an ideal position. Ostomates can wear tight-fitting clothes and not risk the security of their appliance and it is also possible to wear swimwear. Some men choose to wear high waisted trousers to disguise their stoma. These can be purchased from high street stores or there are several companies that specialise in clothing for ostomates. Similarly usual underwear can be worn. However there is also specialised underwear available, some that incorporate internal pockets to hold and support the stoma appliance as it fills (see Chapter 18).

Alcohol

It is possible to drink alcohol with a stoma. It will loosen the faeces if taken in great quantities and may lead to a short-term increase in the faecal output. Care should be taken as always with alcohol to stay within safe limits. Excess may cause many potential problems, such as forgetting to empty or change the appliance.

Support garments

Support garments are available for both men and women. Not all ostomates require abdominal support but during strenuous exercise they can be useful (see Chapter 15 for information on hernias). Support garments can be in the form of underwear or support belts. These are not worn in the immediate post-operative period, but after abdominal wounds have healed.

Travel

It is not generally advisable to fly immediately after surgery. However after the wounds have healed, holidays can be taken. This is further discussed in Chapter 18.

Long-term follow-up

Although an ostomate is never discharged from the stoma care clinic, many do not require or want to have long-term follow-up. It is important to remind the ostomate to periodically remeasure their stoma, particularly if there are changes in weight, although it might be advantageous to visit the clinic yearly to review new products and ensure that all current products are still required and used appropriately (Taylor 2003). However a visit three months after surgery is advisable to ensure that the ostomate is coping with their stoma, as it cannot be assumed that all those that require assistance will request it. Lifelong access to the stoma specialist nurse should enable the patient to retain control over their life and stoma.

References

Adams T, Dufton R, Lamb C & Taylor M (2003) Hospital secondments of community nurses to improve stoma care. *British Journal of Community Nurses.* **8(12)**: 539–43.

Allison M (1996) Discharge planning. In: Myers C (ed) *Stoma Care Nursing: a Patient Centred Approach.* London: Arnold.

Bekkers MJTM, Van Knippenberg FCE, Van Den Borne HW & Van Berge-Henegouwen GP (1996) Prospective evaluation of psychosocial adaptation to stoma surgery: the role of self-efficacy. *Psychosomatic Medicine.* **58(2)**: 183–91.

Berry J (2006) What happens to used colostomy pouches outside the acute setting? *World Council of Enterostomal Therapists Journal.* **26(1)**: 15–18.

Black PK (2000) *Holistic Stoma Care.* London Baillière Tindall.

Black PK (2004) Psychological, sexual and cultural issues for patients with a stoma. *British Journal of Nursing.* **13(12)**: 692–7.

Erwin-Toth P & Doughty DB (1992) Principles and procedures of stomal management. In: Hampton BG & Bryant RA (eds) *Ostomies and Continent Diversions: Nursing Management.* London: Mosby Year Book.

Hunter M (2004) A sense of self. *Gastrointestinal Nursing.* **2(8)**: 12–15.

Kirkwood L (2006) Postoperative stoma care and the selection of appliances. *Journal of Community Nursing.* **20(3)**: 12–18.

Lee J (2001) Nurse prescribing in practice: patient choice in stoma care. *British Journal of Community Nursing.* **6(1)**: 33–7.

McKenzie F, White CA, Kendall S, Finlayson A, Urquhart M *et al.* (2006) Psychological impact of colostomy pouch change and disposal. *British Journal of Nursing.* **15(6)**: 308–16.

Mead J (1994) An emphasis on practical management – discharge planning in stoma care. *Professional Nurse.* **9(6)**: 405–10.

O'Connor G (2003) Discharge planning in rehabilitation following surgery for a stoma. *British Journal of Nursing.* **12(13)**: 800–7.

O'Connor G (2005) Teaching stoma-management skills: the importance of self-care. *British Journal of Nursing.* **14(6)**: 320–4.

Price B (1990) *Body Image. Nursing Concepts and Care.* London: Prentice Hall

Pringle W & Swan E (2001) Continuing care after discharge from hospital for stoma patients. *British Journal of Nursing.* **10(19)**: 1275–88.

Pullen M (2002) The roles of stoma care and colorectal nurses. *Nursing and Residential Care.* **4(10)**: 485–8.

Readding LA (2005) Hospital to home: smoothing the journey for the new ostomist. *British Journal of Nursing.* **14(16)**: S16–S20.

Royal College of Nursing (1994) *Disposal of Health Care Waste in the Community.* London: RCN.

Rust J (2007) Care of patients with stomas: the pouch change procedure. *Nursing Standard.* **22(6)**: 43–7.

Salter M (1999) Stoma care – overcoming the stigma. *Nursing Times.* **86(18)**: 67–71.

Skingley S (2004) Changing practice: the role of the community stoma nurse. *British Journal of Nursing.* **13(2)**: 79–86.

Taylor P (2003) Community aspects of stoma care. In: Elcoat C (ed) *Stoma Care Nursing.* London: Hollister.

White C (1998) Psychological management of stoma-related concerns. *Nursing Standard.* **12(36)**: 35–8.

Williams J (2007) Stoma care nursing: what the community nurse needs to know. *British Journal of Community Nursing.* **12(8)**: 342–6.

Chapter 14

Nutrition

Morag Pearson

Introduction

Nutrition plays an important role in the management of people with stomas and pouches. Their nutritional status approaching surgery varies with their general health and underlying condition. Some will need peri-operative nutritional support to aid recovery and all will require guidance with food reintroduction post-operatively. The location of the stoma or pouch within the gastrointestinal tract may affect fluid, electrolyte or nutrient absorption, which has implications for maintaining adequate nutritional status. Therefore, everyone requires advice on how to take a balanced diet with regular monitoring of their nutritional status to identify potential problems. Some people associate changes in stoma or pouch function with variations in diet and empirically restrict their diet to improve control, but may unwittingly risk nutritional deficiency. Unfortunately, there is little objective evidence to support dietary recommendations but giving information about the relationship between food, the underlying disease and stoma or pouch function will help people to develop an acceptable diet without compromising nutritional adequacy.

Nutrition may be easily overlooked when the focus is on helping people to adapt to the physical and psychological challenges of stoma or pouch formation, yet they frequently express concern about what they should eat. This chapter will help health care professionals to provide dietary information by explaining the nutritional implications of stoma or pouch formation, the development of a balanced diet for health and acceptable function and the provision of peri-operative nutrition support.

Digestion and absorption of nutrients

Understanding the impact of stoma or pouch formation on gastrointestinal function will enable the reader to understand the rationale for dietary advice.

Food is masticated in the mouth, then passed down the oesophagus into the stomach, where it is mixed with gastric juice and churned to a liquid chyme, which is slowly released into the duodenum. There, it is mixed with bile and pancreatic enzymes, which break down protein, fats and carbohydrate into simple nutrients, suitable for absorption and utilisation by the body. The small bowel (duodenum, jejunum and ileum) varies in length from three to eight metres and it is of relevance to stoma and pouch forma-tion that most protein, carbohydrate, vitamins and minerals are absorbed within the first two metres of jejunum. Fats are absorbed throughout the jejunum and ileum, whilst vitamin B_{12} and bile acids can only be absorbed at specific receptor sites in the terminal ileum (Nightingale & Spiller 2001).

The jejunum, ileum and colon differ markedly in their ability to absorb water and sodium, which has implications for function and dietary advice. Daily, in addition to food and drink, approximately four litres of digestive juices, comprising 0.5 l saliva, two litres gastric juices and 1.5 l pancreatico-biliary secretions, enter the jejunum (Nightingale & Woodward 2006). The intra-luminal contents of the jejunum are maintained iso-osmolar with plasma at approximately 300 milliosmoles per litre (mosmol/l) and at a sodium concentration of approximately 100 millimoles per litre (mmol/l) through passive diffusion (Nightingale *et al.* 1990). Sodium absorption is dependent on its luminal concentration, water movement and is coupled with the absorption of glucose and amino acids. In contrast, the ileum actively absorbs water and sodium against a concentration gradient to reduce the effluent volume passing through the ileocaecal valve to about one litre containing approximately 100 mmol sodium. The ascending colon readily absorbs water and sodium to produce approximately 100–150 g faeces per day (Nightingale & Spiller 2001).

Food residues like fibre and resistant starch escape digestion in the small bowel and pass through into the colon where they are fermented by colonic bacteria. Fermentation produces short chain fatty acids (utilised for energy) and gases, which are either absorbed and excreted via the lungs or passed as flatus (Englyst & Hudson 2000).

'The Balance of Good Health'

People with stomas or pouches can maintain good health by taking a bal-anced diet. However, they may need advice on how to adapt the healthy eating recommendations to suit their particular type of stoma or pouch.

A balanced diet is one which provides all the nutrients required by the body to function effectively and to prevent deficiency diseases. It also helps to maintain a healthy weight and to reduce the risk of developing disorders such as heart disease and some forms of cancer. The main nutrients required by the body include carbohydrate (a source of energy), fat (a source of energy and essential fatty acids), protein (the material for growth and repair of the body; a component of enzymes, hormones and antibodies; a source of energy), vitamins (used in the regulation of chemical processes within the body including energy release from food) and minerals (help control the composition of body fluids; essential components of enzymes, proteins such as haemoglobin, bones and teeth).

Healthy eating guidance recommends a diet based on carbohydrate-rich foods like bread, potatoes, rice, pasta and cereals, which is rich in fruit and vegetables, moderate in amounts of milk, dairy products, meat, fish or alternatives, low in fat and sugar with reduced salt. No single food can provide all the essential nutrients so it is important to eat a wide variety of foods to achieve a balanced diet (see Table 14.1). 'The Balance of Good

Table 14.1 Choosing a balanced diet

Food group	What's included	Main nutrients	Message
Bread, other cereals & potatoes	Bread, breakfast cereals, pasta, rice, oats, noodles, maize, millet, cornmeal & starchy vegetables e.g. potatoes, yams & plantains	Carbohydrate Fibre (non-starch polysaccharide or NSP) Some calcium & iron B vitamins	• Base meals around foods from this group. Avoid frying or adding too much fat to these foods • Good energy source • Manipulate fibre for acceptable stoma or pouch function
Fruit & vegetables	Fresh, frozen, dried & canned fruit & vegetables. Unsweetened fruit juice. Beans and pulses can also be eaten as part of this group	Vitamin C Carotenes Folate Fibre (NSP) Some carbohydrate	• Try to eat at least five portions of a variety of fruit & vegetables every day, where a portion is one medium fruit, three tablespoons cooked/tinned fruit, 150 ml unsweetened fruit juice, three tablespoons vegetables, beans or pulses or one dessert bowl of salad (see further reading) • Good source of antioxidant vitamins, which help lower the risk of heart disease & some cancers • Manipulate fibre for acceptable stoma or pouch function
Milk & dairy foods	Milk, cheese, yoghurt, fromage frais & calcium-enriched soya alternatives	Calcium Protein Vitamin B_{12} Vitamins A & D	• Take moderate amounts & choose lower fat versions (see further reading) • Good source of calcium to maintain healthy bones & prevent osteoporosis
Meat, fish & alternatives	Meat, poultry, fish, eggs, nuts, seeds, beans, pulses, tofu, textured vegetable protein (TVP) & mycoprotein	Protein Iron B vitamins Vitamin B_{12} (in foods of animal origin) Zinc Magnesium Some fibre (NSP)	• Eat moderate amounts, choose lower fat versions & avoid adding fat in cooking • Good sources of protein for growth & repair of body tissues & of iron for healthy blood • Aim to eat at least two portions of fish a week, including one portion of oily fish like salmon, mackerel, trout, herring, fresh tuna, sardines or pilchards to help reduce the risk of heart disease

Foods containing fats	Margarine, butter, low-fat spreads, cooking oils, oil-based salad dressings, mayonnaise, cream, chocolate, crisps, biscuits, pasties, cakes, puddings, ice cream, rich sauces & gravies	Fat Some vitamins & essential fatty acids	• Eat sparingly – small amounts, less often & choose low-fat alternatives to avoid becoming overweight • Reduce saturated fats & replace with small amounts of unsaturated fats to reduce cholesterol & lower risk of heart disease (see further reading)
Foods containing sugars	Soft drinks, sweets, jam, sugar, cakes, puddings, biscuits, pastries & ice cream	Sugar, with minerals in some products & fat in others	• Limit foods containing sugar to prevent weight gain & to reduce the risk of tooth decay
Foods containing salt	Processed foods, ready meals, tinned foods, breakfast cereals, soups, sauces, pickles, stock cubes, crisps, crackers, bacon, cheese, smoked fish & shell fish	Sodium	• Take no more than six grams of salt per day – use less in cooking or added to food & choose lower salt foods to reduce blood pressure & the risk of stroke or heart disease (see further reading) • When stoma or pouch losses high, increase intake to prevent deficiency
Fluid	Water, tea, coffee, fruit juices, sugar-free squashes or fizzy drinks	Fluid	• Take plenty of water (six to eight glasses or 1.5 l) or other fluid a day. Sugar-containing drinks should not be drunk too often and limited to mealtimes to reduce the risk of tooth decay • Moderate alcohol to prevent liver damage & weight gain (up to two to three units/day for women & three to four units/day for men – see further reading)

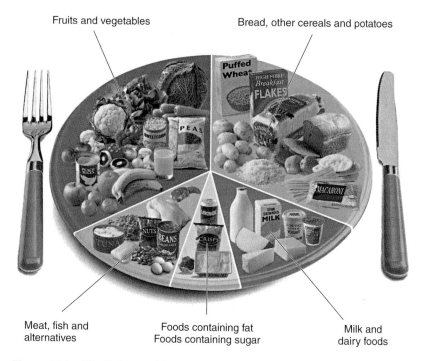

Fruits and vegetables

Bread, other cereals and potatoes

Meat, fish and
alternatives

Foods containing fat
Foods containing sugar

Milk and
dairy foods

Figure 14.1 'The Balance of Good Health'. (Reproduced with kind permission of the controller of HMSO).

Health' is a pictorial guide, which can be used to help people make healthy food choices (see Figure 14.1). Food is divided into five groups relating to their main nutrient content and the plate shows the proportions of food from each group required to build up a balanced diet. 'The Balance of Good Health' applies to healthy individuals over the age of five, except those with special dietary requirements, and can be used to guide the food choices of people with stomas or pouches. However, people with an ileostomy or ileoanal pouch may need to moderate their fibre intake for acceptable function and may need extra salt to replace losses and prevent deficiency. Additional information and resources may be found in the further reading section.

Colostomy

Nutritional implications of colostomy formation

Stool consistency depends on the location of the stoma within the colon. The more distal the stoma, the more opportunity there is for fluid absorption and the more solid the stool formed. People with a descending or sigmoid colostomy tend to pass stool once or twice a day with a consistency similar to normal faeces, while those with a transverse or ascending colostomy pass stool more frequently, with a mushy consistency (Cummings 2000). Thus like the general population, colostomates can maintain adequate hydration by taking about 1.5 litres of fluid per day (see Table 14.1).

Nutrients are absorbed normally in the small bowel but there is little objective research of nutritional status or dietary habits post colostomy formation. Most attain a healthy body weight (Bulman 2001), take a normal diet and whilst some do associate certain foods with adverse symptoms such as flatus, malodour or loose stool, they continue to consume the food in moderation (Floruta 2001; Gazzard *et al*. 1978; Giunchi *et al*. 1988). Colostomates should, therefore, take a balanced diet in line with guidelines for the general population (see Table 14.1 and Figure 14.1) with adequate fibre to prevent constipation (Cummings 2000; DOH 1991). Eating regular meals will promote regular stoma function. Maintenance of a healthy weight helps prevent stoma retraction, which may occur when weight gain causes tension on the bowel.

Dietary management of functional problems post-colostomy formation

Constipation

Constipation is usually caused by lack of dietary fibre, an inadequate fluid intake or from the side effects of medications such as analgesics, antimotility drugs, antimuscarinics, beta-blockers or tricyclic antidepressants (Carter 1999) rather than by mechanical obstruction (Cummings 2000). Dietary fibre, known scientifically as non-starch polysaccharide (NSP), refers to plant materials, which resist digestion in the small bowel and pass in to the colon, where they increase faecal bulk by holding water and stimulating bacterial growth. This bulk quickens transit through the colon, leaving less time for water absorption, thereby producing a softer stool, which is easier to pass. Therefore, constipation may be prevented or treated by increasing fibre containing foods (DOH 1991) like wholemeal or granary bread, wholegrain cereals, brown rice or pasta, fruit, vegetables, pulses, nuts or seeds to a level which achieves acceptable stoma function for the individual. Fibre should be introduced slowly to allow the gut time to adjust to the increased flatus production in order to prevent symptoms such as abdominal distension, bloating or pain. A daily fluid intake of 1.5 to 2 litres is required to support the bulking action of fibre.

Diarrhoea

Diarrhoea may be caused by infection, lactose intolerance, stress or from the side effects of medications such as antibiotics, magnesium containing antacids, iron preparations, proton pump inhibitors, metaclopramide and domperidone (Carter 1999). However, just like people with an intact bowel, colostomates may experience loose stool with individual foods, particularly those which increase faecal bulk or stimulate the bowel and especially if eaten in large quantities. People with stomas in the ascending colon may experience loose stool more frequently due to their proximal location within the colon. Foods commonly implicated include fibrous foods, spicy foods, fried foods, alcohol, beverages containing caffeine and sweets or medications containing sorbitol (Bulman 2001; Floruta 2001; Giunchi *et al.* 1988). Keeping a food and symptom diary will help identify the culprit. If fibre is suspected, then switching to a lower fibre alternative (white bread, refined breakfast cereals, white rice or pasta, removing skins, seeds, pips or stalks from fruit/vegetables or reducing intake of pulses, nuts and dried fruits) may reduce symptoms. If other foods are suspected then eating them in smaller quantities may be sufficient to reduce symptoms. Alternatively the food may be omitted when avoidance of loose stool is important. Anti-diarrhoeal medication may be taken to slow transit and thicken the stool.

Flatus

Colostomates have no voluntary control over when they pass flatus, which may prove embarrassing and therefore a major source of concern. Flatus is produced as a normal part of digestion from swallowed air and the bacterial fermentation of fibrous and other food residues in the colon (Bolin & Stanton 1998). Flatus is passed when gas production exceeds the colonic absorptive capacity (Englyst & Hudson 2000). Studies in people with intact bowels have found significant individual variation in both the volume and composition of flatus (Tomlin *et al.* 1991). Swallowed air may be reduced by:

- eating small regular meals in a relaxed environment;
- eating slowly, chewing food carefully, avoiding talking while eating or eating with mouth open;
- avoiding smoking, gum chewing or taking drinks through a straw;
- stirring fizzy drinks to allow the bubbles of gas to dissipate before drinking.

Colonic fermentation may be decreased by (Cummings 2000; Rumessen & Gudmand-Hoyer 1988):

- reducing fibre through changing to white bread, refined cereals, white rice or pasta, removing skins, seeds, pips or stalks from fruit/ vegetables or reducing intake of pulses, nuts and dried fruits;
- reducing non-absorbable sugars such as raffinose and stacchyose found in beans and peas;
- reducing fructo-oligosaccharides and inulin found in artichokes, onions, leeks, chicory and salsify;
- reducing resistant starch found in unmilled grains and seeds, unripe banana, incompletely cooked potato and maize, cooked and cooled starches other than cereal starches; most starch should be freshly cooked and eaten hot or as white bread or rice;
- reducing milk in those with lactase deficiency;
- reducing sorbitol from sugar-free sweets or medications.

Summary of dietary advice for colostomates

- Take a balanced diet in line with healthy eating guidance for the general population (see Table 14.1 and Figure 14.1).
- Develop a regular eating pattern for acceptable stoma function.
- Ensure an adequate fibre and fluid intake to prevent constipation.
- Control flatus by reducing swallowed air and foods known to increase colonic fermentation.
- Moderate intake of any foods which repeatedly cause diarrhoea.

Ileostomy

Nutritional implications of ileostomy formation

The location of the stoma within the ileum depends on the underlying disorder and extent of any previous resections, but generally it is placed as distally as possible to maximise absorption. Loss of the colon, and its function of absorbing water and sodium, results in higher losses and, on average, ileostomates empty their bags four to five times per day, passing 400–800 ml of a mushy consistency stool, containing 40–80 mmol sodium (McNeil *et al.* 1982). They maintain adequate fluid and sodium balance by compensating for these higher losses through renal conservation (Svaninger *et al.* 1991), increased absorption in the remaining small bowel (Kennedy *et al.* 1983) and increased dietary intake (Bingham *et al.* 1982; Hill 1982; Kennedy *et al.* 1982). However, even modest ileal resections can increase fluid loss leading to chronic dehydration and an increased risk of developing renal stones (Bambach *et al.* 1981). In people with stoma losses of less than 1200 ml daily, dehydration may be prevented by taking daily 1.5–2 litres (8–10 cups) of fluid like water, tea, coffee, unsweetened fruit juice or sugar-free squashes, and sodium depletion prevented by taking half to one level teaspoon of salt added to food, used in cooking or from regular inclusion of salty foods (see Table 14.1) (Nightingale & Woodward 2006). This contradicts healthy eating guidance to reduce salt so it is important to explain the rationale that extra salt is required to replace losses and prevent depletion. Once the stoma adapts, additional salt may not be needed, provided the diet includes some salty or processed foods.

Nutrients are absorbed normally in the upper small bowel and most attain good health with little evidence of nutritional deficiency. When compared with a control group matched for age, sex and occupation, ileostomates had normal haematological and biochemical indices of nutritional status but weighed on average 4.1 kg less, which was attributed to loss of the colon, water depletion and loss of the colonic energy salvaging system (McNeil *et al.* 1982). The two groups had similar energy and nutrient intakes but the ileostomates ate more salt, less dietary fibre, mainly due to lower fruit and vegetable intakes, and had lower iron, vitamin A and C intakes (Bingham *et al.* 1982). Vitamin B_{12} deficiency is rare unless more than 80 cm terminal ileum is removed, when three-monthly intramuscular replacement becomes necessary (Lenz 1975; Thompson & Wrathell 1977).

Once the stoma adapts (after six to eight weeks) and people become familiar with its usual function, they feel more confident to experiment with food and many find that they can enjoy the freedom of a varied and balanced diet in line with current healthy eating guidance (see Table 14.1 and Figure 14.1). Most take low-fibre starchy foods (white bread, white rice and pasta, refined cereals, potato without skin) to avoid increasing output or flatus but should be encouraged to include fruit and vegetables for their protective vitamins. These should be well chewed, to reduce the risk of a blockage and may be better tolerated if skins, seeds, pips and stalks are removed, or if taken in tinned, well cooked, puréed or juice formats. Red meats, liver, kidney, oily fish, eggs and pulses are good sources of iron and should be included two to three times per week. Weight, haematological and biochemical indices of nutritional status should be regularly monitored to prevent deficiencies.

Dietary management of functional problems post-ileostomy formation

Obstruction

Fibrous food residues resist digestion in the small bowel so have the potential to cause a blockage if eaten in large quantities or if not properly chewed as they may form a food plug that can stick at the point where the ileum narrows as it passes through the abdominal wall to form the stoma, particularly if tissue is oedematous post-operatively. Thus people with new stomas are advised to avoid physically indigestible foods like nuts, seeds, fruit and vegetable skins, raw vegetables, salad, peas, sweetcorn, mushrooms, celery, dried fruit, coconut, pineapple and mango for the first six weeks post-operatively. Thereafter, if desired, these foods may be reintroduced in small portions, well chewed (Wood 1998). A blockage may cause pain, bloating, temporary reduction in stoma function or vomiting. If conservative management (withholding food whilst continuing oral fluids) fails to resolve symptoms then hospital admission is required for intravenous hydration and to exclude other causes such as adhesions, parastomal hernia or recurrent disease (Burch 2005).

High output

A high output may be caused by temporary, early post-operative functional problems, the proximal placement of the stoma to defunction an ileoanal pouch or as a result of previous small bowel resections, active Crohn's disease, abdominal sepsis, partial small bowel obstruction, infective enteritis or medication side effects (Tsao *et al.* 2005). Once outputs exceed two litres, increased dietary intake of salt and water will not keep up with losses, precipitating the risk of dehydration, sodium depletion and potentially life-threatening metabolic disturbances if not adequately managed (Nightingale & Woodward 2006). Dehydration is indicated by a low urine output (less than one litre/24 hrs), rapid weight loss (one kg in 24 hrs indicates fluid depletion by one litre) and in the absence of renal disease by a raised urea and creatinine (Nightingale & Woodward 2006). Because of the influence of the renin–angiotensin mechanism, the plasma sodium concentration will remain normal until body stores are severely depleted (Ladefoged & Olgaard 1985), so a random urinary sodium test provides a better indicator of sodium status (less than 20 mmol/litre indicates maximal renal conservation in response to sodium depletion). Physical signs of depletion become apparent before major changes in blood chemistry, providing important warning signs and include thirst, dry mouth, loss of appetite, nausea, lethargy, muscle cramps, sunken dark-ringed eyes, reduced skin tone, rapid low volume pulse and dizziness on standing due to postural hypotension (confirmed by lying and standing blood pressure) (Nightingale 2003).

Management includes treatment of the underlying cause and repletion with intravenous saline (Nightingale & Woodward 2006). When thirsty, the patient's natural response is to drink fluids like water, tea, coffee, juice or squash. However, these are low in sodium and they dilute the jejunal sodium concentration below 100 mmol/l, causing sodium to diffuse from the tissues into the luminal fluid to raise its concentration back to 100 mmol/l. Although normally reabsorbed in the ileum, when the output is high, much of this sodium-enriched fluid is lost via the stoma, increasing the patient's thirst and perpetuating the cycle. The remedy is to reduce the jejunal secretion of sodium, by restricting the patient's intake of hypotonic fluids to one litre and meeting their fluid requirements with a glucose–saline solution containing 90–120 mmol/l sodium (Newton *et al.* 1985; Nightingale *et al.* 1992). A modification of the World Health Organisation's cholera solution, which contains 90 mmol sodium per litre, is suitable (20 g glucose, 3.5 g sodium chloride, 2.5 g sodium bicarbonate added to one litre of tap water) (Nightingale & Woodward 2006). It tastes like sweet seawater so its palatability may be improved by chilling and flavouring with small amounts of squash or fruit juice. Patients should sip one litre of this solution slowly throughout the day. It has a higher sodium concentration than most commercial preparations used to treat infective or traveller's diarrhoeas.

Alternative solutions include replacing sodium bicarbonate with sodium citrate to increase palatability or giving a glucose polymer solution to allow more energy absorption (Nightingale *et al.* 1992). People should include salt to the limit of palatability in cooking or added to food after serving to utilise the coupled absorption of sodium with glucose and amino acids in the jejunum (Fordtran 1975). Alternatively they may take salty foods like cheese, bacon, ham, sausages, smoked fish, shell fish, canned fish, meat or fish pastes, tinned or processed foods, meat or yeasts extracts, salted crisps and crackers. Anti-diarrhoeal medication (loperamide, 4 mg taken four times a day or codeine phosphate, 60 mg taken four times a day) may be given 30–60 minutes before food and at bedtime to slow gastrointestinal transit and allow more time for absorption (Nightingale & Woodward 2006). Anti-secretory medication (omeprazole, 40 mg taken once or twice daily) may be given to those with outputs exceeding two litres to reduce gastric acid secretion (Nightingale & Woodward 2006). A low-fibre diet will also help to slow transit and thereby promote absorption (white bread, refined breakfast cereals, white rice or pasta, small portions of fruit or vegetables with skin, seeds, pips or stalks removed, small portions of pulses if vegetarian and avoidance of nuts and dried fruits).

Relationship between eating pattern and ileostomy function

Eating regular meals helps to establish regular ileostomy function. An ileostomy tends to be most active after the biggest meal of the day, which for many is the evening meal, but this can disturb sleep with the need to empty the appliance during the night. This may be overcome by experimenting with the timing or size of the evening meal by, for example, eating at least two hours before bedtime or by switching the largest meal to midday with a smaller snack meal in the evening (Bingham *et al.* 1982). Anyone concerned with daytime activity, for example in relation to a journey, should keep a food and symptom diary to evaluate individual stoma function in relation to meal pattern.

Relationship between individual foods and ileostomy function

Ileostomy formation results in loss of control over evacuation and understandably people fear any food which may increase output, odour or flatus, so seek advice about which foods to avoid. Unfortunately, the available information is often inconsistent due to a lack of objective evidence from the literature to support dietary recommendations (Floruta 2001).

When the food choice of 79 ileostomates was compared with 70 controls from the normal population, significant differences were noted (Bingham *et al.* 1982). More than half the ileostomates either avoided or took smaller portions of foods, which appeared unchanged in their faeces including nuts, pips, seeds, onions, beetroot, lettuce, raw cabbage and carrot, peas, sweetcorn, mushrooms and dried fruit. Odour was less of a problem than had been expected, but onions did increase odour and onions, peas and carbonated beverages increased flatus. Beetroot discoloured the effluent; although not avoided, this was alarming for those who had not been forewarned. Bingham noted that the ileostomates varied in their sensitivity to individual foods and that no single food affected all those interviewed, a finding supported by other authors (Gazzard *et al.* 1978; Thomson *et al.* 1970).

Kramer (1987) attempted to obtain more objective data by investigating the effect of 37 individual foods on ileostomy output in seven people with long established, normal functioning stomas, each acting as their own control, who took a self-selected baseline diet and tested each food over a three-day experimental period. He tested foods which are frequently avoided by ileostomates and again noted that subjects varied in their response to individual foods. Only five fruits (grapes, peaches, raisins, strawberries and bananas), one vegetable (baked beans) and prune juice significantly increased ileostomy output. Alcohol, fried foods and spices did not increase output. Although only a small number of foods were investigated, Kramer concluded that many foods are probably unnecessarily forbidden or avoided relative to their effect on ileostomy output.

This supports the importance of advising ileostomates to make food choices based on their own individual tolerance rather than simply following lists of foods to avoid. Whilst the experience of others may serve as a guide, people should be encouraged to try all foods and only avoid those which repeatedly cause unacceptable symptoms for them. Tolerance may change with time so they should periodically retry any problem foods. If they experience difficulty with this process or there is concern that the resulting diet may be nutritionally unbalanced then a registered dietitian can provide more detailed assessment and advice.

Summary of dietary advice for ileostomates

- Post-operatively, take a soft, low-fibre diet, well chewed for the first six weeks to avoid blockages.
- Take a balanced diet for good health (see Table 14.1 and Figure 14.1).
- For outputs less than 1200 ml daily, take adequate fluid and salt to prevent dehydration.
- For outputs of 1200–2000 ml daily or more, start anti-diarrhoeal and anti-secretory medication, reduce intake of hypotonic fluids to one litre, introduce one litre of a glucose–saline solution containing 90 to 120 mmol sodium/litre and add salt to food to reduce losses and prevent fluid and sodium depletion.
- Develop a regular eating pattern and experiment with the timing or size of meals for acceptable stoma function.
- Try all foods and only avoid those which repeatedly cause unacceptable symptoms.
- Monitor weight, biochemical and haematological indices of nutritional status at follow-up.
- If difficulty is experienced with establishing a balanced diet or acceptable function, refer to a registered dietitian for assessment and advice.

Ileoanal pouch

Nutritional implications of ileoanal pouch formation

Proctocolectomy with formation of an ileoanal pouch from 30–60 cm of terminal ileum restores intestinal continuity in people with familial adenomatous polyposis or ulcerative colitis. They open their pouch three to seven times per day, passing on average 650 g stool of semi-solid, mushy or liquid consistency (Nicholls *et al.* 1981; Pemberton 1993), and their daily faecal weight, urinary volume and sodium excretion are similar to those of ileostomates (Santavirta *et al.* 1991). They also maintain fluid and sodium balance through renal conservation (Christie *et al.* 1990) and increased absorption within the ileum (Lerch *et al.* 1989), although this increases their incidence of renal stones (Christie *et al.* 1996). They too should take adequate fluid (1.5–2 litres) and salt (half to one level teaspoon of salt added to food, used in cooking or from regular inclusion of salty foods) to replace losses. Once the pouch adapts, extra salt may not be needed provided the diet includes some processed or salty foods. If they experience an increased output from the pouch, vomiting or increased sweating then extra fluid and salt is required to prevent dehydration. If the problem is severe or symptoms of dehydration are experienced, then medical help should be sought.

The pouch is formed from terminal ileum, which does not affect nutrient absorption in the upper small bowel, but, as the specific absorptive site, may have implications for vitamin B_{12} and bile acids. Most demonstrate good health with normal nutritional status (Chartrand-Lefebvre *et al.* 1990; Fiorentini *et al.* 1987; Lerch *et al.* 1989; O'Connell *et al.* 1986). Up to a third experience low haemoglobin or iron deficiency anaemia, although it is unclear whether this is due to inadequate intake, increased requirements or blood loss (Lerch *et al.* 1989; M'Koma 1994; O'Connell *et al.* 1986). The ileum normally contains very little bacteria, but when the pouch takes on its new role of storing faeces, its bacterial population increases to a level which is intermediate between that of ileostomy effluent and normal faeces. This increases flatus production and the potential for bacterial degradation of vitamin B_{12} and bile acids within the pouch (Nasmyth & Williams 1993).

In a study of 83 people three years after ileoanal pouch formation, 11% had low serum vitamin B_{12} levels and 36% had impaired B_{12} absorption (M'Koma 1994). This finding is supported by other studies (Hojlund Pederson *et al.* 1985; Hylander *et al.* 1991) although it is unclear whether this is due to reduced absorption across the pouch mucosa or the bacterial binding of vitamin B_{12} within the pouch, rendering it unavailable for absorption (M'Koma 1994; Nasmyth & Williams 1993). Similarly, several studies have demonstrated a malabsorption of bile acids (Bain *et al.* 1995; Fiorentini *et al.* 1987; Hylander *et al.* 1991; Lerch *et al.* 1989; Salemans *et al.* 1993), which may reduce the enterohepatic circulation and cause fat malabsorption, a finding confirmed by some (Fiorentini *et al.* 1987; M'Koma *et al.* 1994) but not by others (Heppel *et al.* 1982; Nicholls *et al.* 1981). While more research is needed, these studies highlight the importance of encouraging people to take a balanced diet (see Table 14.1 and Figure 14.1) and monitoring their nutritional status at follow-up to prevent deficiencies.

Dietary management of functional problems post-ileoanal pouch formation

Functional disturbances following loop ileostomy closure

Following loop ileostomy closure, intestinal function may be impaired by smooth muscle and villous atrophy in the distal ileal limb, caused by loss of mucosal contact with trophic luminal nutrients and pancreatico-biliary secretions during faecal diversion (Williams *et al.* 2007). Intestinal obstruction occurs in up to 29%, mainly at the temporary ileostomy closure site, especially if tissue is oedematous (Salemans & Nagengast 1995). Obstruction may be prevented by introducing a soft, low-fibre diet, which is well chewed. Once the swelling subsides (after two to four weeks) and the pouch begins to adapt, then the diet may be slowly broadened. Motility may take up to six months to return to normal (Williams *et al.* 2007) and increased stool frequency is common until the pouch adapts to its new role of storing faeces. Stool frequency may be reduced by taking a low fibre diet and introducing anti-diarrhoeal medication.

Relationship between eating pattern and ileoanal pouch function

Developing a regular eating pattern helps to establish acceptable pouch function. In a study of 69 people, one year after ileostomy closure, the majority opened their pouch five to eight times per day and within 30 minutes to four hours after a meal (Tyus *et al.* 1992). Pouch frequency increased with the number of meals eaten and stool output increased after the largest meal of the day. The authors concluded that people concerned with pouch output should:

- consume no more than three meals per day;
- experiment with the timing and size of their evening meal to reduce pouch frequency at night for example by eating their last meal at least two hours before bedtime or by switching their largest meal to midday and taking a smaller meal in the evening;
- evaluate daytime meal and pouch pattern by keeping a diary.

Steenhagen *et al.* (2006) noted that the urge to defaecate was stronger after a cooked meal (45% within half an hour) than after sandwiches (15% within half an hour), which may reflect the larger weight, volume or caloric content of a cooked meal.

Relationship between individual foods and ileoanal pouch function

People with ileoanal pouches associate changes in pouch function with variations in diet, but there is little documented data to support dietary recommendations for this group. Studies of the relationship between individual foods and pouch function have relied on questionnaires, which produce subjective results, since it may be difficult to accurately identify the effect of specific foods when eaten as part of a mixed diet. Perceptions are, however, important modifiers of eating habits, because people will experiment with diet in an attempt to improve pouch function and their quality of life (Coffey *et al.* 2002). Up to one-third of people associate symptoms with specific foods (Chartrand-Lefebvre *et al.* 1990; Fujita *et al.* 1992; Goldberg 1987; Steenhagen *et al.* 2006) but food intolerances are highly variable between people. Rather than suggesting a stringent diet, it is helpful to give people general guidance about possible food intolerances and encourage them to plan food choices around their own individual tolerance. Symptoms have been associated with the following foods (Chartrand-Lefebvre *et al.* 1990; Coffey *et al.* 2002; Fujita *et al.* 1992; Lerch *et al.* 1989; Steenhagen *et al.* 2006; Tyus *et al.* 1992; Wexner *et al.* 1989):

- increased stool output: fibrous foods, e.g. pulses, leafy green vegetables, raw vegetables, raw fruits, wholegrain cereals, nuts and sweetcorn; spicy foods, alcohol, caffeine-containing beverages, fruit juices, fried foods, chocolate, milk;
- decreased stool output: white bread, rice, pasta, potato, banana;
- anal irritation: spicy foods, nuts, seeds, coconut, citrus fruits and juices, raw fruit and vegetables;
- increased flatus: broccoli, sprouts, cabbage, cauliflower, onion, garlic, leeks, asparagus, beans, spicy foods, beer, milk, fizzy drinks;
- increased faecal odour: fish, onions, garlic, eggs.

People should try all foods and only avoid those which repeatedly cause unacceptable pouch function. Tolerance may change with time, so they should periodically retry any problem foods. If people report difficulty with this process or exclude multiple foods, then a registered dietitian can supervise an exclusion diet or provide advice on nutritional adequacy.

Fibre

People report variable responses to fibre, with some finding it beneficial and others reporting an adverse effect (Wexner *et al.* 1989). Insoluble fibre (wholemeal bread, wholegrain cereals, fruits and vegetables) has water holding and stool bulking properties which may help thicken the faeces, but if taken in large quantities may increase pouch frequency (Faller *et al.* 1986; Raymond & Becker 1986). Soluble fibre (oats, pulses, fruit and vegetables) absorbs fluid to form a viscous gel, which delays gastric emptying and may slow and thicken stool output (Wendland 1996) but not all sources are well tolerated (Coffey *et al.* 2002) and supplementary fibre in the form of pectin or methylcellulose did not reduce stool frequency (Thirlby & Kelly 1997). People should experiment with fibre to find out which type and what quantity suits them best. If flatus causes discomfort then reducing swallowed air and foods which may increase bacterial fermentation within the pouch (see colostomy section) is helpful.

Pouchitis

Pouchitis is an acute inflammation of the ileal pouch, which occurs in approximately 50% of people whose original diagnosis was ulcerative colitis. Its cause is thought to be multifactorial; involving a dysregulated immune response to altered luminal bacteria in a genetically susceptible host (Cheifetz & Itzkowitz 2004). Diagnosis is based on symptoms (watery diarrhoea, abdominal discomfort, urgency, incontinence with occasionally bleeding and fever) plus endoscopic and histological criteria. Treatment with antibiotics is successful, but five to 15% experience refractory or frequent recurrent pouchitis. A relatively new and exciting therapy is probiotics, which are living microorganisms that when ingested in adequate amounts exert health benefits beyond basic nutrition. VSL#3 is a probiotic, which contains four strains of lactobacilli, three strains of bifidobacteria and one strain of streptococcus. It has been shown to be effective in maintaining remission from chronic pouchitis (Gionchetti *et al.* 2000; Mimura *et al.* 2004) and in preventing acute pouchitis (Gionchetti *et al.* 2003). However, the role of probiotics in clinical practice needs to be better defined in terms of mode of action, most appropriate type, dose and timing of treatment and whether prebiotics (dietary products that promote growth of beneficial bacteria) may have additive or synergistic effects, before they become regular therapy.

Summary of dietary advice for people with ileoanal pouches

- Post conversion, take a soft, low-fibre diet, well chewed for the first two to four weeks to prevent blockage at the ileostomy closure site.
- Take a balanced diet for good health (see Table 14.1 and Figure 14.1).
- Take adequate fluid and salt to prevent dehydration.
- Develop a regular eating pattern and experiment with the timing or size of meals for acceptable pouch function.
- Try all foods and only avoid those which repeatedly cause unacceptable symptoms.
- Monitor weight, biochemical and haematological indices of nutritional status at follow-up.
- If difficulty is experienced with establishing a balanced diet or acceptable function, refer to a registered dietitian for assessment and advice.

Urostomy

Nutritional implications of urostomy formation

A urostomy is formed, following resection of the bladder, from an isolated section of ileum, which is used to pass urine from the ureters out through the stoma. A short (15–25 cm) section of terminal ileum is taken, to preserve vitamin B_{12} and bile acid absorption and the remaining ends of the ileum are joined to restore gastrointestinal continuity. Urostomates absorb fluid and nutrients normally and can maintain nutritional health by taking a balanced diet in line with current healthy eating guidance (see Table 14.1 and Figure 14.1).

Dietary management of functional problems following urostomy formation

Urinary infections

Bacteria like *Escherichia coli* are natural inhabitants of the gut, including the section used to form the ileal conduit, which means small quantities will be passed in the urine, introducing the risk of a urinary infection. This may be prevented by daily drinking at least two litres of fluid to maintain urine flow, prevent stasis and thereby prevent bacterial growth

(Fillingham 1999). More fluid may be required during hot weather or exercise to maintain urine flow.

Mucus is produced by the ileal conduit, which provides an ideal medium for bacterial growth. Although there is no published evidence, cranberry juice is often recommended to prevent urinary infection in urostomates, because it is thought to inhibit the adhesion of bacteria to the uroepithelium (Busuttil 1996). The optimal dosage is unknown, but Busuttil suggests urostomates should take up to 250 ml twice per day. Cranberry products are not recommended in people on warfarin as they may cause an adverse reaction (Drugs and Therapeutic Bulletin 2005). Those with diabetes should choose low sugar versions.

Urinary odour or colour

It is important to warn people that certain foods such as oily fish, onions, garlic and some spices may change the odour of urine. Beetroot may colour urine pink or red, which should not be mistaken for blood (Watson 1987).

Dietary advice

- Take a well balanced diet for good health (see Table 14.1 and Figure 14.1).
- Ensure a high fluid intake to prevent urinary infections.

Peri-operative nutrition

Nutritional risk

Adequate nutrition is vital to recovery from surgery and the nutritional status of people approaching stoma or pouch surgery will depend on their general health and underlying condition. Malnutrition develops when people do not get sufficient nutrients to meet their requirements, as a result of reduced food intake, impaired ability to absorb or metabolise nutrients or when requirements are increased by the metabolic consequences of inflammation, infection, surgery or cachexia (Bond 1997).

When intake is inadequate, fat and muscle stores are utilised for energy resulting in weight loss. Malnutrition slows post-operative recovery and contributes to the development of complications such as wound dehiscence, infection, loss of physical strength, reduced cardiovascular or respiratory function and low morale (Bond 1997). However, pre-operative nutritional support (Smith *et al.* 1997; Walsh 2001) and early post-operative feeding improves clinical outcome (Edington *et al.* 1997; Lewis *et al.* 2001).

Nutrition screening

Health care professionals play a central role in identifying and supporting patients who are malnourished. Ideally, nutritional care should be considered when planning elective surgery (Fulham 2004). All patients require screening at their first outpatient appointment and on hospital admission by assessing weight, body mass index (BMI), the degree of any unintentional weight loss or reduced food intake and the time period over which this occurred (NICE 2006). This process can be easily undertaken using a validated tool such as the 'Malnutrition Universal Screening Tool' ('MUST') for adults (Elia 2003), which identifies people who are:

- nutritionally at risk (eaten little for more than five days, poor absorptive capacity, high nutrient losses, increased nutritional needs) and who require support with eating and drinking; or
- malnourished (BMI less than 18.5 kg/m^2; unintentional weight loss of more than 10% in the last three to six months; BMI less than 20 kg/m^2 with unintentional weight loss of more than 5% in the last three to six months) and who require dietetic assessment and advice.

Screening should be repeated weekly for inpatients and when there is clinical concern for outpatients.

Provision of nutrition support

Health care professionals can help people to maximise their nutrient intake by advising on food choice. Post-operatively people may experience a reduced appetite and loose frequent stool until the remaining bowel adapts. It can be difficult to motivate them to eat and drink, particularly if they are afraid that this will increase their output so it is important to reassure them that reintroducing food will help to slow and thicken output as well as aid overall recovery. People will need much reassurance and encouragement during this phase.

Those with poor appetite should be advised to take small nutritious meals, supplemented with in-between meal snacks:

- Ensure each meal contains protein for tissue repair (meat, fish, cheese, eggs, milk, yoghurt or pulses) and starchy carbohydrate for energy and stool thickening (bread, cereal, potato, rice or pasta).
- Choose nutritious desserts such as milk puddings, custard, blancmange, yoghurt or cheese.
- Take nutritious snacks such as sandwiches, cheese and crackers, cereal, milky drinks or energy dense snacks such as chocolate, biscuits, cakes, ice cream or crisps.
- Fortify foods with energy from extra butter, margarine, cream, mayonnaise, sugar, jam, honey or marmalade.

Hospital catering services are developing to better meet patient needs by providing a wider range of meal choices. Snacks are now often available outside normal food service hours (NHS Estates 2001).

Those with very poor intake may benefit from a commercial sip-feed to increase nutrient intake. Depending on local policy, these may be given by nursing staff or prescribed by the dietitian or doctor. These milk, juice or yoghurt tasting supplements should be sipped slowly in between meals and different types offered if the first option is unacceptable. Alternatively overnight enteral tube feeding may optimise intake until oral intake improves. Parenteral feeding may be considered if the gastrointestinal gut is non-functional, inaccessible, perforated or if intestinal tolerance persistently limits enteral tube feeding in malnourished surgical or critical care patients (NICE 2006).

Monitoring

Monitoring patients' food or supplement intake and their weekly weight is crucial in assessing the effectiveness of nutritional support. Those who deteriorate may be referred to the dietitian or nutrition team for further assessment and advice.

Initiatives such as 'Essence of Care' (DOH 2001) play an important role in developing quality, patient-focused nutritional care. They provide health care professionals with a framework for identifying local training needs, developing care protocols and monitoring tools for auditing nutritional care against national standards.

Conclusion

People with stomas or pouches often request advice on what to eat and health care professionals play a vital role in providing nutritional information. This helps people understand the relationship between food, their underlying disease and stoma or pouch function so they can develop a balanced diet for health, acceptable function and, above all, so they can enjoy their food.

References

Bain IM, Mostafa AB, Harding LK, Neoptolemos JP & Keighley MRB (1995) Bile acid absorption from ileoanal pouches using enema scintigraphy. *British Journal of Surgery.* **82**: 614–17.

Bambach CP, Robertson WG, Peacock M & Hill GL (1981) Effect of intestinal surgery in the risk of urinary stone formation. *Gut.* **22**: 257–63.

Bingham S, Cummings JH & McNeil NI (1982) Diet and health of people with an ileostomy (1). Dietary assessment. *British Journal of Nutrition.* **47**: 399–405.

Bolin TD & Stanton RA (1998) Flatus emission patterns and fibre intake. *European Journal of Surgery.* **582(suppl)**: 115–18.

Bond S (1997) *Eating Matters: A Resource for Improving Dietary Care in Hospitals.* Newcastle: University of Newcastle Centre for Health Services Research.

Bulman J (2001) Changes in diet following the formation of a colostomy. *British Journal of Nursing.* **10**: 179–86.

Burch J (2005) The pre- and postoperative nursing care for patients with a stoma. *British Journal of Nursing.* **14**: 310–18.

Busuttil R (1996) Cranberry juice. *Professional Nurse.* **11**: 525–6.

Carter N (1999) Drugs and the effect on stomas: In: Taylor P (ed) *Stoma Care in the Community.* London: Nursing Times Books.

Chartrand-Lefebvre C, Heppell J, Davignon I, Dubé S & Pomp A (1990) Dietary habits after ileal pouch-anal anastomosis. *Canadian Journal of Surgery.* **33**: 101–5.

Cheifetz A & Itzkowitz S (2004) The diagnosis and treatment of pouchitis in inflammatory bowel disease. *Journal of Clinical Gastroenterology.* **38**: S44–S50.

Christie PM, Knight GS & Hill GL (1990) Metabolism of body water and electrolytes after surgery for ulcerative colitis: conventional ileostomy versus J pouch. *British Journal of Surgery.* **77**: 149–51.

Christie PM, Knight GS & Hill GL (1996) Comparison of relative risks of urinary stone formation after surgery for ulcerative colitis: conventional ileostomy versus J-pouch. *Diseases of Colon and Rectum.* **39**: 50–4.

Coffey JC, Winter DC, Neary P, Murphy A, Redmond HP *et al.* (2002) Quality of life after pouch-anal anastomosis: an evaluation of diet and other factors using the Cleveland global quality of life instrument. *Diseases of the Colon and Rectum.* **45**: 30–8.

Cummings JH (2000) Nutritional management of diseases of the gut. In: Garrow JS, James WPT & Ralph A (eds) *Human Nutrition and Dietetics.* 10th edn. London: Churchill Livingstone.

Department of Health (1991) *Dietary Reference Values for Food Energy and Nutrients for the United Kingdom. Report of the Panel on Dietary Reference Values of the Committee on Medical Aspects of Food Policy. Report on Health and Social Subjects 41.* London: HMSO.

Department of Health (2001) *Essence of Care, Patient Focused Benchmarking for Health Care Practitioners.* London: Department of Health.

Drugs and Therapeutic Bulletin (2005) *Cranberry and Urinary Tract Infection.* **43**: 17–19.

Edington J, Kon P & Martyn CN (1997) Prevalence of malnutrition after major surgery. *Journal of Human Nutrition and Dietetics.* **10**: 111–16.

Elia M (2003) *The 'MUST' Report: Nutritional Screening of Adults: A Multidisciplinary Responsibility. Development and Use of the 'Malnutrition Universal Screening Tool' ('MUST') for Adults.* Redditch: Malnutrition Advisory Group of the British Association for Parenteral and Enteral Nutrition (BAPEN).

Englyst HN & Hudson GH (2000) Carbohydrates. In: Garrow JS, James WPT & Ralph A (eds) *Human Nutrition and Dietetics.* 10th edn. London: Churchill Livingstone.

Faller MC, Welling RE & Lambert CE (1986) Nutritional implications and dietary management postproctocolectomy and ileal reservoir construction. *Journal of the American Dietetic Association.* **86**: 1235–6.

Fillingham S (1999) Caring for patients with urological stomas. *Journal of Community Nursing.* **12**: 29–34.

Fiorentini MT, Locatelli L, Ceccopieri B, Bertolino F, Ostellino O *et al.* (1987) Physiology of ileoanal anastomosis with ileal reservoir for ulcerative colitis and adenomatosis coli. *Diseases of Colon and Rectum.* **30**: 267–72.

Floruta CV (2001) Dietary choices of people with ostomies. *Journal of Wound, Ostomy and Continence Nursing.* **28**: 28–31.

Fordtran JS (1975) Stimulation of active and passive sodium absorption by sugars in the jejunum. *Journal of Clinical Investigation.* **55**: 728–37.

Fujita S, Kusunoki M, Shoji Y, Owado T & Utsunomiya J (1992) Quality of life after total proctocolectomy and ileal J-pouch-anal anastomosis. *Diseases of Colon and Rectum.* **35**: 1030–9.

Fulham J (2004) Improving the nutritional status of colorectal and surgical patients. *British Journal of Nursing.* **13**: 702–8.

Gazzard BG, Saunders B & Dawson AM (1978) Diets and stoma function. *British Journal of Surgery.* **65**: 642–4.

Gionchetti P, Rizzello F, Venturi A, Brigidi P, Matteuzzi D *et al.* (2000) Oral bacteriotherapy as maintenance treatment in patients with chronic pouchitis: a double-blind, placebo-controlled trial. *Gastroenterology.* **119**: 305–9.

Gionchetti P, Rizzello F, Helwig U, Venturi A, Lammers KM *et al.* (2003) Prophylaxis of pouchitis onset with probiotic therapy: a double-blind, placebo-controlled trial. *Gastroenterology.* **124**: 1202–9.

Giunchi G, Cacciaguerra G, Borlotti ML, Pasini A & Giulianini G (1988) Bowel movement and diet in patients with stomas. *British Journal of Surgery.* **75**: 722.

Goldberg SM (1987) Proctocolectomy and ileoanal anastomosis with an S pouch: functional results. *Canadian Journal of Surgery.* **30**: 359–61.

Heppel J, Kelly KA, Phillips SF, Beart RW, Telander RL *et al.* (1982) Physiological aspects of continence after colectomy, mucosal proctectomy and endorectal ileoanal anastomosis. *Annals of Surgery.* **195**: 435–43.

Hill GL (1982) Metabolic complications of ileostomy. *Clinics in Gastroenterology.* **11**: 260–7.

Hojlund Pederson B, Simonson L, Kuld Hansen L, Giese B, Justesen T *et al.* (1985) Bile acid malabsorption in patients with an ileum reservoir with a long efferent leg to an anal anastomosis. *Scandinavian Journal of Gastroenterology.* **20**: 995–1000.

Hylander E, Rannem T, Hegnhoj J, Kirkegarrd P, Thale M *et al.* (1991) Absorption studies after ileal J-pouch anastomosis for ulcerative colitis. A prospective study. *Scandinavian Journal of Gastroenterology.* **26**: 65–72.

Kennedy HJ, Lee ECG, Claridge G & Truelove SC (1982) The health of subjects living with a permanent ileostomy. *Quarterly Journal of Medicine.* **203**: 341–57.

Kennedy HJ, Al-Dujaili EAS, Edwards CRW & Truelove SC (1983) Water and electrolyte balance in subjects with a permanent ileostomy. *Gut.* **24**: 702–5.

Kramer P (1987) Effect of specific foods, beverages and spices on amount of ileostomy output in human subjects. *American Journal of Gastroenterology.* **82**: 327–32.

Ladefoged K & Olgaard K (1985) Sodium homeostasis after small bowel resection. *Scandinavian Journal of Gastroenterology.* **20**: 361–9.

Lenz K (1975) The effect of the site of lesion and extent of resection on duodenal bile acid concentration and vitamin B12 absorption in Crohn's disease. *Scandinavian Journal of Gastroenterology.* **10**: 241–8.

Lerch MM, Braun J, Harder M, Hofstadter F, Schumpelick V *et al.* (1989) Postoperative adaptation of the small intestine after total colectomy and J-pouch-anal anastomosis. *Diseases of Colon and Rectum.* **32**: 600–8.

Lewis SJ, Egger M, Sylvester PA & Thomas S (2001) Early enteral feeding versus 'nil by mouth' after gastrointestinal surgery: systematic review and meta-analysis of controlled trials. *British Medical Journal.* **323**: 1–5.

McNeil NI, Bingham S, Cole TJ, Grant AM & Cummings, JH (1982) Diet and health of people with an ileostomy (2). Ileostomy function and nutritional state. *British Journal of Nutrition.* **47**: 407–15.

M'Koma AE (1994) Follow-up results of haematology data before and after restorative proctocolectomy: clinical outcome. *Diseases of Colon and Rectum.* **37**: 932–7.

M'Koma AE, Lindquist K & Liljeqvist L (1994) Biochemical laboratory data in patients before and after restorative proctocolectomy. *Annales de Chirurgie.* **48**: 525–34.

Mimura T, Rizzello F, Helwig U, Poggioli G, Schreiber S *et al.* (2004) Once daily high dose probiotic therapy (VSL#3) for maintaining remission in recurrent or refractory pouchitis. *Gut.* **53**: 108–14.

Nasmyth DG & Williams NS (1993) Pouch ecology. In: Nicholls J, Bartolo D & Mortensen N (eds) *Restorative Proctocolectomy.* Oxford: Blackwell Scientific.

National Institute for Health and Clinical Excellence (NICE) (2006) *Nutrition Support in Adults. Clinical Guideline 32.* London: Department of Health.

Newton CR, Gonvers JJ, McIntyre PB, Preston DM & Lennard-Jones JE (1985) Effect of different drinks on fluid and electrolyte losses from a jejunostomy. *Journal of Royal Society of Medicine.* **78**: 27–34.

NHS Estates (2001) *Better Hospital Food Programme*. Department of Health: London.

Nicholls RJ, Belliveau P, Neill M, Wilks M & Tabaqchali S (1981) Restorative proctocolectomy with ileal reservoir: a pathophysiological assessment. *Gut.* **22**: 462–8.

Nightingale JMD (2003) The medical management of intestinal failure: methods to reduce the severity. *Proceedings of Nutrition Society.* **62**: 703–10.

Nightingale JMD & Spiller RC (2001) Normal intestinal anatomy and physiology. In: Nightingale JMD (ed) *Intestinal Failure*. London: Greenwich Medical Media.

Nightingale JMD & Woodward JM (2006) Guidelines for management of patients with a short bowel. *Gut.* **55**, supplement IV: iv1–iv12.

Nightingale JMD, Lennard-Jones JE, Walker ER & Farthing MJG (1990) Jejunal efflux in short bowel syndrome. *The Lancet.* **336**: 765–8.

Nightingale JMD, Lennard-Jones JE, Walker ER & Farthing MJG (1992) Oral salt supplements to compensate for jejunostomy losses: comparison of sodium chloride capsules, glucose-electrolyte solution, and glucose-polymer-electrolyte solution (Maxijul). *Gut.* **33**: 759–61.

O'Connell PR, Rankin DR, Weiland LH & Kelly KA (1986) Enteric bacteriology, absorption, morphology and emptying after ileal pouch–anal anastomosis. *British Journal of Surgery.* **73**: 909–14.

Pemberton JH (1993) Complications, management, failure and revisions. In: Nicholls J, Bartolo D & Mortensen N (eds) *Restorative Proctocolectomy*. Oxford: Blackwell Scientific.

Raymond JL & Becker JM (1986) Ileoanal pull-through: a new surgical alternative to ileostomy and a new challenge in diet therapy. *Journal of the American Dietetic Association.* **86**: 663–5.

Rumessen JJ & Gudmand-Hoyer E (1988) Functional bowel disease: malabsorption and abdominal distress after ingestion of fructose, sorbitol and fructose-sorbitol mixtures. *Gastroenterology.* **95(3)**: 694–700.

Salemans JMJI & Nagengast FM (1995) Clinical and physiological aspects of ileal pouch-anal anastomosis. *Scandinavian Journal of Gastroenterology.* **30**, supplement 212: 3–12.

Salemans JMJI, Nagengast FM, Tangerman A, Van Schaik A, De Haan AFJ *et al.* (1993) Postprandial conjugated and unconjugated serum bile acid levels after proctocolectomy with ileal pouch-anal anastomosis. *Scandinavian Journal of Gastroenterology.* **28**: 786–90.

Santavirta J, Harmoinen A, Karvonen AL & Matikainen M (1991) Water and electrolyte balance after ileoanal anastomosis. *Diseases of Colon and Rectum.* **34**: 115–18.

Smith IC, Walker LG, Eremin O & Heys SD (1997) The value of nutritional support in the peri-operative period: an analysis of randomised controlled trials. *British Journal of Surgery.* **84**, supplement 1: 41.

Steenhagen E, de Roos NM, Bouwman CA, Van Laarhoven JHM & Van Staveren WA (2006) Sources and severity of self-reported food intolerance after ileal pouch-anal anastomosis. *Journal of the American Dietetic Association.* **106**: 1459–62.

Stelzner M, Fonkalsrud EW, Buddington RK, Phillips JD & Diamond JM (1990) Adaptive changes in ileal mucosal nutrient transport following colectomy and endorectal ileal pull-through with ileal reservoir. *Archives of Surgery.* **125**: 586–90.

Svaninger G, Nordgren S, Palselius IRN, Fasth S & Hulten L (1991) Sodium and potassium excretion in patients with ileostomies. *European Journal of Surgery.* **157**: 601–5.

Thirlby RC & Kelly R (1997) Pectin and methylcellulose do not affect intestinal function in patients after ileal pouch-anal anastomosis. *American Journal of Gastroenterology.* **92**: 99–102.

Thompson WG & Wrathell E (1977) The relationship between ileal resection and vitamin B12 absorption. *Canadian Journal of Surgery.* **29**: 461–4.

Thomson TJ, Runcie J & Khan A (1970) The effect of diet on ileostomy function. *Gut.* **11**: 482–5.

Tomlin J, Lewis C & Read NW (1991) Investigation of normal flatus production in healthy volunteers. *Gut.* **32**: 665–9.

Tsao SKK, Baker M & Nightingale J (2005) High output stoma after small-bowel resections for Crohn's disease. *National Clinical Practice in Gastroenterology and Hepatology.* **2**: 604–8.

Tyus FJ, Austhof SI, Chima CS & Keating C (1992) Diet tolerance and stool frequency in patients with ileoanal reservoirs. *Journal of the American Dietetic Association.* **92**: 861–3.

Walsh CJ (2001) Perioperative feeding: does it reduce complications? *Colorectal Disease.* **3**, supplement 2: 18–22.

Watson D (1987) Drug therapy – colour changes to faeces and urine. *Pharmaceutical Journal.* **236**: 68.

Wendland B (1996) Nutrition matters for pouch patients. *Quarterly Journal of the Ileostomy and Internal Pouch Support Group.* **150**: 17.

Wexner SD, Jensen L, Rothenberger DA, Wong WD & Goldberg SM (1989) Long-term functional analysis of the ileoanal reservoir. *Diseases of Colon and Rectum.* **32**: 275–81.

Williams L, Armstrong M, Finan P, Sagar P & Burke D (2007) The effect of faecal diversion on human ileum. *Gut.* **56**: 796–801.

Wood S (1998) Nutrition and stoma patients. *Nursing Times.* **94**: 65–7.

Further reading

British Association for Parenteral and Enteral Nutrition, http://www.bapen.org.uk

British Dietetic Association, http://www.bda.uk.com

British Heart Foundation, http://www.bhf.org.uk

British Nutrition Foundation, http://www.nutrition.org.uk

Food Standards Agency, http://www.eatwell.gov.uk, http://www.salt.gov.uk

National Osteoporosis Society, http://www.nos.org.uk

Scientific Advisory Committee on Nutrition, http://www.sacn.gov.uk

Chapter 15

Complications

Jennie Burch

Introduction

There are many complications that can affect the care of a patient's stoma. These are discussed and some solutions offered. The statistics on complications vary, in one study there was found to be an increase in problematic stomas from 14% to 30% in the period from 1996 to 2003 (Cottam 2005). More recently, audits found that one in three ostomates experienced stoma management difficulties in the immediate post-operative period (Cottam & Richards 2006) compared to 16% of ostomates at their two-month follow-up (Ratcliff *et al.* 2005). Urostomies are associated with a 17% complication rate (Wood *et al.* 2003), whereas for children and infants the number of stoma complications was a quarter for colostomates (Nour *et al.* 1996).

Short-term complications

In the first few days following stoma formation a number of complications can occur. The three most common problems identified in an audit of almost 4000 newly formed stomas were retraction (40%), separation (24%) and necrosis (9%) (Cottam & Richards 2006).

Long-term complications

Long-term stoma complications may occur many years after the stoma is formed. Complications related to stomas have been recognised for many years (Brooke 1952) and include parastomal herniae that can lead to problems such as appliance leakage due to difficulty in maintaining a secure appliance.

Allergy and skin sensitivities

A true allergy is actually rare (0.6%) (Lawson 2003), but varying degrees of skin sensitivity may occur. Ostomates with a peristomal rash often mistakenly believe that an allergy is responsible (Lyon *et al.* 2000). In the presence of an allergy the skin will generally be inflamed to the size and shape of the appliance or the bag (Collett 2002). Acute allergic contact dermatitis can be recognised as erythema with indistinct and blurred margins (Lyon & Smith 2001). First-line treatment is usually to change the appliance manufacturer, as there are variations in the appliance constituents (Vujnovich 2004). A patch test may be required, for a few days, to monitor the skin's response to other flanges/base plates (Erwin-Toth 2003). The low incidence of allergic reactions can be seen as an indication of the good quality of stoma products (Smith *et al.* 2002).

Even less common is a skin reaction to topical substances such as soap, deodorant or talc and discontinuation of the product may resolve the problem. It is advisable for ostomates to cleanse their skin with warm tap water only (Lawson 2003). If the skin problem does not resolve the patient should be referred to a dermatologist (Meadows 1997).

Bleeding

There are a number of reasons that a stoma may bleed, therefore it is important to determine the cause and site of the bleeding. Bleeding can occur during cleaning from the surface of the stoma, due to the very vascular mucosa of the bowel (Collett 2002). Bleeding may occur with even the gentlest cleaning, particularly if ostomates are on warfarin for example. Patients should be advised to clean gently and ideally not to clean the stoma itself.

However, if bleeding occurs from the bowel lumen, this needs an urgent review by a health care professional as it could indicate a tumour (Taylor 2001). Trauma at the mucocutaneous junction may also cause bleeding (Blackley 1998). Damage to the stoma may be the result of an improperly sized (Rust 2007) or applied bag. Bleeding may also be the result of varices, granulomas or ulceration (Lawson 2003). Often treatment is to apply pressure to the area and stop the bleeding, but review is necessary to determine if any other treatment is needed.

Cancer recurrence locally

Although it is rare, it is possible to have a cancer on the stoma or at the stoma site. If the stoma or peristomal skin has any nodules or growths they should be carefully assessed. Surgery may be necessary if a malignancy is discovered (Earhart *et al.* 1998).

Crohn's disease

Crohn's disease can affect any part of the gastrointestinal tract and may affect the stoma or peristomal area (Lyon *et al.* 2000). There may be a peristomal fistula or ulceration, which can make appliance adhesion problematic. It might be appropriate if the fistula is close to the stoma to include it in the appliance aperture, while protecting the peristomal skin. If there is skin ulceration a topical steroid preparation might be appropriate (Black 2002). Adhesion of a stoma appliance may prove difficult and this can be overcome by applying a secondary film dressing to the area prior to adhering the stoma appliance.

Constipation

Constipation can be seen as two or fewer bowel motions a week (Powell & Rigby 2000) and may be a problem for colostomates. A balanced diet and sufficient fluids (Collett 2002) helps to prevent constipation (see Chapter 14 on nutrition). The causes of constipation may also include immobility or some analgesics, particularly those with codeine or opiate derivatives (Lawson 2003). If a patient requires these types of analgesics in the short term then a prophylactic laxative may be advisable in conjunction with the pain relief (Teahon 1999). If constipation does occur laxatives may be useful (see Chapter 18).

Diarrhoea

Diarrhoea is the frequent passage of watery motions from the bowel. Some people are prone to diarrhoea with certain foods, such as beer or spicy foods (Meadows 1997). It can also be expected that the more bowel that is surgically removed, particularly the ileum, the looser the stoma output will be. Other causes of diarrhoea include drugs, such as antibiotics (Taylor 2003), infection such as gastroenteritis, anxiety, diseases such as active Crohn's disease, radiotherapy or malabsorption. Antidiarrhoeal medication may be necessary to reduce bowel motility, but should not be used until the cause of the loose stool has been identified. A colostomate may need to wear a drainable bag when they experience loose stool.

Discolouration of the stoma

The stoma may be pale or dark in appearance. A pale stoma may indicate anaemia. If the stoma is bluish there may be some degree of anoxia (Hyland 2002). Infants who cry excessively may develop a purple coloured stoma, which returns to normal when the infant settles. Necrosis will be discussed later.

Flatus

Flatus can be embarrassing in any situation, but with a stoma there is no control (Collett 2002). In a study by Pringle and Swan (2001) 79% of ostomates reported flatus as an issue, reducing to 54% at a year after surgery, showing adaptations by the ostomates. Flatus can be the result of ingested air, thus ostomates can be advised to avoid:

- smoking
- talking while eating
- chewing gum
- using drinking straws.

The colonic bacteria also produce flatus (Meadows 1997). Additionally ostomates can be advised to avoid foods that induce flatus, such as cabbage or greens at times when flatus may cause embarrassment. Colostomy irrigation, a method used to empty the colon, can also assist the colostomate in reducing flatus.

Ballooning

Ballooning can be a problem for some colostomates and occurs when the appliance fills with flatus and becomes visible under clothing. Appliances now have filters that are designed to release flatus but not the odour (Black 2000). However the use of a two-piece appliance can allow the ostomate to release wind by 'burping' their appliance.

Granulomas/overgranulation

Granulomas or overgranulation have a cauliflower appearance and are friable and bleed easily. Overgranulation occurs at the mucocutaneous junction of the stoma and skin (Blackley 1998). Overgranulation occurs more frequently in shorter spouted colostomies (Lyon *et al*. 2000) with 10% reported around colostomies and 2% around ileostomies (Persson *et al*. 2005). Granulomas may be the result of repeated trauma, such as friction from the stoma flange (Lawson 2003) or an irritant reaction to faeces (Smith *et al*. 2002).

Often patients will enlarge the aperture in the appliance to include the overgranulation area in an attempt to reduce appliance leakage, but this perpetuates the problem. It is therefore essential to ensure that the stoma appliance is cut to the correct size, too small may cause rubbing and too large may lead to faeces touching the skin, both of which cause granulomas in some patients. Treatment is usually silver nitrate (Wondergem 2007) two or three times weekly (Collett 2002), but no research substantiates this practice (Johnson & Porrett 2005). Unfortunately recurrence of overgranulation is likely. Surgery may be necessary in extensive cases (Meadows 1997).

The author has met a patient who had overgranulation across the entire surface of his stoma. These were surgically removed and silver nitrate was subsequently used periodically, to prevent recurrence. A medical or surgical review is recommended to ensure that the growths are not cancerous (Blackley 1998).

Hernia

A hernia occurs when part of the abdominal contents protrude beyond the normal confines of the abdominal wall (Snell 2000). Additionally a parastomal hernia is the peritoneum bulging through the weakened muscle wall around the stoma. Parastomal hernias can vary from a slight bulge to a large unsightly swelling (Lawson 2003).

There are no accurate figures on the occurrence of parastomal herniae. Lyon and Smith (2001) consider that 2–3% of all patients will develop a hernia whereas Ratcliff *et al.* (2005) found about 2% had a parastomal hernia at two months post-operation. Pringle and Swan (2001) found 20% of ostomates at one year had a parastomal hernia, whereas in another study herniation occurred in 58% of ostomates within six months of surgery (Thompson & Trainor 2007). End colostomates are most commonly affected (Black 1997).

Siting the stoma through the rectus abdominus muscle is thought to reduce the risk of herniation, but this is not proven (Carmignani & Sugarbaker 2002). Herniation may be the result of a loss of muscle tone in the older person for example (Collett 2002).

There are a number of problems that a hernia can cause an ostomate:

- aching/dragging sensation
- change in abdominal shape
- difficulty visualising the stoma
- sore skin
- obstruction.

(Burch & Sica 2005)

Due to a change in the abdominal shape the appliance may leak (Blackley 1998). The hernia can also stretch the peristomal skin, distorting the shape and making the skin more friable and susceptible to breakdown at each appliance removal. Gentle appliance changes possibly with the use of a skin barrier/protection wipe or spray may help to resolve this problem. Skin creases may also appear and the use of stoma paste and/or washers or seals can help to provide a smooth skin surface for the pouch to stick to. Some ostomates find two-piece appliances to be beneficial as the flange/base plate is left in situ for a few days and the pouch attached to the flange, however most two-piece system do not provide flexibility. The thin adhesive coupling systems address this problem. For some a one-piece system may be preferred. Some patients find they need a larger flange to aid adhesion. Flange extenders or tape may also be used to secure the flange.

If the problem is being unable to see the stoma, a mirror can be used when positioning the appliance. The stoma may become sunken and weight loss may help. Colostomy irrigation may no longer be an appropriate method of management and then a suitable appliance will be required. There is a risk of obstruction, due to the bowel kinking or twisting (Lawson 2003). Obstruction can be identified by colicky abdominal pain (Meadows 1997) and patients need to be advised of this.

Convex pouches should be used with caution for ostomates with a parastomal hernia (Kane *et al.* 2004). Convexity can cause the skin to break down due to the pressure it exerts (Boyd *et al.* 2004): consider soft convex appliances or the use of washers/seals if convexity is necessary.

An abdominal support can help to relieve psychological problems by concealing the hernia and in many situations may prevent other problems.

These are available as panty girdles, support belts or SASH belts (Collett 2002). For some ostomates a surgical repair may be required but results are often poor (Carne *et al.* 2003) with 50% of parastomal hernias reoccurring (Martin & Foster 1996). However newer surgical techniques and the use of synthetic prosthetic mesh appears to be the best method of repair (McGrath *et al.* 2006). It has also been suggested that hernia incidence may be reduced if a mesh is used at the time of stoma formation (Gray *et al.* 2005).

Lifting and exercise advice is required to try and prevent hernia formation either at the stoma formation or following a surgical repair. A study found that ostomates wearing a hernia support belt, starting three months post-operatively and worn for at least one year and used in conjunction with abdominal exercises, appeared to significantly reduce the incidence of parastomal herniation in the first year after surgery (Thompson & Trainor 2005). The herniation rate at two years was 14% but rose to 17% at three years. However, the authors discovered that many ostomates were no longer using the belts or performing the exercises at three years (Thompson & Trainor 2007).

High-output stoma

A faecal output from a stoma of over one litre daily requires careful review. It is important to carefully observe the fluid balance, ensuring that the input exceeds the output. Blood results also need to be monitored, as there is a risk of sodium or magnesium depletion (Collett 2002). The patient may require rehydration, which could include an oral electrolyte solution (see Chapter 16) (Forbes & Myers 1996). Antidiarrhoeal medication may also be necessary to reduce the faecal output that is ideally taken one hour before food (Small 2003). Patients should also be advised to take salt with their meals (Meadows 1997). If the faecal output is fairly liquid it may be collected using a urostomy or a high-output bag. Prevention of sore skin is also essential as the enzymes in the faeces may damage the skin. Protection of the skin can be achieved by use of barrier wipes, sprays or creams and seals/washers for example. Practical tips can include changing the appliance first thing in the morning before eating or drinking. This reduces the risk of the stoma being active during the change.

Ileus (paralytic ileus)

After surgery the peristalsis action of the bowel can cease (Erwin-Toth 2003). This may be for a few hours to several days and nausea and/or vomiting may occur. A post-operative ileus is not often a problem but if nausea or vomiting occurs intravenous fluids and nil orally may be appropriate. However, in line with early discharge after enhanced recovery, generally early oral intake is not contraindicated or problematic (Fearon & Luff 2003).

Infection

Infections of the peristomal skin may be the result of a bacterial, fungal or viral infection (Black 2002). The incidence of infection is about 6% (Lyon *et al.* 2000) and may occur in ostomates with immunosuppression due to chemotherapy (Williams 2007). A common bacterial infection is folliculitis. A fungal infection could be candida for example. Viral infections are less common, such as herpes but should be treated quickly to reduce the attack. Folliculitis, fungal infection and urine infection are discussed separately.

Folliculitis

Folliculitis is inflamed hair follicles. This may be as a result of trauma when removing the appliance or inadequate or too frequent shaving (Blackley 1998). Folliculitis is more common in males with abdominal hair. It is recommended that shaving or clipping (Trainor *et al.* 2003) the peristomal area should only be undertaken once a week (Smith *et al.* 2002). The inflammation may be caused by streptococci or *Staphylococcus aureus* and thus can be treated by antibiotics (Black 2002).

Fungal infection

Fungal infections around a stoma are reasonably uncommon. Candida is rare with about 1% of ostomates at two months having a fungal infection (Ratcliff *et al.* 2005). However, patients with problems of excessive moisture due to leakage, sweating, antibiotics or immunosuppression therapy (Blackley 1998) may experience localised infections. These appear as a macular and papular rash with erythema, often under the stoma flange, and may cause problems with appliance adhesion. Fungal infection can be treated with an antifungal powder (Ziegler & French 2005) or cream (Hess 2003).

Urine infection

A urinary infection is one of the most common problems associated with a urostomy. A urine infection can occur due to a shortened urinary tract system (Taylor 2001). The signs of a urinary infection are malodorous urine or increased sediment or mucus in the urine. The cause may be due to urine not passing through the ileal conduit, due to stenosis, kinking of the bowel or a stricture (Lawson 2003). The bowel that is used as the conduit makes the mucus, but a change in smell may indicate an infection.

Investigations should include a urine test. A specimen should not be obtained from the appliance, but by gently inserting a urinary catheter a few centimetres into the urostomy (Baxter & Lloyd 2004). Antibiotics may be necessary and advice is often to increase oral fluids to two to three litres in a 24-hour period (Blackley 1998) and a daily glass of cranberry juice can be useful (Leaver 1996). However, cranberry juice is contraindicated for patients on warfarin. Adding a few drops of vinegar to the urostomy bag can reduce the odour of the infected urine (Lawson 2003). In the early post-operative days additional vitamin C (ascorbic acid 100 mg daily) can reduce the mucus production (Black 2000). Two-piece appliances can be beneficial if mucus blocks the non-return valve, then the pouch can be replaced on a daily basis without causing skin trauma.

Melanosis coli

Melanosis coli is very rare but visually can be confused with a necrotic bowel due to the stoma discolouration, however the bowel will feel warm. The discolouration is due to long-term laxative use. The stoma will remain discoloured and the ostomate needs to be reassured that this is normal for them.

Mucocutaneous separation

Mucocutaneous separation is seen as the stoma edges detaching from the surrounding skin (Collett 2002). The separation can range from superficial to total dehiscence when the stoma separates from the deeper tissues (Blackley 1998). Mucocutaneous separation may be the result of infection, necrosis or tension on the sutures (Lee & Morris 2003) and may lead to stomal retraction or stenosis. Treatment for superficial wounds may include using protective paste or powder in the cavity (Boyd-Carson *et al.* 2004) and incorporating the cavity into the stoma appliance aperture. If the cavity is heavily exuding or deep it can be filled with alginate rope and the wound covered. Rarely is resuturing required (Lee 2001a). A seal/washer or belt may also be necessary to reduce the risk of leakages (Hess 2003).

Necrosis

It is important in the immediate post-operative period to regularly check the stoma. The stoma should be warm, red and wet, but it may become cool and a purple, dusky colour if there is impaired blood supply (Collett 2002) or black if necrotic (Lawson 2003). However, necrosis is rare at about 1% for ileostomates (Leong *et al.* 1994) and 4% of colostomates (Persson *et al.* 2005). Necrosis in the immediate post-operative period is usually due to a surgical problem, such as difficulty mobilising the bowel (Taylor 1999), and generally develops within one to two days of surgery (Myers 1996). Necrosis occurring later may be due to a tightly fitting appliance or pressure. Necrosis requires urgent surgical review (Meadows 1997).

Superficial necrotic areas often require no action and the surface may slough off (Cronin 2005). To promote the separation of the necrotic tissue, protective powder or debridement may be useful (Blackley 1998). There may also be odour associated with the necrotic tissue and the ostomate needs to be advised of this (Taylor 2001). If the necrotic area is deeper, surgery may be necessary. Unfortunately necrosis may lead to a flush or stenosed stoma, which may in turn cause appliance leakage problems. A case study describes using a GTN patch to prevent ischaemia following surgery for a necrotic bowel, but this cannot be recommended until further research has been undertaken (Johnson & Porrett 2006a).

Obstruction

Bowel obstruction may be a potential problem for ileostomates due to:

- a food bolus blockage;
- adhesions as a result of surgery;
- strangulated hernia;
- volvulus;
- a stricture (narrowing) due to recurrent disease, such as Crohn's disease.

(Lawson 2003)

Obstruction occurs in about 20% of ileostomates (Leong *et al.* 1994). Obstruction in the post-operative period can be a result of oedema from the surgery. Thus immediately after surgery dietary advice is essential, with important issues being to thoroughly chew foods for example. High-fibre foods should also be slowly reintroduced back into the diet.

The signs of a partial obstruction are cramping, abdominal pains, with an offensive watery faecal output, abdominal distension or a swollen stoma (Meadows 1997). Treatment can include drinking to dislodge the blockage, if nausea is not present. The patient can also try gentle abdominal massage or a warm bath. If the symptoms become more severe or if there is a complete blockage and oral fluids cannot be tolerated, hospitalisation and intravenous fluids with a nasogastric tube, to aspirate gastric secretions, may be required (Lawson 2003). Only very rarely if the obstruction persists is surgery required.

Odour

A common worry of ostomates is the thought that they may smell (Baxter & Lloyd 2004). In a study by Pringle and Swan (2001) odour troubled 37% of ostomates. However, odour should only be detected when the appliance is emptied or changed. An air freshener or ostomy deodorant can be used to combat smell and is ideally used before the appliance is emptied or changed. Some foods cause greater odour than others, such as fish, and can be avoided if the smell is unacceptable to the ostomate (Nazarko 2007). Treatment includes capsules, drops or gel placed directly into the appliance (Black 2000). Careful assessment of the bag and its application may reveal a simple solution to the problem; for example, if the appliance is incorrectly positioned it may leak.

Pancaking

Pancaking is a term used when the faeces sits around the top of the stoma appliance. Pancaking may occur with colostomates (Taylor 1999) and cause the appliance to leak, potentially leading to sore skin. There are a number of methods that can be tried to resolve this problem. Some modern appliances have flatus filters that are designed to prevent pancaking. Alternatively the filter can be covered to keep some air within the appliance (Taylor 1999): this assists the faeces to fall to the base of the appliance (Pullen 2002). Other treatment options include stoma bridges, applied externally, or foam blocks that can be stuck inside the bag. Alternatively, using a small amount of oil, talcum powder or a scrunched up tissue inside the bag can be effective (Blackley 1998). There are also specialised solutions that are added to clean, empty pouches that lubricate and deodorise the faeces.

It is, however, important to explore other possible contributing factors. The consistency of the faeces can be too thick or not sufficiently soft (Myers 1996), thus dietary changes can alter the faecal consistency and prevent pancaking. On further assessment it may be evident that inadequate fluids are being taken.

Phantom bladder/rectum

In rare situations a phenomenon known as the phantom bladder or phantom rectum can occur. This is a sensation that there is discomfort in an area that has been surgically removed. However, it can be difficult to treat. Medications that may be effective are analgesia or sometimes drugs to treat epilepsy or depression, which work on the nerves that cause the pain. Some ostomates report benefit from sitting on the toilet and pretending to pass urine or faeces. Nothing will pass if this area has been removed but it is anecdotally effective. On the other hand others consider alternative therapy, such as acupuncture, to be effective (Biley 2001). However, if the pain is new it is advisable to see the doctor to exclude other potential causes, such as infection or disease recurrence, and to give the patient peace of mind.

Prolapse

A prolapsed stoma is observed when the bowel intussuscepts (telescopes) out of the skin opening, becoming longer, and can frequently occur with a transverse colostomy (Collett 2002). Two per cent of ileostomates reported a prolapse in a Swedish study (Persson *et al.* 2005). A prolapsed stoma can occur abruptly without any apparent reason (Myers 1996). A prolapse is often due to the inadequate fixing of the stoma to the abdominal wall during surgery (Lawson 2003), increased abdominal pressure or pregnancy. If the stoma is sited through the rectus muscle there are suggestions that this can minimise the risk of prolapse (Meadows 1997). If a prolapse occurs, the ostomate needs to be reassured that it is not generally serious

(Taylor 1999). However, as the bowel is oedematous there is a risk of trauma or necrosis if the stoma becomes constricted. Thus ostomates need to observe the stoma for changes in colour and signs of obstruction. To contain the prolapsed stoma a larger appliance can be used (Hess 2003). Some ostomates 'feather' the edge of their flange by making small incisions around the flange aperture which will allow slight movement to accommodate the oedema. Some prolapses are fairly minor and can be manipulated back into the body, with the use of a cold compress (Colwell & Beitz 2007) or sugar sprinkled on the bowel to reduce oedema; however, sugar in particular tends to be messy (McErlain *et al.* 2004). Sugar needs to be used with caution in the presence of diabetes, or even avoided. A surgical refashioning can be performed if the patient cannot tolerate the prolapse or if there are complications (Lee 2001a).

Pyoderma gangrenosum

Pyoderma gangrenosum is a non-infectious, ulcerative, inflammatory skin disorder with irregular, undermined, purple edges (Morison & Moffatt 1997) of unknown cause. However, convex appliances have been linked to the development of pyoderma gangrenosum. Lyon and Smith (2001) suggest that pyoderma gangrenosum is rare with an incidence of 0.6% of all reported peristomal skin problems. Pyoderma gangrenosum is associated with active disease, predominantly inflammatory bowel disease. However, diagnosis of pyoderma gangrenosum is difficult as there is no definitive diagnosis and exclusion of other causes is generally required. Pyoderma gangrenosum is most common on the lower extremities (Bennett *et al.* 2000), but can occur around the stoma (Sheldon *et al.* 2000), causing appliance leakage. The lesions can be painful (Ronnau *et al.* 2000) and may enlarge rapidly. Unfortunately pyoderma gangrenosum can be difficult to treat and often takes many months to heal, recurring in about a third of patients.

Therapy can be to treat the underlying disease (Romero-Gomez & Sanchez-Munoz 2002). Most commonly steroids are taken orally (Braun-Falco *et al.* 2002) with daily dosages of up to 120 mg being discussed (Dunwoody *et al.* 2000), but steroids have significant toxicity (Friedman *et al.* 2001) and require tapering after disease control. Steroids may also be given topically, including steroid cream, steroid tape (Rozen *et al.* 2001) or steroid soaked gauze, but this is seldom sufficient without concurrent systemic therapy. Other immunosuppressant therapy, such as tacrolimus in orabase paste (Lyon & Smith 2001), is effective but it is usually reserved for resistant cases (Ma *et al.* 2002) due to the associated toxicity. There are no trials to support steroid usage, but multiple articles discuss their efficacy. Unfortunately, once healing occurs there may be cribriform (sieve like) scarring (Burton 2005), which can cause appliance leakage.

Retraction

A retracted stoma occurs when the bowel pulls back into the abdomen (Mckenzie & Ingram 2001). Statistics vary from about one-quarter of patients at 12 months after surgery (Arumugam *et al.* 2003) to 2% in another study (Persson *et al.* 2005). Retraction can cause appliance leakage due to the effluent seeping under the adhesive (Myers 1996), especially if the faeces are loose. The causes of retraction may be due to weight gain, premature rod removal or the bowel being under too much tension. Retraction may also be the result of previous stoma-related problems such as necrosis or mucocutaneous separation. Although surgery may be required, it can be useful to try a seal, convexity, a stoma belt or to lose weight. Convex products should be used with caution due to the risk of peristomal ulcers (Wyss 2004).

Skin problems

There are a number of parastomal skin problems that can occur. Figures are varied ranging from 27% (Persson *et al.* 2005) to two-thirds of patients reporting skin problems, with 58% suffering with the problem for more than six months, despite many ostomates trying to resolve their problems without assistance (Smith *et al.* 2002). Skin inflammation is common particularly for ileostomates (Lyon *et al.* 1999). This topic is broken down into:

- dermatitis
- existing skin problems
- sore skin.

Dermatitis

Irritation as a result of faeces or urine on the skin (Smith *et al.* 2002) is termed irritant contact dermatitis and is the most common peristomal skin problem (Lyon & Beck 2001). This is most commonly due to the appliance aperture being too large (Lee 2001b), if the stoma is not remeasured after post-operative oedema has reduced, for example. At two months about 10% of ostomates had irritant contact dermatitis (Ratcliff *et al.* 2005). Resizing the appliance aperture usually resolves this and the appliance should be cut no more than 3 mm larger than the stoma (Lawson 2003).

Existing skin problems

Many ostomates have pre-existing skin disorders such as psoriasis and this can also occur on the peristomal skin (Lyon *et al.* 1999); 42% of those with pre-existing skin problems reported that this had affected their appliance adhesion (Lyon *et al.* 2000). The usual therapy for skin conditions such as psoriasis is greasy and this will therefore prevent appliance adherence. However, effective treatment can be to use topical scalp lotions, ideally without alcohol which will sting (Smith *et al.* 2002). Alternatively, apply the lotion to the stoma appliance adhesive and leave it for 15 minutes; this allows the alcohol to evaporate, before adhering it to the skin.

Sore skin

Excoriated skin is the destruction and removal of the surface of the skin. Excoriated skin is most common for ileostomates due to the proteolytic enzymes used in digestion that can lead to denuded skin (Hyland 2002) and urostomates (Collett 2002). For urostomates strongly acidic or alkaline urine can cause excoriation (Lawson 2003). Smith *et al*. (2002) discuss the effective use of sucralfate powder for skin erosion when applied topically. The powder is applied prior to the appliance and forms a sticky paste over the excoriated skin.

The most common complication for an ostomate is sore skin and it affects about one-third of colostomates (Herlufsen *et al*. 2006). An extensive questionnaire study found that 73% of ostomates had skin problems that had affected their appliance, both for pre-existing conditions and new problems (Lyon *et al*. 2000). Leong *et al*. (1994) found that after 20 years the risk of sore skin for an ileostomate was about 30%. Late excoriation was most commonly associated with diabetes and early excoriation associated with emergency surgery (Arumugam *et al*. 2003). Sore skin may be as a result of retraction (Mckenzie & Ingram 2001), stenosis, prolapse, appliance leakage, herniation or a high faecal output. The stomal output can be affected by diet, medication or a bowel resection, the more proximal the stoma, the more fluid and corrosive the faeces. High volumes of liquid effluent can cause maceration if skin isn't adequately protected or if leaks occur. Maceration may become ulcerated if not treated (Blackley 1998). A change in abdominal shape can also cause appliance leakage as a result of weight loss or gain, causing for example skin creases (Myers 1996). To stop the appliances from leaking as a result of the sore skin the ostomates will often cut the appliance aperture larger: this resolves the leaks in some cases but perpetuates the sore skin (Hyland 2002). Careful assessment will usually guide the treatment plan.

Pregnancy may also cause changes in the shape of the skin as may a parastomal hernia. Thus treatment for excoriated skin depends upon the cause. Broken skin in the peristomal area compromises the adhesion and therefore the security of the bag. A cool hairdryer can be used to dry any wet or oozing skin. The use of a protective skin barrier wipe or spray can also assist, preventing the effluent contacting the skin, if an appliance leak does occur. Other skin protectors may be protective paste or powders (Blackley 1998). If the cause of the leaks is a skin crease the use of belts, paste, seals or convexity may help to prevent leakages.

It should be remembered that many flanges are made from a hydrocolloid that has wound healing properties and protects the peristomal skin from the stoma output and bacteria (Hyland 2002). Thus if correctly sized and applied, the appliance flange may resolve the sore skin without additional treatment.

The cause of sore skin may be as a result of changing of the appliance too frequently, causing physical damage to the skin (Trainor *et al*. 2003). In this situation a colostomate may find a two-piece appliance or a drainable pouch beneficial. Often reviewing the application or removal technique can resolve problems (Meadows 1997). However, modern appliances made from hydrocolloid cause fewer problems than older stoma appliances, which some patients may still use. Sore skin may be due to mechanical trauma from harsh cleaning agents or creams (Blackley 1998), which should be stopped.

Stenosis

Stenosis is when the lumen of the bowel narrows at the fascial or cutaneous level, due to scarring (Lawson 2003) and may close completely (Meadows 1997) causing problems with the faecal flow from the body (Johnson & Porrett 2007). About 7% of ileostomates report stenosis of their stoma (Persson *et al.* 2005), although stenosis is less common than herniation or a prolapsed stoma (Black 1997). If the stenosis occurs in the early post-operative period it may be due to surgical technique or mucocutaneous separation (Collett 2002). Stenosis may cause pain on defaecation for colostomates, but keeping the bowel motions soft can help. For ileostomates it may lead to a partial obstruction. For a urostomate, stenosis may result in recurrent urine infections. Treatment may involve daily dilation (Taylor 2001) with a specialised stoma dilator. It is advisable to start with a small size and increase in diameter gradually. Dilators should be used with care, as splitting the skin can cause further scarring. If dilation is ineffective surgery may be required (Taylor 1999).

Stoma trauma

Trauma to the stoma is rare, but is more likely to occur to an ileostomy or urostomy as they are both spouted. There are a number of reasons for a stomal laceration such as the aperture of the appliance being too small or incorrectly fitted and causing trauma to the stoma. This can be resolved by careful assessment of the stoma and appliance change technique. If the trauma is due to an accidental cut during shaving of the peristomal skin it can be useful to shave away from the stoma. There may also be deliberate self-harm of the stoma. If the laceration occurred as a result of a car accident (Taylor 2001) or sporting injury then a stoma shield may be advisable. Lacerations of the stoma are often superficial although they can penetrate the bowel wall (Johnson & Porrett 2006b), but due to the lack of nerve endings in the bowel there is often no pain reported.

Immediate treatment includes stopping the bleeding; this is generally achieved by applying pressure. Healing will generally occur spontaneously within about six weeks. However it is advisable not to clean the stoma itself when replacing appliances but only the peristomal skin, or bleeding may restart. If there is swelling of the stoma the appliance may need to be cut larger initially to prevent any further damage.

Urine crystal formation

Due to the alkaline urine there may be the formation of oxalate crystals (phosphate deposits) on or around the urostomy (Lawson 2003). These may cause irritation, bleeding or possibly ulceration (Leaver 1996). White vinegar can be diluted, in equal proportions with water, and used to dissolve the crystals by direct application to the stoma. Cranberry juice can then be drunk regularly to try and restore the acidic pH and thus reduce the subsequent formation of crystals (Fillingham 1999).

Varices

Peristomal varices or caput medusae can be the result of portal hypertension or liver disease (McCann 2003). The appearance is visible veins through the peristomal skin. There are a number of treatments that might be effective including epinephrine-soaked gauze or injection sclerotherapy (Colwell & Beitz 2007). Simple treatment can be pressure on the bleeding area, should this occur. Ostomates should also be advised to ensure gentle appliance changes.

Conclusion

It can be seen that the ostomate may encounter a large number of complications. However, most ostomates will not encounter many of those listed above and some patients do not report any problems at all with their stoma. Many ostomates will try and resolve these problems themselves but review by the stoma specialist nurse is ideal.

References

Arumugam PJ, Bevan L, Macdonald L, Watkins AJ, Morgan AR *et al.* (2003) A prospective audit of stomas – analysis of risk factors and complications and their management. *Colorectal Diseases.* **5(1)**: 49–52.

Baxter A & Lloyd PA (2004) Elimination: stoma care. In: Dougherty L & Lister S (eds) *The Royal Marsden Hospital Manual of Clinical Nursing Procedures.* 6th edn. London: The Royal Marsden.

Bennett ML, Jackson JM, Jorizzo JL, Fleischer AB, White WL *et al.* (2000) Pyoderma gangrenosum: a comparison of typical and atypical forms with an emphasis on time to remission. Case review of 86 patients from 2 institutions. *Medicine.* **79(1)**: 37–46.

Biley FC (2001) Phantom bladder sensations: a new concern for stoma care workers. *British Journal of Nursing.* **10(19)**: 1290–6.

Black P (1997) Practical stoma care. *Nursing Standard.* **11(47)**: 49–55.

Black P (2000) *Holistic Stoma Care.* London: Baillière Tindall.

Black P (2002) Treating peristomal skin problems in the community. *British Journal of Community Nursing.* **7(4)**: 212–17.

Blackley P (1998) *Practical Stoma, Wound and Continence Management.* Australia: Victoria, Australia Research Publications Pty Ltd.

Boyd K, Thompson MJ, Boyd-Carson W & Trainor B (2004) Use of convex appliances. *Nursing Standard.* **18(20)**: 37–8.

Boyd-Carson W, Thompson MJ, Trainor B & Boyd K (2004) Mucocutaneous separation. *Nursing Standard.* **18(17)**: 41–3.

Braun-Falco M, Stock K, Ring J & Hein R (2002) Topical platelet-derived growth factor accelerates healing of myelodysplastic syndrome-associated pyoderma gangrenosum. *British Journal of Dermatology.* **147(4)**: 829–31.

Brooke BN (1952) The management of an ileostomy including its complications. *The Lancet.* **2(3)**: 102–4.

Burch J & Sica J (2005) Frequency, predisposing factors for and treatment of parastomal hernia. *Gastrointestinal Nursing.* **3(6)**: 29–32.

Burton J (2005) Case study: diagnosis and treatment of pyoderma gangrenosum. *British Journal of Nursing.* **14(16)**: S10–13.

Carmignani C & Sugarbaker PH (2002) Parastomal hernias. *Problems in General Surgery.* **19(4)**: 65–72.

Carne PWG, Robertson GM & Frizelle FA (2003) Parastomal hernia. *British Journal of Surgery.* **90(7)**: 784–93.

Collett K (2002) Practical aspects of stoma management. *Nursing Standard.* **17(8)**: 45–55.

Colwell JC & Beitz J (2007) Survey of wound, ostomy and continence (WOC) nurse clinicians on stomal and peristomal complications. *Journal of Wound, Ostomy and Continence Nursing.* **34(1)**: 57–69.

Cottam J (2005) Audit of stoma complications within three weeks of surgery. *Gastrointestinal Nursing.* **3(1)**: 19–23.

Cottam J & Richards K (2006) National audit of stoma complications within 3 weeks of surgery. *Gastrointestinal Nursing.* **4(8)**: 34–9.

Cronin E (2005) Problem stomas and the use of convexity. *Gastrointestinal Nursing.* **3(10)**: 33–40.

Dunwoody CJ, McCann SA & Zumbo M (2000) Pyoderma gangrenosum: a case study for pain management in dermatology nursing. *Dermatology Nursing.* **12(5)**: 313–26.

Earhart K, Mueller V & Murray D (1998) Stoma care during cancer therapy: special people/special needs. *World Council of Enterostomal Therapists Journal.* **18(3)**: 21–2.

Erwin-Toth P (2003) Ostomy pearls. *Advances in Skin and Wound Care.* **16(3)**: 146–52.

Fearon KCH & Luff R (2003) The nutritional management of surgical patients: enhanced recovery after surgery. *Proceedings of the Nutrition Society.* **6**: 807–11.

Fillingham S (1999) Caring for patients with urological stomas. *Journal of Community Nursing.* **13(12)**: 29–34.

Forbes A & Myers C (1996) Enterocutaneous fistula and their management. In: Myers C (ed) *Stoma Care Nursing: A Patient-Centred Approach.* London: Arnold.

Friedman S, Marion JF, Scherl E, Rubin PH & Present DH (2001) Intravenous cyclosporin in refractory pyoderma gangrenosum complicating inflammatory bowel disease. *Inflammatory Bowel Disease.* **7(1)**: 1–7.

Gray M, Colwell JC & Goldberg MT (2005) What treatments are effective for the management of parastomal hernia? *Journal of Wound, Ostomy and Continence Nursing.* **32(2)**: 87–92.

Herlufsen P, Olsen AG, Carlsen B, Nybaek H, Karlsmark T et al. (2006) Study of peristomal skin disorders in patients with permanent stomas. *British Journal of Nursing.* **15(16)**: 854–62.

Hess CT (2003) Ostomy pearls. *Advances in Skin and Wound Care.* **16(3)**: 146–52.

Hyland J (2002) The basics of ostomies. *Gastroenterology Nursing.* **25(6)**: 241–4.

Johnson A & Porrett T (2005) Developing an evidence base for the management of stoma granulomas. *Gastrointestinal Nursing.* **3(8)**: 26–8.

Johnson A & Porrett T (2006a) The application of GTN in managing stomal ischemia. *Gastrointestinal Nursing.* **4(6)**: 28–32.

Johnson A & Porrett T (2006b) Stomal lacerations and trauma – strange things do happen. *Gastrointestinal Nursing.* **4(4)**: 16–18.

Johnson A & Porrett T (2007) Stomal stenosis, a complex stoma complication: case study. *Gastrointestinal Nursing*. **5(1)**: 17–22.

Kane M, McErlean D, McGrogan M, Thompson MJ & Haughey S (2004) Management of parastomal hernia. *Nursing Standard*. **18(19)**: 43–4.

Lawson A (2003) Complications of stomas. In: Elcoat C (ed) *Stoma Care Nursing*. London: Hollister.

Leaver RB (1996) Cranberry juice. *Professional Nurse*. **11(8)**: 525–6.

Lee J (2001a) Common stoma problems: a brief guide to community nurses. *British Journal of Community Nursing*. **6(8)**: 407–13.

Lee J (2001b) Nurse prescribing in practice: patient choice in stoma care. *British Journal of Community Nursing*. **6(1)**: 33–7.

Lee J & Morris O (2003) Stoma complications: a case of cooperation. *British Journal of Community Nursing*. **8(7)**: 302–6.

Leong APK, Londono EE & Phillips RKP (1994) Life-long analysis of stomal complications following ileostomy. *British Journal of Surgery*. **81**: 727–9.

Lyon CC & Beck MH (2001) Dermatitis. In: Lyon C & Smith A (eds) *Abdominal Stomas and Their Skin Disorders. An Atlas of Diagnosis and Management*. London: Martin Dunitz.

Lyon CC & Smith A (2001) *Abdominal Stomas and Their Skin Disorders. An Atlas of Diagnosis and Management*. London: Martin Dunitz.

Lyon CC, Griffiths CEM & Beck MH (1999). Psoriasis in abdominal stoma patients: presentation and treatment. *British Journal of Dermatology*. **141**(supplement 55): 28.

Lyon CC, Smith AJ, Griffiths CEM & Beck MH (2000) The spectrum of skin disorders in abdominal stoma patients. *British Journal of Dermatology*. **143(6)**: 1248–60.

Ma G, Jones G & MacKay G (2002) Pyoderma gangrenosum: a great marauder. *Annuals of Plastic Surgery*. **48(5)**: 546–52.

McCann EM (2003) Common ostomy problems. In: Milne CT, Corbett LQ & Dubuc DL (eds) *Wound, Ostomy and Continence Nursing Secrets*. Philadelphia: Hanley & Belfus.

McErlain D, Kane M, McGrogan M & Haughey S (2004) Prolapsed stoma. *Nursing Standard*. **18(18)**: 41–2.

McGrath A, Porrett T & Heyman B (2006) Parastomal hernia: an exploration of the risk factors and the implications. *British Journal of Nursing*. **15(6)**: 317–21.

Mckenzie FD & Ingram VA (2001) Dansac invent convex in the management of flush ileostomy. *British Journal of Nursing*. **10(15)**: 1005–9.

Martin L & Foster G (1996) Parastomal hernia. *Annals of the Royal College of Surgeons of England*. **78(2)**: 81–4.

Meadows C (1997) Stoma and fistula care. In: Bruce L & Finlay TMD (eds) *Nursing in Gastroenterology*. London: Churchill Livingstone.

Morison M & Moffatt C (1997) Leg ulcers. In: Morison M, Moffatt C, Bridel-Nixon J & Bale S (eds) *Nursing Management of Chronic Wounds*. 2nd edn. London: Mosby.

Myers C (1996) Appliance leakage. In: Myers C (ed) *Stoma Care Nursing*. London: Arnold.

Nazarko L (2007) Colostomy: complications and effective management. *Nursing and Residential Care*. **9(3)**: 104–8.

Nour S, Stringer MD & Beck J (1996) Colostomy complications in infants and children. *Annals of the Royal College of Surgeons of England*. **78(6)**: 526–30.

Persson E, Gustavsson B, Hellström A-L, Lappas G & Hultén L (2005) Ostomy patients' perceptions of quality of care. *Journal of Advanced Nursing*. **49(1)**: 51–8.

Powell M & Rigby D (2000) Management of bowel dysfunction: evacuation difficulties. *Nursing Standard*. **12(47)**: 47–54.

Pringle W & Swan E (2001) Continuing care after discharge from hospital for stoma patients. *British Journal of Nursing*. **10(19)**: 1275–88.

Pullen M (2002) Management of difficult stomas. *Nursing and Residential Care.* **4(2)**: 76–80.

Ratcliff CR, Scarano KA & Donovan AM (2005) Descriptive study of peristomal complications. *Journal of Wound, Ostomy and Continence.* **32(1)**: 33–7.

Romero-Gomez M & Sanchez-Munoz D (2002) Infliximab induces remission of pyoderma gangrenosum. *European Journal of Gastroenterology & Hepatology.* **14(8)**: 907.

Ronnau AC, Schmeideberg SV, Bielfeld P, Ruzicka T & Schuppe H (2000) Pyoderma gangrenosum after cesarean delivery. *American Journal of Obstetrics and Gynaecology.* **183(2)**: 502–4.

Rozen SM, Nahabedian MY & Manson PN (2001) Management strategies for pyoderma gangrenosum: case studies and review of literature. *Annals of Plastic Surgery.* **47(3)**: 310–15.

Rust J (2007) Care of patients with stomas: the pouch change procedure. *Nursing Standard.* **22(6)**: 43–7.

Sheldon DG, Sawchuck LL, Kozarek RA & Thirlby RC (2000) Twenty cases of peristomal pyoderma gangrenosum. Diagnostic implications and clinical management. *Archives of Surgery.* **135**: 564–9.

Small M (2003) Management of intestinal failure. *Nursing Times.* **99(3)**: 52–3.

Smith AJ, Lyon CC & Hart CA (2002) Multidisciplinary care of skin problems in stoma patients. *British Journal of Nursing.* **11(5)**: 324–30.

Snell R (2000) *Clinical Anatomy for Medical Students.* 6th edn. London: Lippincott Williams & Wilkins.

Taylor P (1999) Stomal complications. In: Taylor P (ed) *Stoma Care in the Community: A Clinical Resource for Practitioners.* London: NT Books.

Taylor P (2001) Care of patients with complications following formation of a stoma. *Professional Nurse.* **17(4)**: 252–4.

Taylor P (2003) Clinical issues in stoma care practice. *Nursing and Residential Care.* **5(8)**: 366–70.

Teahon E (1999) Constipation. In: Porrett T & Daniels N (eds) *Essential Coloproctology for Nurses.* London: Whurr.

Thompson MJ & Trainor B (2005) Incidence of parastomal hernia before and after a prevention programme. *Gastrointestinal Nursing.* **3(20)**: 23–7.

Thompson MJ & Trainor B (2007) Prevention of parastomal hernia: a comparison of results 3 years on. *Gastrointestinal Nursing.* **5(3)**: 22–8.

Trainor B, Thompson MJ, Boyd-Carson W & Boyd K (2003) Changing an appliance. *Nursing Standard.* **18(13)**: 41–2.

Vujnovich A (2004) Peristomal faecal/urine dermatitis and allergy. *Gastrointestinal Nursing.* **2(5)**: 25–31.

Williams J (2007) A guide to maintaining healthy parastomal skin. *Gastrointestinal Nursing.* **5(7)**: 18–22.

Wondergem F (2007) Stoma care – a guide to daily living. *JCN.* **21(4)**: 18–22.

Wood DN, Allen S, Greenwell TJ & Shah PJR (2003) Stomal complications of ileal conduit diversion. *British Journal of Urology.* **91**(supplement 2): 92.

Wyss H (2004) Retracted stomas and the optimisation of convex ostomy products. *World Council of Enterostomal Therapists Journal.* **24(3)**: 26–8.

Ziegler M & French ET (2005) How do we manage difficult ostomy pouching in the rehabilitation setting? *Rehabilitation Nursing.* **30(3)**: 84.

Chapter 16

Fistulae and Intestinal Failure

Jennie Burch

Introduction

This chapter will discuss enterocutaneous fistulae and intestinal failure, both of which are rare but associated with considerable morbidity (Lloyd *et al.* 2006). The care and causes of fistulation will be discussed and practical skills provided. It is also possible to have a urinary fistula. This is much less common than faecal fistulae and can result following radiotherapy to the bladder. The surgical repair of urinary fistulae is often problematic but the appliance care is the same as for faecal fistulae. Intestinal failure (IF) can have devastating effects on the patient and the care will briefly be discussed. Parenteral nutrition (PN) is a method of feeding that can be for the short or long term and is often required by patients with intestinal failure. The need for parenteral nutrition is only undertaken after careful assessment due to the considerable risks associated with it, namely infection.

Defining fistulae

A fistula is an abnormal communication between two epithelial surfaces (Forbes & Myers 1996). An enterocutaneous fistula can be seen as an abnormal passage between the gastrointestinal tract and the skin (Lloyd *et al.* 2006). This should not be confused with a fistula in ano or anal fistula, which is a tract between the skin and the anal canal (Forbes 2001).

Aetiology

There may be a number of causes of enterocutaneous fistulae, but they always have sepsis or abscess related origins (Forbes 2001). The formation of a faecal fistula usually occurs following abdominal surgery, with 75–85% occurring in the post-operative period (Falconi & Pederzoli 2001).
  Fistulae can occur due to:

- surgery
  - poor technique
  - poor blood supply to the bowel ends

   o   tension on the sutures
   o   distal obstruction
   o   malnutrition
   o   sepsis
- Crohn's disease
- cancer
- irradiation damage
- diverticular disease
- trauma
   o   gunshot
   o   childbirth
   o   ingested foreign bodies.
         (Forbes & Myers 1996; Lloyd *et al.* 2006; Makhdoom *et al.* 2000)

Of all enterocutaneous fistulae 20–30% are associated with Crohn's disease (Keighley & Williams 1993). However, fistulation following surgery for Crohn's disease can often heal with conservative therapy.

Of patients with diverticular disease 2% will fistulate but it is found in 20% who have surgery (Sher *et al.* 1999). Only in very limited situations, such as for an infant with an imperforate anus, will there be a congenital enterocutaneous fistula. Medication, such as steroids, may also be associated with an increased risk of colonic fistulae (Keighley & Williams 1993).

Classification of enterocutaneous fistulae

There is no universally accepted classification of enterocutaneous fistulae; however, fistulae can be classified as simple, multiple or complex (Forbes 2001). The faecal output can also be used to classify fistulae.

Simple and complex enterocutaneous fistulae

A simple enterocutaneous fistula has a single bowel perforation without associated complications (see Figure 16.1). There may be a short tract from the enterotomy to the skin (Keighley & Williams 1993). Simple fistulae have a better prognosis and are more likely to heal spontaneously than complex enterocutaneous fistulae.

Complex fistulae (see Figure 16.2) include those in which there is complete disruption of the bowel and seepage into the surrounding areas (Forbes 2001). There may be long or multiple tracts and distal obstruction.

High- and low-output fistulae

A high-output fistula is defined as having an output of more than 500 ml daily (Blackley 1998). This differs from a high-output stoma where the output exceeds one litre daily. The high output is often due to reduced bowel length or ineffective absorption capabilities of the bowel, due to Crohn's disease or radiation damage. High-output fistulae generally have a worse prognosis and are less likely to heal spontaneously than those with low outputs (Keighley & Williams 1993).

A colonic fistula may be classified as a low faecal output and may pass 200–500 ml daily. Colonic fistulae may pass only flatus or minimal amounts

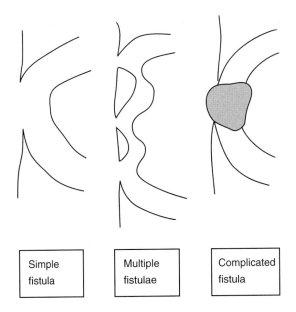

| Simple fistula | Multiple fistulae | Complicated fistula |

Figure 16.1   Types of enterocutaneous fistulae.

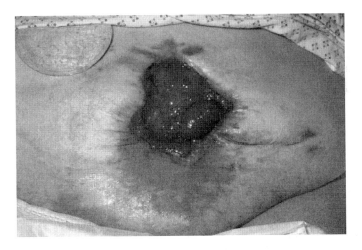

Figure 16.2   Complex enterocutaneous fistula.

of faeces, particularly if the majority of the bowel content is passed either via a stoma or rectally.

Post-operative and spontaneous fistulae

A post-operative fistula is most commonly due to an anastomotic leak. Factors that may affect the healing of an anastomosis are age, nutritional status, blood supply and intra-abdominal sepsis. Fistulae occurring after a stoma closure generally resolve spontaneously but drainage of an abscess may be required (Keighley & Williams 1993).

The diseases that are most likely to result in a spontaneous fistula are Crohn's disease, diverticular disease and colorectal cancer. Spontaneous fistulae associated with Crohn's disease are most likely to originate from the ileum and there is usually distal obstruction (Keighley & Williams 1993).

Signs and symptoms

Prior to a fistula formation there may be fever, colicky abdominal pain and localised erythema. This is followed by purulent discharge for a few days and finally faecal matter (Keighley & Williams 1993).

Imaging fistulae

To be able to plan treatment it is important to determine the anatomy of the enterocutaneous fistula. Thus imaging is required. Contrast studies such as computed tomography (CT) scans and magnetic resonance imaging (MRI) are most commonly used (Lloyd *et al.* 2006). CT scans are useful, but frequently fail to identify the fistulous opening. However, CT does demonstrate associated abscesses and retroperitoneal disease. MRI can show 75% of all fistulous orifices and can discriminate normal and abnormal tissue (Forbes & Myers 1996). Fistulograghy can also be crucial in fistula management to demonstrate any abnormal communications (Bartram & Halligan 1997). Fistulography is performed by catheterising the cutaneous opening and inserting a water-soluble contrast through the foley catheter. Barium should never be used to investigate fistulae of unknown origin, due to the risk of barium peritonitis if the fistula discharges inside the abdomen. Abdominal ultrasound can show abnormal areas and abscesses, but not usually the fistula tract. Abdominal x-rays are not particularly useful either, although they may demonstrate a fluid level within an abscess cavity.

It was previously thought to be important how much bowel was resected, but it is now realised that the length remaining is of consequence and this needs to be assessed to plan treatment.

Immediate management

Management for high output fistulae should focus on the correction of any fluids and electrolyte imbalances and abscess drainage (Forbes & Myers 1996). Aggressive treatment and prompt drainage of intra-abdominal collections can be performed under ultrasound or CT guidance (Lloyd *et al.* 2006). Fluid replacement may be in the form of oral supplements (such as electrolyte solution), subcutaneous (Forbes 2003) or intravenous fluids.

Fistula management

Other considerations are the patient's nutritional status, skin care and psychological support (Lloyd *et al.* 2006), as malnutrition may occur in the longer term (Nightingale 2001). Surgery should not be an initial consideration except in life-threatening situations. The area of fistulated bowel will dictate the treatment required. It is important to realise that a bowel disrupted by a fistula will only absorb fluids and nutrients to the point of exit from the body. However in some cases feeding by fistuloclysis is possible.

Patients with a distal enterocutaneous fistula may be suitable for enteral feeding and have adequate absorption. However, patients with proximal enterocutaneous fistulae may need to be nil by mouth initially (Nightingale 2003). For a very short bowel, with a length before the fistulae or stoma of less than 100 cm of small bowel, parenteral nutrition is usually required (Nightingale *et al.* 1992). Parenteral nutrition is required if patients are unable to obtain sufficient nutrition from their diet, but if possible enteral feeding is preferred (Forbes 2007). Care is the same as for patients with intestinal failure. Even if parenteral nutrition is required it is often beneficial to eat, as this maintains a healthy gut lining (Forbes 1997). The type of diet that is usually advisable for this patient group is high calorie and salt, but low fibre. Fibre may block the fistula appliance; therefore care must be taken to ensure that the patient chews their food thoroughly.

High faecal outputs can result in rapid dehydration, reduced circulating blood volume, oliguria, electrolyte imbalance, acidosis and severe skin excoriation around the fistula. Ideally urine output should be at least 800 ml daily (Nightingale & Woodward 2006).

Long-term use of intravenous fluids or parenteral nutrition should be given via a dedicated feeding line to help to reduce the risk of infection. An intravenous infusion may be useful to replace the essential elements lost via the fistula. Parenteral nutrition is required if energy is also required via the parenteral route. Patients may be able to cope simply on subcutaneous fluids, generally overnight, on a daily basis or less frequently. This reduces some of the risks associated by intravenous methods. However, the area used to give the subcutaneous fluids, for example the thigh or abdomen, can remain oedematous with the fluid for a period of time. It has also been noticed that the time taken for the fluids to be absorbed into the body depends on the level of dehydration and is quicker if the patient is dehydrated.

An accurate fluid balance and monitoring of blood results can assist the clinician in planning the patient's care (Phillips & Walton 1992). Dehydration can be seen by a sudden weight reduction. Reduction of a high faecal output is ideal and often achieved with medication or fluid restriction. Medication such as loperamide, codeine phosphate or proton pump inhibitors may be necessary (Small 2003a).

Spontaneous fistula closure

About half of uncomplicated post-operative fistulae heal spontaneously (Anderson 1998) and closure is usually within six weeks of the fistula opening. The chances of spontaneous healing are increased if the fistula occurs following surgery and there is no distal obstruction. The rates of spontaneous fistula closure in studies are very varied as patient groups are different. A study by Hollington *et al.* (2004) found that the spontaneous closure rate was about 20%.

There are a number of factors that adversely affect the chances of spontaneous fistula closure:

- high faecal output
- spontaneous fistulation
- sepsis
- distal obstruction
- complex fistula
- co-morbidity
- colorectal cancer
- radiation enteritis
- Crohn's disease
- discontinuity of the bowel.
                    (Lloyd *et al.* 2006)

Surgical management

Fistulae that do not heal spontaneously may require surgical intervention. If a fistula occurs within ten days of surgery, the fistula can be defunctioned with a stoma. This is achieved by diverting the faecal path proximal to the fistula (Carlson 2003). Some surgeons at this stage may resect the fistula or there may be spontaneous closure, after the fistula is defunctioned.

If the fistula occurs more than ten days after surgery it can be dangerous to re-enter the peritoneal cavity due to the dense adhesions and the risk of multiple enterotomies. The adhesions are generally most dense between three weeks and three months after the surgery (Lloyd *et al.* 2006). To improve surgical results it is usually advisable to wait a minimum of three months, but some surgeons prefer to delay surgery until six months to a year following the last operation. This allows the body time to strengthen. Surgical repair is less likely to be effective if there is diseased bowel, such as Crohn's disease. For low-output Crohn's disease related fistulae where surgery is contraindicated, drugs such as azathioprine and ciclosporin may assist in fistula closure (Strong 1997). In some situations it is not possible to undertake a surgical repair, due to co-morbidity for example, and some people learn to live with and manage their fistula successfully.

Morbidity and mortality

There are a number of factors that may affect the survival rates of a patient with a fistula:

- malignancy
- radiotherapy
- high fluid losses
- electrolyte imbalance
- sepsis

- malnutrition
- intestinal ischaemia.
    (Nightingale 2001)

Sepsis is the most common reason for death in the early stages of an intestinal fistulation. Sepsis increases the risk of thromboembolism and respiratory failure (Keighley & Williams 1993). The highest mortality rates are associated with malignancy or radiotherapy, but these are very rare (Anderson 1998). Mortality also increases in patients over 65 years. However, there may be a good prognosis for colonic fistulae, if there is no ischaemia.

Mortality in the past was very high but appears to be decreasing as experience is gained in the management of fistulae. This may be due to a number of factors, such as parenteral nutrition (Falconi & Pederzoli 2001), control of sepsis or prompt replacement of fluids and electrolytes. Mortality rates vary from about 5% (McIntyre *et al.* 1984) up to a third (Lloyd *et al.* 2006).

Unless sepsis is eradicated by early drainage there is a high risk of continued malnutrition, leading to organ failure and thromboembolism that may be fatal (Keighley & Williams 1993). Other morbidity could be seen as bleeding gums, candidiasis, loss of hair, malnutrition, depression, excoriated skin, immobility, isolation from family and friends and possible financial problems. A multidisciplinary team approach can help to alleviate the patients' problems related to a long hospitalisation.

Fistula appliances

In the past fistulae were managed with the use of dressings: these held the bowel content in contact with the skin, causing excoriation. A fistula appliance (see Figure 16.3) is useful to collect the fistula output, which can then be used to calculate the fluid requirements required (Burch & Buchan 2004) and prevents skin excoriation. Skin integrity can be maintained by careful application of an appropriate stoma or fistula appliance (Burch 2003). The appliance will also contain the faecal odour (Benbow & Losson 2002), an important issue to patients. Containment of the faeces and/or urine passed from the fistula can be difficult (Benbow 2001), due to the unpredictable positions in which fistulae can occur and the potential corrosive nature of the output. Thus skin care is of the utmost importance.

There are a variety of fistula appliances available (Benbow 2001). To determine which appliance would be the most suitable the fistula requires assessing for size and output. It would seem logical that having faeces on the wound that surrounds the fistula would lead to infection and erosion of the wound (Meuleneire 2003) but this has not been the author's experience and granulation at the base of the wound does occur.

Continual suction (Westrate 1996) has also been used to prevent excoriated skin, but this restricts the patient's mobility (Kordasiewicz 2004). This is the principle of the VAC dressings (Benbow 2006). VAC therapy is controversial, but some consider it useful for fistula care (Wild *et al.* 2007), whereas others consider it may lead to fistulation when used on abdominal

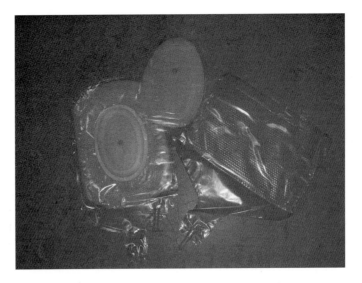

Figure 16.3 Fistula appliances.

wounds (Rao *et al.* 2007). This has been used on fistulae as well as highly exudating wounds, but use remains experimental.

Low-output fistula appliances

If the output from the fistula is very low or simply flatus and the skin opening is small, a dressing may be appropriate. However, due to the risk of excoriation a skin protector is required, such as wipes/sprays or a non-absorbent dressing, for example a protective wafer can be used around the fistula and dressings used on top of this. However the use of an ileostomy bag may be more appropriate for a drain site for example (Burch 2004). An ileostomy appliance allows containment and monitoring of the fistula output and can be useful for small, low-output fistulae.

If the output is low but the fistula is within a large dehisced wound, a dressing may still be appropriate. A wound/fistula manager from one of the various manufacturers may be useful for outputs of a few hundred millilitres.

High-output fistula appliances

For high output from a small skin opening a urostomy appliance can be used to contain the faeces. If the output is over one litre, connecting a night drainage bag (those used in conjunction with a urinary catheter) can be beneficial. Connecting extra drainage capacity can reduce the strain on the appliance and eliminates the need for frequent appliance emptying. If the output is too thick to pass through a urostomy appliance a high-output appliance or ileostomy bag may be suitable: often as the output thickens the volume also reduces. If the output is below one litre daily an ileostomy appliance is usually effective.

If there is a high output and a large wound one of the fistula appliances may be required. A higher faecal output is more likely to cause excoriated skin, so careful fistula bag application is required as well as meticulous skin care.

Application of a fistula appliance

A practical guide for using a fistula appliance:

- Collect the required equipment; this may include warm tap water, cleaning cloths (kitchen roll can be useful in the community), rubbish bag and appliance. Additional equipment may include skin protector wipes, paste, seals, suction machine, hairdryer and/or air freshener.
- Gently remove the old appliance.
- Carefully clean the skin around the fistula with warm tap water (there is no need for sterile water as the faeces touching the wound is not sterile).
- Carefully dry the skin around the fistula.
- Assess the skin integrity.
- If the skin is intact no action needs to be taken.
- If the skin is broken and oozing it may be useful to leave the wound open to the air for a while (preparation of the appliance can be performed in this time). Some patients leave the skin to dry in the air for 20 minutes to one hour and no infections have been noted by the author with this method of care.
- If after leaving the fistula open to the air there is still oozing skin, a small amount of stoma powder may be useful. This should be applied sparingly and dusted off for best effect.
- If the skin is damp or very oozy then a cool hairdryer may be used to dry the skin. There are no studies to support the use of a hairdryer, but the author and others have used this with good results. Care must be taken not to burn the skin and the hairdryer should be kept moving and not be positioned too close to the skin. Up to five minutes is usually adequate, but if the skin dries with the hairdryer and then becomes wet again quickly repeated use may be required. Up to three repetitions will dry most excoriated skin.
- Measure and record the wound size; a template can be made for future appliance changes (the backing of the fistula appliance can be kept and dated for subsequence usage).
- If skin protection is required, apply it.
- If further skin protection is necessary the use of seals to border the wound edges can be useful; this is often necessary when the fistula output is corrosive.
- If the skin is uneven the use of a stoma paste (Frost 1991) or seals may be required. Paste is useful in very shallow dips, but most contain alcohol, which will sting (for about 30–60 seconds) if used on broken

skin, so the patient needs to be aware of this. If there are deeper creases then using a small amount of seal, strip paste or similar may be useful. The aim of paste and seals is to provide a level surface upon which to place the appliance. However, paste takes a while to 'dry' and therefore needs to be used sparingly, as the more paste that is used the longer the drying time and the longer the patient will need to be confined to bed following the appliance change. Even for the biggest fistula no more than half a tube should be used per appliance.

- Once the surface around the fistula is level, the hole in the appliance can be cut, usually about two or three millimetres larger than the wound and to the shape of the wound.
- Remove the appliance backing and apply a thin line of paste to the inner edge of the appliance to further help with adhesion.
- The appliance should be carefully placed around the fistula, onto the skin (or seals).
- Gently but firmly press the inner edges down, working to the outer edges of the appliance. Hold the appliance, or ask the patient to hold the appliance for several minutes to aid adhesion. Pay particular attention to any areas that are prone to leaks.
- Ask the patient to rest on the bed for 45 minutes to one hour and keep the appliance still and flat.
- Ideally the patient should not eat or drink immediately prior to the appliance change, to reduce the amount of faeces being passed during the change procedure. It is also useful not to eat or drink for one hour following the change, as some fistulae will pass the oral intake quickly and if the appliance is not completely adhered there may be seepage under the appliance reducing the wear time and potentially causing skin excoriation.
- Some patients have reported that if a small leak occurs, cleaning the tract that the leakage has formed, to remove any bowel motion, and then using paste to re-stick the edges can be useful, if the appliance is newly applied.
- *Note*: Tape should never be used to secure a leaking appliance (unless for a very short time in an emergency situation and then perform an appliance change as soon as possible) as this holds the faeces to the skin and will potentially cause excoriation.

It may take some time to establish the best plan of care that is effective for a particular patient and the patient needs to be informed of this. An appliance should ideally be left on for two days up to a maximum of one week but replaced sooner if leakage occurs. A good plan of care is to establish how long an appliance lasts and change the appliance according to each patient's own 'wear time' which is often preferable to waiting until it leaks. This can help increase the patient's confidence in the fistula appliance, allows planning to be made and prevents excoriation. The digestive enzymes in the faecal matter may cause severe alkaline burns to the skin (Moore 2002) within three to four hours (Meadows 1997). Excoriated skin is painful and the appliance does not adhere as well to wet, broken skin as to intact skin, potentially leading to further leaks.

Other issues

There are a number of issues that may affect a patient with an enterocutaneous fistula. While the patient is in the hospital situation they may be isolated from their family and friends for a long period of time. On discharge home, which may be possible prior to a surgical repair, there should be multidisciplinary team involvement, including the GP and community nurses.

Intestinal failure

Intestinal failure and short bowel syndrome are used synonymously. However there are subtle differences between the two. Short bowel syndrome is encompassed within the definition of intestinal failure. One definition of intestinal failure can be seen as reduced intestinal absorption so that macronutrients and/or water and electrolyte supplementation are required to maintain health (Nightingale 2003). This means that there is only a short length of bowel, or an adequate bowel length but a poor absorptive function. Severe intestinal failure requires parenteral nutrition and possibly additional fluids, whereas mild intestinal failure will require oral supplements or dietary manipulation.

Short bowel, as its name suggests, is a physically shortened length of bowel. Short bowel syndrome is rare with an incidence of less than one case per 100 000 of the population in the UK and an incidence of one case per 1 000 000 (Forbes 2003).

Intestinal failure can also be classified as acute (temporary) and chronic. Acute intestinal failure is potentially reversible and the most commonly seen intestinal failure. More than 90% of patients with severe intestinal failure are within the peri-operative period (Kennedy *et al.* 2002). Chronic intestinal failure tends to be associated with a short bowel and is less common. Another description of patients with intestinal failure is net secretors or net absorbers. Net secretors often have less than 100 cm of small bowel, with a faecal output of more than the oral intake. This leads to a negative fluid and sodium balance and requires parenteral nutrition (Nightingale 2003). Net absorbers conversely tend to have one to two metres of jejunum and a positive fluid and sodium balance and can generally manage with a strict oral therapy. In critically ill patients in the intensive care setting, it is critical to provide nutrition and enteral is preferred to parenteral, if possible (Kutayli *et al.* 2005).

Signs and symptoms of intestinal failure

The signs and symptoms of short bowel syndrome include:

- electrolyte imbalance
- dehydration
- deficiencies in:
  - calcium
  - magnesium

- o   zinc
- o   iron
- o   vitamin B_{12}
- o   fat soluble vitamin deficiency
- malabsorption of:
  - o   carbohydrates
  - o   lactose
  - o   protein
- gastric acid hypersecretion
- formation of cholesterol biliary calculi and renal oxalate calculi
- steatorrhoea (oily, malodorous faeces)
- diarrhoea
- weight loss.
            (Nightingale & Woodward 2006; Sundaram *et al.* 2002)

Causes of intestinal failure

Intestinal failure may be the result of large resections of the bowel or a disease process such as Crohn's disease. Patients with intestinal failure generally fall into one of three groups, i.e. patients with:

- stoma
- enterocutaneous fistula
- enterocolic anastomosis.
            (Small 2003b)

The most common causes of chronic intestinal failure are:

- Crohn's disease
- bowel infarct resulting in extensive bowel resection
- radiation damage
- bowel motility disorders
  - o   pseudo-obstruction
  - o   scleroderma.
            (Sundaram *et al.* 2002; Wood 1996)

Treatment of intestinal failure

The aims of intestinal failure management are to:

- provide nutrition, fluids and electrolytes;
- reduce the severity of the intestinal failure;
- prevent and treat any complications;
- try and achieve a good quality of life;
- reduce gut secretions;
- slow intestinal transit.
            (Forbes 2003; Nightingale 2003)

Treatment for intestinal failure can range from parenteral nutrition given daily, to infusions three times weekly or daily fluids without nutrients.

Some patients require no additional intravenous fluids (Forbes 2003). Patients with intestinal failure can reduce water and electrolyte losses by careful fluid balance management and appropriate drug use (Nightingale 2003).

Thorough assessment and nutritional management is required to achieve optimum outcomes. Parenteral or total parenteral nutrition is required in the early stages, as is replacement of electrolytes and fluids lost (Sundaram *et al.* 2002).

To establish hydration the patient is initially kept nil by mouth and given intravenous saline, sometimes with additional magnesium. Monitoring of serum magnesium and urine sodium concentrations should be undertaken (Nightingale 2003); however, the latter test is of no value to patients with renal failure (Forbes 2003). It is also advised to add salt to meals (Forbes 2001).

Treatment for the patient with a jejunostomy or high-output fistula will include oral rehydration solution and a restriction of oral hypotonic fluids, such as water or tea, that contain no sodium (Small 2003a) often limited to 500 to 1000 ml (Forbes 2001). However it can be difficult to cope with the fluid restrictions and the extreme thirst (Small 2003b) which may lead to patients not complying with the restrictions. It is important to reinforce the importance to patients as non-compliance can lead to electrolyte imbalance and death in extreme cases.

Compliance with oral fluid restriction is often difficult for patients to understand, particularly when they feel thirsty, and explaining it to the patient can assist comprehension (Forbes 2003). It seems illogical but fluid is restricted because the first part of the small bowel is designed to have a luminal sodium concentration of about 90 mmol. If oral hypotonic fluids are taken that contain no sodium, the body recognises a drop in the sodium levels. To correct this, sodium and fluids are transferred from the body into the bowel. For those with an intact bowel this additional sodium and fluid are reabsorbed further along the gastrointestinal tract and pose no problem. For those with a short bowel this sodium is potentially lost via a fistula or stoma for example. This can lead to two potential complications, firstly an electrolyte imbalance resulting from the loss of sodium but also a loss of fluid. Thus it is possible to drink a small amount of fluid and subsequently pass more than was consumed.

To alleviate this problem a rehydration solution can be taken, often one litre daily. Preparations are available at the chemist, which can be useful for those without intestinal failure for holiday diarrhoea, for example dioralyte. A stronger concentration is described by the World Health Organisation, which has been modified for the intestinal failure patient to:

- one litre of tap water
- 3.5 g sodium chloride
- 20 g glucose
- 2.5 g sodium bicarbonate.
            (Small 2003b)

Ideally the best way to take rehydration solution is to sip it throughout the day. This solution is anecdotally more palatable if the drink is kept cold or a small amount of juice is added (Forbes 2003). Some patients have reported that when they are very dehydrated the solution tastes better than when they are well hydrated.

Medications in intestinal failure

There are a number of medications that may potentially be useful for treating patients with intestinal failure. It is important to remember that the jejunum does not absorb bile salts or vitamin B_{12} and supplementation will be necessary if the ileum has been removed (Nightingale 2003). There are a variety of drugs that can be useful for patients with intestinal failure. Those used will depend upon the section of bowel removed. For example, small bowel resections often lead to increased incidence of peptic ulcer disease, thus the use of H_2 receptor blockers and proton pump inhibitors such as omeprazole can be beneficial to regulate gastric acid production and can also reduce diarrhoea. However, octreotide is less useful than would be expected, as fewer than 5% of patients gain prolonged benefit of reduction in secretions (Forbes 2003). Metronidazole can be taken to effectively treat bacterial overgrowth (Sundaram *et al.* 2002).

Loperamide and codeine phosphate can be used to slow bowel transit and these are often used in higher than normal levels, up to 64 mg of loperamide and 480 mg of codeine phosphate daily (Forbes 2003). These high doses are only used in patients with a very short bowel when lower doses have failed and under careful supervision. Loperamide is ideally taken before meals and before bed. It is suggested that for best effects loperamide should be taken 30–60 minutes prior to food (Forbes 2001). Liquid and syrup forms of loperamide are not generally advised, as they have a high sugar content that can increase the faecal output. However, if capsules or tablets pass in the stoma bag they can be opened or crushed. Anti-secretory drugs can be effective if stomal outputs exceed intake (Nightingale 2003).

A number of tips may help those with intestinal failure. Regular oral intake of food should be encouraged, little and often is generally best. Separation of fluids and solid foods tends to reduce faecal output. Although some foods may cause problems and should be avoided, this can vary between patients and there are no foods that must be excluded in all patients, although a high-energy diet is ideal. Fatty diets may be problematic for those with colon and cause steatorrhoea (Forbes 2003). Oral supplementation may be useful or a polymeric diet may be required given by tube feeding such as nasogastric or gastrostomy.

In summary enteral therapy for patients with intestinal failure is to:

- limit hypotonic fluids to 500 ml daily;
- take oral rehydration solution;
- use antisecretion drugs;
- encourage oral feeding;
- consider additional feeding;
- consider additional supplements.

(Forbes 2003)

Complications associated with intestinal failure

The reduced absorptive surface area leads to rapid transit of the intestinal contents through the gastrointestinal tract and prognosis will depend upon the length of bowel that remains. Most nutrients are absorbed in the first 100–150 cm of the small bowel. Some areas are more efficient than others at absorption and other sections of bowel specifically absorb certain nutrients, for example, the terminal ileum absorbs vitamin B_{12}. Therefore, if specific areas are resected this may alter the patient's ability to absorb certain nutrients. If the duodenum is removed there may be dumping syndrome, where there is less control over the stomach emptying into the bowel. If the jejunum is resected the jejunal secretions are altered, including the gastric inhibitory peptide. This can lead to increased gastric secretions and may potentially adversely affect protein and lipid digestion (Thibodeau & Patton 2007). This and other factors can compound the diarrhoea associated with intestinal failure. Those with a jejunostomy absorb less than 35% of the energy available from their diet (Sundaram *et al.* 2002). Ileal resections can also alter transit through the stomach and proximal small bowel. Bacterial overgrowth can cause malabsorption (Sundaram *et al.* 2002).

If there is more than 100 cm of small bowel to the jejunostomy, this will allow most jejunostomates to survive without parenteral nutrition and its associated risks (Nightingale 2003).

All patients with short bowel tend to develop gallstones and require cholecystectomy within two years following extensive intestinal resection (Sundaram *et al.* 2002). Steatorrhoea leads to a deficiency in fat-soluble vitamins that can lead to night blindness (lack of vitamin A), osteomalacia (softening of the bones due to lack of vitamin D) and bleeding (vitamin K deficiency).

The presence of a colon can be beneficial but can also cause several problems, including diarrhoea and formation of calcium oxalate renal stones (Sundaram *et al.* 2002). It has been found that 25% of adults with less than 200 cm of jejunum anastomosed to the colon develop symptomatic renal stones (Nightingale *et al.* 1992). There is an advice leaflet available called *Intestinal Failure (IF) – Understanding IF* (see www.stmarkshospital. org.uk).

Bowel adaptation

It has been found that the bowel can adapt for up to two years following resection. This adaptation can include increased mucosal surface area through enterocyte hyperplasia (Sundaram *et al.* 2002). The colon can also adapt if it is present and can convert unabsorbed carbohydrates into absorbable short chain fatty acids, partially as a result of changes in the colonic bacteria.

Future options for intestinal failure

Potential treatment in the future may include drugs that might be useful to promote intestinal adaptation (Lloyd *et al.* 2006). Future surgical options that have a limited use currently include reversal of bowel segments but this remains controversial (Carlson 2003). Another option for patients with intestinal failure is bowel transplantation. However mortality is currently high (at one year it is 25%) and therefore home long-term parenteral nutrition is preferable (Forbes 2003).

Parenteral nutrition (PN)

Parenteral nutrition is feeding not via the enteral route, such as intravenously. The decision to give parenteral nutrition is not taken lightly due to the risks associated with this method of feeding, with the most serious being sepsis that has led to death (Forbes 2007).

Parenteral nutrition is specifically made for each patient to include their prescription of calories and other dietary requirements. Parenteral nutrition is infused under the control of a pump often over 12–16 hours at night and the nurse or patient needs to care for the line aseptically to prevent infection. Parenteral nutrition needs to be refrigerated prior to use, which can make travel problematic for patients who require home parenteral nutrition. However, it is possible, with careful planning, for patients to travel abroad. Parenteral nutrition is often incorrectly named TPN (total parenteral nutrition) (Kitchen & Forbes 1999). TPN is actually when a patient gains all their fluid and dietary requirements from the parenteral nutrition, however most patients are also able to eat.

Parenteral nutrition is likely to be required long term for patients with:

- very short bowel (less than 80 cm ending in a stoma or less than 50 cm of small bowel anastomosed to colon);
- a proximal fistula;
- outputs greater than 1.5 litres daily, despite full drug therapy;
- patients with intestinal failure who have pain with eating.

(Forbes 2003)

Parenteral nutrition should ideally be used in conjunction with enteral feeding and this should be commenced as soon as possible to allow bowel adaptation to occur (Sundaram *et al.* 2002). If no enteral nutrients are taken there can be atrophy of the bowel mucosa, which will decrease absorption when oral feeding is recommenced.

There are several complications associated with parenteral nutrition. The cost of parenteral nutrition is high and funding needs to be agreed with the patient's PCT (primary care trust). However, risks are significant, with a survival rate of patients requiring parenteral nutrition at three years of 70% (Nightingale 1999). For patients that require lifelong parenteral nutrition it is ideal for the patient to be taught how to provide the parenteral nutrition and other aspects of its care, although home care nurses can give the feed to those that are unable to be independent (Davidson 2005). It is also possible that there will be hospital admissions to treat line infections.

There are a number of other problems that may be encountered when using parenteral nutrition. Sepsis is the most common long-term problem that is prevented by using sterile procedures when connecting and disconnecting the feed. Other potential problems include refeeding syndrome, rebound hypoglycaemia, fluid overload, hyperglycaemia and an electrolyte imbalance.

Refeeding syndrome

Refeeding syndrome can lead to severe and potentially life-threatening electrolyte fluctuations that can cause metabolic, neuromuscular and haematological problems. Refeeding syndrome can occur as a result of the body of those with malnutrition attempting to use the energy from the artificial nutritional support (Duncan & Silk 2001). As a preventative method, when patients with malnutrition start parenteral feed their electrolyte and fluid levels are regularly monitored. Initially feeds require very careful prescription and review by a specialist multidisciplinary team. Refeeding syndrome may also occur in patients that are enterally fed (Bloch & Mueller 2000).

Rebound hypoglycaemia

Rebound hypoglycaemia can occur once the parenteral feed infusion is completed as a result of changes in insulin levels. This can be prevented by tapering the infusion rate before stopping the infusion (Thomas 2001).

Fistuloclysis

Fistuloclysis is a relatively new concept of feeding patients with an enterocutaneous fistula. While the idea is good, the management can be difficult. Early attempts to infuse directly into the fistula were to re-infuse the effluent passed from the proximal limb of the fistula. However, this method proved unpopular and has evolved to fistuloclysis with polymeric feed. Fistuloclysis can be defined as the insertion of feed into the distal opening of the enterocutaneous fistula to provide nutritional benefit and to improve/maintain gut integrity. However this is only effective if there is 75 cm or more of healthy bowel length distal to the fistula (Carlson 2003). Fistuloclysis is only suitable to those who have been proved by investigation to have no internal openings of the bowel into the abdominal cavity, as internal leakage of the feed would lead to sepsis. A nasogastric feed is inserted into the distal bowel via a catheter (Sathyanarayana *et al.* 2005). The body produces waste as it processes this feed, which will exit the body via a stoma or anus. Fistuloclysis can in a select group of patients prevent the need for parenteral nutrition (Teubner *et al.* 2004).

There are, however, a number of problems that may be encountered with fistuloclysis, such as abdominal bloating. In order to prevent this, it is advised to slowly increase the infusion rate. Alternatively the feeding tube can fall out. This may be as a result of the inflated catheter balloon becoming dislodged by the peristalsis action of the bowel and is difficult to resolve. Conversely a rare complication has been reported, where the peristaltic activity has pulled the entire feeding catheter into the bowel, which in one situation required surgical removal (Mettu 2004). It is therefore essential to carefully secure the catheter into position. The distal output will increase once feed is commenced, which can initially lead to management problems. However, loperamide can be used with effect when inserted directly into the fistuloclysis tube prior to the feed. Another potential problem may be that the feed can backtrack into the fistula appliance, thus not effectively providing nutrition and causing management problems. This is usually resolved by slowing the feed down. One of the most problematic issues related to fistuloclysis is passing the feeding tube through the appliance without causing leakage. Specialised equipment is available which can resolve this problem. Details of this and the instructions on fistuloclysis are provided in a booklet by Farrer & Teubner (2003).

Conclusion

Caring for patients with enterocutaneous fistulae and intestinal failure is an ongoing challenge to the multidisciplinary team. There have, however, been some improvements in patient care, with the use of parenteral nutrition. However, mortality and morbidity rates are high and living with a fistula and/or intestinal failure is difficult, requiring care and support from the multidisciplinary team to make the necessary life changes.

References

Anderson KN (1998) *Mosby's Medical and Nursing Dictionary*. 5th edn. London: Mosby-Year Book Inc.

Bartram CI & Halligan S (1997) Imaging. In: Nicholls RJ & Dozois RR (eds) *Surgery of the Colon and Rectum*. London: Churchill Livingstone.

Benbow M (2001) The use of wound drainage bags for complex wounds. *British Journal of Nursing*. **10(19)**: 1298–301.

Benbow M (2006) An update on VAC therapy. *Journal of Community Nursing*. **20(4)**: 28–32.

Benbow M & Losson G (2002) Fistula management following appendectomy: nursing challenges. *Journal of Wound Care*. **11(2)**: 59–61.

Blackley P (1998) *Practical Stoma, Wound and Continence Management*. Australia: Research Publications Pty Ltd.

Bloch AS & Mueller C (2000) Enteral and parenteral nutrition support. In: Mahan LK & Escott-Stump S (eds) *Krause's Food, Nutrition and Diet Therapy*. 10th edn. Pennsylvania: W.B. Saunders.

Burch J (2003) The nursing care of a patient with enterocutaneous fistulae. *British Journal of Nursing*. **12(12)**: 736–40.

Burch J (2004) Priorities in nursing management of fistulas in a community setting. *British Journal of Community Nursing*. 9(6 supplement): S6–S14.

Burch J & Buchan D (2004) Support and guidance for intestinal failure and enterocutaneous fistula care. *Gastrointestinal Nursing*. **2(7)**: 25–32.

Carlson GL (2003) Surgical management of intestinal failure. *Proceedings of the Nutrition Society*. **62(3)**: 711–18.

Davidson A (2005) Management and effects of parenteral nutrition. *Nursing Times*. **101(42)**: 28–31.

Duncan HD & Silk DBA (2001) Enteral feeding. In: Nightingale JMD (ed) *Intestinal Failure*. London: Greenwich Medical Media Ltd.

Falconi M & Pederzoli P (2001) The relevance of gastrointestinal fistulae in clinical practice: a review. *Gut.* **49**(supplement IV): iv2–iv10.

Farrer K & Teubner A (2003) *Fistuloclysis Distal Feeding: Information and Guidance for Patients and Health Care Professionals.* Manchester: Salford Royal Hospital.

Forbes A (1997) *Clinician's Guide to Inflammatory Bowel Disease.* London: Chapman & Hall.

Forbes A (2001) *Inflammatory Bowel Disease: A Clinician's Guide.* 2nd edn. London: Arnold.

Forbes A (2003) Intestinal failure and short bowel syndrome. *Medicine.* **31**(3): 98–100.

Forbes A (2007) Parenteral nutrition. *Current Opinions in Gastroenterology.* **23**: 183–6.

Forbes A & Myers C (1996) Enterocutaneous fistulae. In: Myers C (ed) *Stoma Care Nursing: A Patient-Centred Approach.* London: Arnold.

Frost S (1991) Managing high output fistulas. *Nursing Standard.* **11**(51): 25–7.

Hollington P, Mawdsley J, Lim W, Gabe SM, Forbes A *et al.* (2004) An 11-year experience of enterocutaneous fistula. *British Journal of Surgery.* **91**: 1646–51.

Keighley MRB & Williams NS (1993) *Surgery of the Anus, Rectum and Colon.* Vol. 2. London: W.B. Saunders.

Kennedy JF, Baker ML & Nightingale JMD (2002) Appropriate parenteral nutrition – the role of the hospital nutrition support team. *Clinical Nutrition.* **21**(suppl 1): 35.

Kitchen P & Forbes A (1999) Parenteral nutrition. *Current Opinions in Gastroenterology.* **15**(2): 167–75.

Kordasiewicz LM (2004) Abdominal wound with a fistula and large amount of drainage status after incarcerated hernia repair. *Journal of Wound and Ostomy Nursing.* **31**(3): 150–3.

Kutayli ZN, Domingo CB & Steinberg SM (2005) Intestinal failure. *Current Opinions in Anaesthesiology.* **18**(2): 123–7.

Lloyd DAJ, Gabe SM & Windsor ACJ (2006) Nutrition and management of enterocutaneous fistula. *British Journal of Surgery.* **93**: 1045–55.

McIntyre PB, Ritchie JK, Hawley PR, Bertram CI & Lennard-Jones JE (1984) Management of enterocutaneous fistulas; a review of 132 cases. *British Journal of Surgery.* **71**: 293–6.

Makhdoom ZA, Komar MJ & Still CD (2000) Nutrition and enterocutaneous fistulas. *Journal of Clinical Gastroenterology.* **31**(2): 195–204.

Meadows C (1997) Stoma and fistula care. In: Bruce L & Finlay TMD (eds) *Nursing in Gastroenterology.* London: Churchill Livingstone.

Mettu SR (2004) Fistuloclysis can successfully replace parenteral feeding in the nutritional support of patients with enterocutaneous fistula – correspondence. *British Journal of Surgery.* **91**(9): 1203.

Meuleneire F (2003) Enterocutaneous fistulas following oncological surgery: a challenge for nurses. ECET congress München poster presentation.

Moore S (2002) Practical issues in the management of patients with a jejunostomy. *World Council of Enterostomal Therapists Journal.* **22**(2): 39–41.

Nightingale JMD (1999) Management of patients with a short bowel. *Nutrition.* **15**: 633–7.

Nightingale JMD (2001) The short bowel. In: Nightingale J (ed) *Intestinal Failure.* London: Greenwich Medical Media.

Nightingale JMD (2003) The medical management of intestinal failure: methods to reduce the severity. *Proceedings of the Nutrition Society.* **62**(3): 703–10.

Nightingale JMD & Woodward JM (2006) Guidelines for management of patients with a short bowel. *Gut.* **55**(suppl IV): iv1–iv12.

Nightingale JMD, Lennard-Jones JE, Gertner DJ, Wood SR & Bartram CI (1992) Colonic preservation reduces need for parenteral therapy, increases incidence of renal stones, but does not change high prevalence of gall stones in patients with a short bowel. *Gut.* **33**: 1493–7.

Phillips J & Walton M (1992) Caring for patients with enterocutaneous fistulae. *British Journal of Nursing.* **1(10)**: 496–500.

Rao M, Burke D, Finan PJ & Sagar PM (2007) The use of vacuum-assisted closure of abdominal wounds: a word of caution. *Colorectal Diseases.* **9(3)**: 266–8.

Sathyanarayana N, Shenoy KR, Alvares JF & Pai SB (2005) Enteral feeding by fistuloclysis in a midjejunal fistula. *Indian Journal of Gastroenterology.* **24(3)**: 124–5.

Sher ME, Cheney L & Ricciardi J (1999) Diverticular disease. In: Porrett T & Daniel N (eds) *Essential Coloproctology for Nurses.* London: Whurr.

Small M (2003a) Management of intestinal failure. *Nursing Times.* **99(3)**: 52–3.

Small M (2003b) Living with intestinal failure. *Nursing Times.* **99(3)**: 54.

Strong SA (1997) Crohn's disease. In: Nicholls RJ & Dozois RR (eds) *Surgery of the Colon and Rectum.* London: Churchill Livingstone.

Sundaram A, Koutkia P & Apovian C (2002) Nutritional management of short bowel syndrome in adults. *Journal of Clinical Gastroenterology.* **34(3)**: 207–20.

Teubner A, Morrison K, Ravishankar HR, Anderson ID, Scott NA *et al.* (2004) Fistuloclysis can successfully replace parenteral feeding in the nutritional support of patients with enterocutaneous fistula. *British Journal of Surgery.* **91(5)**: 625–31.

Thibodeau GA & Patton KT (2007) *Anatomy and Physiology.* 6th edn. Missouri: Mosby Elsevier.

Thomas B (2001) *Manual of Dietetic Practice.* 3rd edn. Oxford: Blackwell Science.

Westrate JTM (1996) Care of the open wound in abdominal sepsis. *Journal of Wound Care.* **5(7)**: 325–8.

Wild T, Goetzinger P & Telekey B (2007) VAC and fistula formation. *Colorectal Disease.* **9(6)**: 572–6.

Wood S (1996) Nutrition and the short bowel syndrome. In: Myers C (ed) *Stoma Care Nursing: A Patient-Centred Approach.* London: Arnold.

Chapter 17

Bowel Irrigation

Jennie Burch and Julie Duncan

Introduction

Irrigation is becoming an increasingly used form of management for bowel dysfunction, such as chronic faecal incontinence, constipation or neurological bowel disorders. It can also be useful in colostomy management, in providing a more predictable and controllable faecal output. In this chapter we will provide an overview of various irrigation methods, namely rectal, colonic and colostomy irrigation as well as antegrade colonic enema (ACE) and percutaneous endoscopic colostomy (PEC). We aim to provide a practical guide for all the forms of irrigation.

Rectal irrigation

In recent years rectal irrigation has been increasingly used in the management of chronic constipation and faecal incontinence in patients refractory to other conservative measures. Irrigation is performed retrogradely via the rectum and has been shown to be an effective bowel management tool in patients with a range of underlying conditions including spinal injuries, spina bifida and functional bowel problems. Rectal irrigation has been used less commonly in the United Kingdom (UK) due to a lack of purpose-designed equipment. Recently Coloplast Ltd has introduced such a kit and it can be envisaged that irrigation will become more commonplace.

The new kit, available on prescription, encompasses a rectal catheter with a balloon to keep the catheter in place, an infusion bag and pump to instil the fluid. Irrigation takes place sitting on the toilet. According to the literature most people will irrigate with tepid tap water though laxatives may be added if necessary. Volumes will range from 300 to 1500 ml depending on the individual patient (Tod *et al.* 2007). It has been advised to commence on 750 ml of tap water and titrate this depending on the individual response (Christensen *et al.* 2006). In a Danish study it has been reported that rectal irrigation is successful in up to 91% of people (Krogh *et al.* 1999).

Indications for rectal irrigation

- Neurogenic bowel dysfunction, e.g. spina bifida, multiple sclerosis, spinal injury

- Chronic faecal incontinence
- Chronic constipation
- Evacuation disorders

Contraindications to rectal irrigation

- Obstructing colonic or rectal mass
- Recent anal, rectal or colonic surgery
- Acute active inflammatory disease
- Severe cognitive impairment (unless carer administers)

Relative contraindications

- Spinal cord injury above T6 (observe for autonomic dysreflexia)
- Pregnancy
- Active perianal sepsis
- Painful anorectal conditions e.g. haemorrhoids, anal fissure
- Severe diverticular disease
- Diarrhoea
- Severe cardiac conditions
- Faecal impaction

Autonomic dysreflexia is a potentially life-threatening complication of a spinal cord injury at level T6 and above. It is related to an overactivity of the sympathetic nervous system and can manifest in symptoms including hypertension, bradycardia, shortness of breath, blurred vision and profuse sweating. Anything that would have been painful or uncomfortable before the injury can lead to autonomic dysreflexia. The two most common causes are a full bowel or bladder, e.g. blockage of a catheter. Removal of the stimuli along with head elevation is the main response to resolve an episode. If not treated properly seizures, stroke or death can result.

Benefits of rectal irrigation

- Symptom relief
- Improved quality of life
- Improved independence

Potential complications of rectal irrigation

- Time consuming
- May need assistance to administer
- Abdominal pain or discomfort
- Mild anal bleeding
- Rectal pain or discomfort
- Perforation of the bowel

There have been a small number of case reports detailing bowel perforation as a result of rectal irrigation though one was of a Turkish man who had self-administered a garden hose! Generally, however, it can be assumed the risk will be similar to the insertion of any other invasive rectal procedure.

Full details of the rectal irrigation equipment and procedure can be found on a protocol published by Coloplast Ltd (www.burdettinstitute. org.uk; www.coloplast.co.uk).

In summary, rectal irrigation is a useful bowel management strategy for those refractory to other bowel management techniques. There appear to be limited adverse effects and, as tap water is used, it can be assumed there will be no long-term reduction in efficacy. There is an increasing volume of literature demonstrating its usefulness.

Colonic irrigation

Not to be confused with rectal irrigation, colonic irrigation (or hydro-therapy) is a method of irrigating the entire colon as a complementary therapy for a range of conditions. The conditions colonic hydrotherapy is claimed to benefit include constipation, diarrhoea, halitosis, headaches, acne and 'psychological states' (Anderson 1992). The main proponents of this therapy are alternative practitioners and it is a controversial practice in conventional medicine. The rationale for colonic irrigation has tradition-ally related to the theory of autointoxication: that is, the belief that intes-tinal waste poisons the body and causes many illnesses (Ernst 1997). However, there is no evidence to support this theory. Additionally there have been concerns about potential adverse effects of colonic irrigation. There are documented reports of infection, perforation and electrolyte imbalance (Handley *et al.* 2004; Norlela *et al.* 2004; Richards *et al.* 2006) although these complications are thought to be rare.

Colostomy irrigation

The optimal method of colostomy management is debatable. Currently there are a number of methods used to care for a colostomy. These include a colostomy appliance to collect faeces, a plug (discussed in the appliances chapter) to retain faeces for a period of time, drug or dietary manipulation (Williams & Johnston 1980) and/or colostomy irrigation.

Colostomy irrigation was first described in 1927 in Britain by Lockhart-Mummery, a surgeon at St Mark's Hospital, London. The principle of colostomy irrigation is to provide control of faecal output and continence to the colostomate. Colostomy irrigation involves instilling lukewarm water into the distal colon via the colostomy, resulting in the dilatation of the colon. This is followed by a reflex contraction that expels the faeces, flatus and instilled water (Taylor 1995) usually with good results.

Despite its perceived improvement in the colostomate's quality of life, irrigation is largely under-utilised in the UK, despite the literature discuss-ing merits such as 'able to lead a normal life' (Seargeant 1966). Almost 20 years ago only 5% of colostomates used irrigation (Wade 1989) and this figure is similar today (Woodhouse 2005). Anecdotally, clinicians do not always support the technique due to lack of knowledge/confidence in teaching or the perceived risk of colonic perforation (Macdonald 1991). In addition some colostomates may be unwilling to intubate their stoma.

Use of colostomy irrigation varies throughout the world depending on the availability of equipment and health care provision. For example, in the United States of America about 90% of colostomates irrigate (Stockley 1981) possibly due to the cost of stoma appliances.

Benefits of colostomy irrigation

There are many advantages to irrigating a colostomy including good continence control for the ostomate with planned evacuations and no need to use an appliance in between irrigations. Irrigation is considered to be more cost effective than using colostomy appliances (Macdonald 1991) and may reduce landfill waste. Troublesome symptoms such as skin soreness, gas production and faecal odour can also be reduced (Terranova *et al.* 1979). Ostomates who irrigate often report improvements in their ability, or confidence, to participate in their day-to-day activities such as work, sport or sexual intercourse.

Potential complications of colostomy irrigation

Disadvantages of colostomy irrigation include the time taken to irrigate (Readding 2006) which is approximately one hour daily and the potential of faecal leakage between irrigations. This would often necessitate the wearing of a stoma appliance (O'Bichere *et al.* 2000) that may be an undesirable outcome. Generally, irrigation is considered to be a very safe procedure. However, rare complications have included death due to colonic perforation (although this is very unlikely with modern equipment), colonic burns as a result of hot irrigation fluid (Gattuso *et al.* 1996) and fluid and electrolyte imbalance due to high irrigation volumes (Shollenberger *et al.* 2000).

Assessing suitability for colostomy irrigation

Each colostomate should be individually assessed prior to commencing irrigation. Irrigation is not suitable for all colostomates and should not be used by ileostomates. When assessing the colostomate, written and oral information should be provided. The nurse should evaluate the colostomate's understanding of the information and answer any questions. The surgeon's or GP's opinion should be sought prior to commencing irrigation (Macdonald 1991).

Pringle (2005) suggests that colostomy irrigation can begin as soon as bowel sounds resume or can commence seven days post-operatively. However, Williams & Johnston (1980) recommend waiting three months after surgery before starting irrigation. This allows the bowel function to settle, the wounds, particularly the perineal wound, to heal, thus making irrigation more comfortable.

The colostomates that are most suitable for irrigation have either a sigmoid or descending colostomy. Irrigation is rarely successful on colostomies formed from either the ascending or transverse colon

(Shollenberger *et al.* 2000) due to a higher faecal output (Erwin-Toth & Doughty 1992) and there is more likely to be bowel motion between irrigations. Motivation from the colostomate is also necessary as irrigation is time consuming and may need to be performed daily (at least initially). However, age does not seem to be a problem to irrigation (Venturini *et al.* 1990).

The issues that may adversely affect suitability for irrigation are:

- Physical:
  - poor eyesight
  - poorly visible stoma
  - poor manual dexterity or arthritis
  - irregular colostomy outputs
  - irritable bowel syndrome (may exacerbate other symptoms)
  - insufficient remaining colon
  - renal impairment
  - cardiac impairment
  - stomal complications such as prolapse, stenosis, parastomal herniation, retraction
- Conditions with a risk of perforation:
  - residual or recurrent cancer
  - diverticulitis
  - crohn's disease
  - colostomates receiving pelvic or abdominal radiation
- Environmental/cognitive factors:
  - low motivation
  - cognitive impairment
  - inadequate toilet facilities, preferably with a combined toilet and bathroom
  - inadequate time.

Colostomy irrigation regime

Irrigation is normally performed every 24–72 hours. The majority irrigate on alternate days (McPhail 2003).

Predominantly the literature advocates the use of warm tap water at body temperature (Gattuso *et al.* 1996). Some suggest saline (Erwin-Toth & Doughty 1992) while others consider softened water to be unsuitable due to the sodium content (Macdonald 1991). There have been concerns over the absorption of the irrigation fluid if the patient is dehydrated and therefore the risk of hypernatremia if saline is used. The most commonly and simply used irrigation solution is tap water.

Irrigation fluid is usually instilled into the body rapidly and safely under gravity (Gattuso *et al.* 1996). The volume of fluid used per irrigation is reported as anything from 250 to 1500 ml, with 500 ml as the most appropriate (Meyhoff *et al.* 1990). Anecdotally some colostomates report better outcome from pump-assisted irrigation and consider the whole procedure to be quicker. It can be seen that currently there are no firm guidelines for colostomates in relation to the volume of irrigation fluid.

Time taken to complete irrigation varies dependent on the individual patient and, certainly, the literature reports vary from 30 to over 60 minutes;

usually about 45 minutes is adequate. There have been a limited number of studies on adding medication to the fluid to improve the speed or effects of irrigation. When adding glycerol trinitrate solution (GTN) to irrigation fluid the time taken to perform the irrigation was significantly reduced to about half (O'Bichere *et al.* 2001). However, side effects of fluctuating pulse and blood pressure (both returning spontaneously to baseline values) limit the use and therefore GTN cannot be recommended in this context.

A small study was undertaken using polyethylene glycol solution (an osmotic laxative) compared to water alone (O'Bichere *et al.* 2004). This study found that the washout time was considerably reduced with less between irrigation leakages. Irrigation with the polyethylene glycol solution, however, on such a small study cannot be recommended for use.

Colostomy irrigation equipment

Equipment is available from various companies in the UK and is generally available on prescription (FP10). As irrigation is usually only performed by colostomates with a permanent stoma the equipment is generally free of charge. The equipment for irrigation is:

- water reservoir
- tubing with a flow regulator
- cone
- plastic sleeve (one- or two-piece)
- warm tap water in a jug
- lubricating gel
- hook to hold the water reservoir
- stoma cap.

The irrigation tubing and reservoir can be used for up to two years (Pringle 2005). The tubing may become discoloured, but if it is cleaned with hot, soapy water (not boiling) it is generally considered safe to reuse (Taylor 1995). The cones should be changed every six months (Macdonald 1991). The irrigation sleeves in the UK are single use. However, in countries where equipment needs to be self-funded the two-piece sleeves can be used for four weeks if washed in warm soapy water and dried between uses (Pringle 2005).

Colostomy irrigation procedure

Irrigation can be performed at any time in the day, but it should ideally be at the same time to promote a good bowel regime. After an initial training session the colostomate should practise daily at home and is generally reviewed by the nurse after one week. The patient should contact the nurse prior to this if there are any queries. Individual patient assessment is required but often several nurse-supervised practises are necessary.

Colostomates may eventually be able to irrigate on alternate days. Stockley (1981) suggests daily irrigation for one week, then alternate days.

No irrigation fluid returns from the colostomy

- Water may not leave the colostomy after instillation due to the patient being tense. Relaxation, deep breathing and gentle abdominal massage may be useful. Also try some gentle activity.
- Dehydration may prevent return of the instilled water, i.e. due to pyrexia or a hot climate. In this situation an appliance should be worn until the next irrigation and the colostomate needs to be advised to take more oral fluids to prevent dehydration (Erwin-Toth & Doughty 1992).

Faeces passed between irrigation

- There may have been insufficient time allowed to empty the bowel after the irrigation procedure.
- The volume of irrigation fluid may be too great. Try reducing the irrigation volume, particularly if volumes exceed 1500 ml. High volumes can increase bowel stimulation and peristalsis (Shollenberger *et al.* 2000).
- Review the time between irrigations; perhaps try irrigating more frequently.
- Review the diet as over-eating or a change in diet to more spicy foods, alcoholic drinks, particularly beer/lager, or excessive fresh fruit can alter the faecal output.

General advice

- It may be useful to have a radio or reading matter in the room when irrigating.
- A normal diet can be taken by colostomates who irrigate.
- Only use water for irrigation that is safe to drink. In countries with uncertain water quality it is advisable to use bottled water to irrigate.
- If during instillation the irrigation fluid escapes down the sleeve, gently push the cone into the colostomy to prevent this occurring.
- As diarrhoea can occur at any time, it is useful for the colostomate to keep a small supply of appliances.
- Irrigation should be ceased if diarrhoea occurs until it resolves.
- If irrigation has not been performed for some time, the stoma function can return to normal but may become dependent upon irrigation. However, there is no research to substantiate reduction in transit times following irrigation (Macdonald 1991). Oral laxatives can assist (Erwin-Toth & Doughty 1992).
- If bleeding occurs from the stoma surface it may be that irrigation needs to be performed more gently.
- In rare cases the distension of the colon over-stimulates the vagal nerve causing bradycardia, hypotension and fainting. In this situation irrigation is not appropriate for the colostomate (Blackley 1998).
- Diet and exercise can help to regulate the bowel and can improve the effects of irrigation (Shollenberger *et al.* 2000).

Travel

Irrigation can be successfully performed when away from home as long as there are adequate facilities. There are a number of ways that the colostomate can simplify irrigation when travelling, such as using a coat hanger to hold the water reservoir. As the irrigation kit is contained in a small holdall it is easy to transport, but should be taken as hand luggage in the aeroplane in case of the luggage going astray.

Antegrade colonic enemas (ACEs)

The Malone antegrade colonic enema (ACE/MACE) has been an invaluable addition in the surgical treatment of faecal incontinence, soiling and constipation, since it was introduced in 1990 (Malone *et al.* 1990). Herndon *et al.* (2004) found that an ACE was less beneficial for intractable constipation compared to faecal incontinence. The terms ACE and MACE are used interchangeably in the literature. In an ACE procedure the appendix or a small segment of bowel (Diamond & Pohl 2003) is used to make a conduit through which fluid is inserted. The irrigation fluid enters the colon to cleanse it and leaves via the anus. ACE procedures may be performed for adults but there is more use and experience with children (see www.stmarkshospital.org.uk for a patient information leaflet).

Benefits of an ACE

Success with an ACE can be seen as improved or total faecal continence and is achieved in most children (Barqawi *et al.* 2004). An ACE enables the patients to administer their own enema, thereby having greater independence, self-esteem and reduced toilet time. An ACE is also effective long-term management of adult neurogenic bowel (Teichman *et al.* 2003).

Yerkes *et al.* (2003) found that all patients preferred using the ACE compared to medical management, although children resented the time taken to perform the procedure. Social confidence and hygiene were significantly better for wheelchair users (94%) and ambulatory (87%) patients. Patient satisfaction has been found to be excellent (Tackett *et al.* 2002).

Conditions that may benefit from an ACE procedure

Patients with a relatively normal colonic function but with rectal or anal problems have better results than those with colonic motility dysfunction. Very young children do not function well with an ACE (Curry *et al.* 1999). The conditions for which an ACE has been beneficial include:

- intractable constipation
- neurological disorders, e.g. spina bifida
- spinal cord injury
- anorectal anomaly, e.g. imperforate anus
- Hirschsprung's disease.

ACE is useful for adults with a spinal cord injury that is refractory to conservative methods, although other therapies may also be of benefit. For an ACE procedure to work it is essential to have proper patient selection to ensure appropriate motivation (Teichman *et al.* 2003).

Disadvantages/complications with an ACE

There are a number of disadvantages to the ACE procedure listed below:

- stomal stenosis
- incomplete continence
- stomal leakage
- lack of patient independence.
            (Yerkes *et al.* 2003)

Stoma stenosis at the skin level is the most common complication and rates are reported as being about 30% (Kim *et al.* 2006; Malone 2004). Stenosis may require surgical intervention (Barqawi *et al.* 2004); however, twice daily catheterisation can prevent or treat minor stenosis (Yerkes *et al.* 2003). Stenosis is less of a problem with newer techniques of stoma formation and frequent catheterisation.

Some uncommon, early complications are wound infection in 2% (Tackett *et al.* 2002), small bowel obstruction in 2% (Yerkes *et al.* 2001) and a gangrenous channel in 2% (Curry *et al.* 1999). There are also life-threatening risks associated with the use of different irrigation fluids. Electrolyte imbalance has also been reported causing significant morbidity when using normal saline, hypertonic phosphate and tap water enemas although rarely. Signs and symptoms of water intoxication include weakness, vomiting, mental status changes, seizures, cool skin and large volumes of dilute urine; those particularly at risk are children with congenital megacolon and severe constipation (Yerkes *et al.* 2001). Bloods should be monitored six to eight weeks after surgery and if satisfactory should probably be checked every six months.

The failure rate of ACEs is 24% (Yerkes *et al.* 2003).

Equipment for irrigating an ACE

- catheter
- enema
- bladder syringe
- irrigation kit

Solutions used for irrigation

The irrigation solutions with an ACE are either warm tap water, saline or phosphate-based enemas; 28% of patients used medication instilled through their ACE to improve effects (Yerkes *et al.* 2003).

However, it should be noted that softened water has been associated with elevated sodium and chloride levels in a single case, although these returned to normal quickly when using untreated tap water (Yerkes *et al.*

2001). The volume of irrigation fluid is also variable from 200 to 1000 ml per procedure. Koyle (2001) considers tap water to be a safe, cheap option for irrigation, whereas softened water is an 'unpredictable potential hazard and should be avoided' (Yerkes *et al.* 2001: 1478).

Frequency of ACE irrigation

Irrigation is generally performed daily, but catheterisation of the ACE should be twice daily to dilate the tract (Barqawi 2004).

Time to irrigate an ACE

The amount of time taken to perform the irrigation varies from 20 minutes to over an hour. However, the catheter size and volume of fluid used did not affect the time for irrigation to be completed (Yerkes *et al.* 2003).

Continence with an ACE

About 75% of those with an ACE were either continent or had only mild soiling using an ACE. Most people used an ACE alone but 20% wore a pad just in case of incontinence (Yerkes *et al.* 2003). Irrigation efficacy is maximised if regular oral medication to control constipation is used in conjunction with the ACE. If acceptable continence is not achievable it may be suitable to perform a colostomy (Curry *et al.* 1999). In France a study was performed on 25 patients with an ACE for faecal incontinence; only 18 were still using their ACE but 16 of those judged their result to be excellent and one had converted to a colostomy (Lefèvre *et al.* 2006).

In conclusion, the ACE has been shown to be effective in a carefully selected patient group. However, the patient does need daily commitment and realistic expectations as ACE irrigation may not be a complete solution (Yerkes *et al.* 2003). 'The MACE procedure has come to be accepted as an effective treatment for children and adults with faecal incontinence and constipation' (Curry *et al.* 1999: 339).

Percutaneous endoscopic colostomy (PEC)

A percutaneous endoscopic colostomy is a modification of the PEG (gastrostomy) using the same equipment and technique. A PEC is a simple, outpatient, endoscopic technique that allows access for antegrade colonic irrigation (Heriot *et al.* 2002). A PEC tube is inserted into the colon through which irrigation can be performed. This promotes evacuation of the colon into the toilet improving continence or constipation. The gastrostomy tube does need a sufficiently rigid inner flange to reduce the risk of early tube dislodgement (see www.burdettinstitute.org.uk for a patient information leaflet).

Who is suitable for a PEC?

The patient groups that may benefit from the PEC are those with:

- recurrent sigmoid volvulus (RSV)
- intractable constipation
- diarrhoea
- faecal incontinence
- megacolon
- acute colonic pseudo-obstruction.
                    (Pountney 2005)

RSV is where the sigmoid colon twists upon itself causing pain and bowel obstruction. A PEC is particularly suitable for those not fit for general anaesthetic. In this instance two PEC tube sites are used to secure the colon to the abdominal wall (Daniels *et al.* 2000). PECs inserted to control RSV require no further treatment and are simply used to stop the bowel from twisting.

Patients who have intractable constipation, diarrhoea or incontinence refractory to other therapies may be suitable for a PEC. A PEC is used to perform antegrade distal colonic and rectal irrigation. For those with constipation a PEC can be used instead of or as an adjunct to medical management, i.e. oral laxatives. A PEC may be useful for people with megacolon if the dilated colon causes pain and evacuation difficulties. The PEC can be used to decompress the colon when necessary. A PEC is unsuitable for those with colonic ischaemia or mechanical intestinal obstruction.

The National Institute for Health and Clinical Excellence (NICE 2006) have reviewed the use of a PEC and consider that the safety and efficacy is adequate for elderly and frail patients with recurrent sigmoid volvulus and colonic motility problems. However in children the evidence for use is limited.

The procedure

The PEC is often inserted as an endoscopy procedure without a general anaesthetic. Bowel preparation is advisable but is not mandatory. A light sedative is often given intravenously and a local anaesthetic is used at the insertion site. The colonoscope is passed through the anus to assist in the PEC insertion and a balloon secures it into the colon. The site is not usually marked, as it is not easy to bring the PEC tube to a predictable position. The initial discomfort at the tube insertion site is usually managed with mild analgesia (Pountney 2005).

To reduce the risk of infection IV antibiotics are given immediately before insertion (Heriot *et al.* 2002). Antibiotics are also given at eight and 16 hours post procedure.

After the procedure the patient is allowed to eat, drink and mobilise normally. The tube is connected to a bag for 24 hours to decompress the colon, after which it may be plugged with the attached cap. However, adhesive tape should be used to secure the tube and care should be taken not to dislodge it. In patients with impaired cognitive function the PEC tube should be firmly strapped to the skin to prevent inadvertent displacement.

Light gauze can be placed around the tube after the procedure to absorb any blood from the incision. No dressing should be applied after 24 hours unless there is discharge. The area should be cleansed daily with soap and water (Pountney 2005). After about six weeks, a low profile device like a large button may be used.

Complications

The use of a PEC is still in its infancy, as only a few hundred procedures have been undertaken. There have been a variety of complications:

- infection
- pain
- tube dislodgement
- faecal leakage around the tube.

There is a 15% post-procedure infection rate (Pountney 2005). Superficial infection and discharge around the tube is quite common and requires no treatment except for regular cleaning. There has been a report of treating an infected PEG site with Actisorb Silver 220 (Leak 2002). Serious infections are rare but may require antibiotics or possibly a hospital admission. Signs of an infection include severe abdominal pain and/or a painful, spreading redness on the skin around the tube, necessitating medical review. Pain, however, may be due to excessive tension on the abdominal skin by the PEC.

Dislodgement of the tube may occur. If displacement occurs in the first few days after insertion it may require surgical repair to close the hole in the colon. Once the tube has been replaced by a flat button tube, dislodging is uncommon, but should it occur another tube should be inserted into the opening within a few hours otherwise the aperture will close. In an emergency the doctor can insert a temporary size 14 French foley catheter. There has been a report of the PEC flange becoming embedded in the abdominal wall necessitating a subtotal colectomy and ileostomy (Bertolini *et al.* 2007).

Faecal leakage around the tube occasionally occurs and usually settles in a few days. Dietary manipulation may reduce incidence of leakage.

Some people do not find that a PEC suits them. In this situation as long as the tube is left in situ for at least one month it can be removed by cutting the top off the tube and the inner part will pass in the bowel motion. The skin exit site will discharge for a few days before closing naturally.

Change frequency of tube

The PEC tube should be replaced every six months to stop the balloon disintegrating (Pountney 2005).

Irrigation procedure

If the PEC is for irrigation purposes then the patient should start irrigating 24 hours after the tube is inserted. Initially 30–50 ml of saline should be instilled using a 50 ml bladder syringe. Subsequently irrigation is performed using a PEG feed giving set that consists of a plastic reservoir and tubing. 500 ml of warm tap water (at body temperature) although up to two litres twice daily have been reported (Heriot *et al.* 2002). The patient should sit on the toilet and slowly (over five to ten minutes or more slowly if discomfort is felt) instil the water from the reservoir through the tubing into the PEC. Higher volumes of irrigation fluid may be required to cleanse the distal colon and rectum. The patient should start to evacuate within a few minutes and the bowel should be empty within about 20–30 minutes. Some patients use additives, such as phosphate enema or 5 ml of bisacodyl syrup, through the tube to reduce the amount of warm tap water required and give better results.

Frequency

Most people irrigate on alternate days, but if leakage occurs within this time daily irrigation may be necessary. Dietary manipulation may be useful to alter stool consistency.

Conclusion

There are various ways of irrigating the colon to achieve satisfactory evacuation and continence. The literature is inconclusive on issues such as irrigation fluids, fluid volumes and frequency of irrigation. After a period of experimentation, for the carefully selected patient irrigation can be very effective.

Irrigation is not normally a first-line management strategy but should be considered as an alternative or adjunct therapy to improve symptoms and thus quality of life.

References

Anderson G (1992) Colonic irrigation: beneficial therapy or dangerous fad? *Here's Health.* **2**: 46–7.

Barqawi A, De Valdenebro M, Furness PD III & Koyle MA (2004) Lessons learned from stomal complications in children with cutaneous catherizable continent stomas. *British Journal of Urology.* **94(9)**: 1344–7.

Bertolini D, de Saussure P, Chilcott M, Girardin M & Dumonceau J-M (2007) Severe delayed complication after percutaneous endoscopic colostomy for chronic intestinal pseudo-obstruction: a case report and review of the literature. *World Journal of Gastroenterology.* **13(15)**: 2255–7.

Blackley P (1998) *Practical Stoma, Wound and Continence Management.* Victoria, Australia: Research Publications Pty Ltd.

Christensen P, Bazzocchi G, Coggrave M, Abel R, Hultling C *et al.* (2006) A randomized control trial of transanal irrigation versus conservative bowel management in spinal cord injured patients. *Gastroenterology.* **131**: 738–47.

Curry JI, Osbourne A & Malone PSJ (1999) The MACE Procedure: experience in the United Kingdom. *Journal of Pediatric Surgery.* **34(2)**: 338–40.

Daniels IR, Lamparelli MJ, Chave H & Simson JNL (2000) Recurrent sigmoid volvulus treated by percutaneous endoscopic colostomy. *British Journal of Surgery.* **87(10)**: 1419.

Diamond DA & Pohl HG (2003) Use of a colon based tubularized flap for an antegrade continence enema. *The Journal of Urology.* **168(1)**: 324–6.

Ernst E (1997) Colonic irrigation and the theory of autointoxication: a triumph of ignorance over science. *Journal of Clinical Gastroenterology.* **24(4)**: 196–8.

Erwin-Toth P & Doughty DB (1992) Principles and procedures of stomal management. In: Hampton BG & Bryant RA (eds) *Ostomies and Continent Diversions: Nursing Management.* London: Mosby Year Book.

Gattuso JM, Kamm MA, Myers C, Saunders B & Roy A (1996) Effects of different infusion regimens on colonic motility and efficacy of colostomy irrigation. *British Journal of Surgery.* **83(10)**: 1459–62.

Handley DV, Rieger NA & Rodda DJ (2004) Rectal perforation from colonic irrigation administered by alternative practitioners. *Medical Journal of Australia.* **181(10)**: 575–6.

Heriot AG, Tilney HS & Simson JNL (2002) The application of percutaneous endoscopic colostomy to the management of obstructed defecation. *Diseases of the Colon and Rectum.* **45(5)**: 700–2.

Herndon CDA, Rink RC, Cain MP, Lerner M, Kaefer M *et al.* (2004) In situ Malone antegrade continence enema in 127 patients: a 6-year experience. *The Journal of Urology.* **172**: 1689–91.

Kim J, Beasley SW & Maoate K (2006) Appendicostomy stomas and antegrade colonic irrigation after laparoscopic antegrade continence enema. *Journal of Laparoendoscopic and Advanced Surgical Techniques.* **16(4)**: 400–3.

Koyle MA (2001) Editorial comment. *The Journal of Urology.* **166**: 1478.

Krogh K, Kvitzau B, Jorgensen TM & Laurberg S (1999) Treatment of anal incontinence and constipation with transanal irrigation. *Ugeskrift for Laeger.* **161(3)**: 253–6.

Leak K (2002) PEG site infections: a novel use for Actisorb Silver 220. *British Journal of Community Nursing.* **7(6)**: 321–5.

Lefèvre JH, Parc Y, Giraudo G, Bell S, Parc R *et al.* (2006) Outcome of antegrade continence enema procedures for faecal incontinence in adults. *British Journal of Surgery.* **93**: 1265–9.

Macdonald K (1991) Colostomy irrigation: an option worth considering. *Professional Nurse.* **7(1)**: 15–18.

McPhail J (2003) Irrigation techniques. In: Elcoat C (ed) *Stoma Care Nursing.* London: Hollister.

Malone PSJ (2004) The antegrade continence enema procedure. *British Journal of Urology.* **93(3)**: 248–9.

Malone PS, Ransley PG & Keily EM (1990) Preliminary report: the antegrade continence enema. *Lancet.* **336**: 1217–18.

Meyhoff HH, Andersen B & Levin Neilsen S (1990) Colostomy irrigation: a clinical and scintigraphic comparison between three different irrigation volumes. *British Journal of Surgery.* **77**: 1185–6.

National Institute for Health and Clinical Excellence (2006) *Percutaneous Endoscopy Colostomy.* London: NICE.

Norlela S, Izham C & Khalid BAK (2004) Colonic irrigation-induced hyponatremia. *Malaysian Journal of Pathology.* **26(2)**: 117–18.

O'Bichere A, Sibbons P, Doré C, Green C & Phillips RKS (2000) Experimental study of faecal continence and colostomy irrigation. *British Journal of Surgery.* **87(7)**: 902–8.

O'Bichere A, Bossom C, Gangoli S, Green C & Phillips RKS (2001) Chemical colostomy irrigation with glycerol trinitrate solution. *Diseases of the Colon and Rectum.* **44(9)**: 1324–7.

O'Bichere A, Green C & Phillips RKS (2004) Randomized cross-over trial of polyethylene glycol electrolyte solution and water for colostomy irrigation. *Diseases of the Colon and Rectum.* **47(9)**: 1506–9.

Pountney D (2005) Bowel control with PEC. *Gastrointestinal Nursing*. **3(8)**: 14–16.

Pringle W (2005) Irrigation. In: Breckman B (ed) *Stoma Care and Rehabilitation*. London: Elsevier Churchill Livingstone.

Pullen RL (2006) Teaching your patient to irrigate a colostomy. *Nursing*. **36(4)**: 22.

Readding L (2006) Colostomy irrigation – an option worth considering. *Gastrointestinal Nursing*. **4(3)**: 27–33.

Richards DG, McMillin DL, Mein EA & Nelson CD (2006) Colonic irrigations: a review of the historical controversy and the potential for adverse effects. *Journal of Alternative and Complementary Medicine*. **12(4)**: 389–93.

Seargeant PW (1966) Colostomy management by irrigation technique: reviews of 165 cases. *British Medical Journal*. **2**: 25–6.

Shollenberger D, Spirk M & Small CC (2000) Gastrointestinal care. In: Holmers HN (ed) *Nursing Procedures*. 3rd edn. Pennsylvania: Springhouse Corporation.

Stockley A (1981) Irrigation. In: Breckman B (ed) *Stoma Care*. Beaconsfield, Bucks: Beaconsfield Publishers.

Tackett LD, Minevich E, Benedict JF, Wacksman J & Sheldon CA (2002) Appendiceal versus ileal segment for antegrade continence enema. *The Journal of Urology*. **167**: 683–6.

Taylor P (1995) Colostomy irrigation – a safe practice? *Journal of Clinical Nursing*. **4(3)**: 203–4.

Teichman JMH, Zabihi N, Kraus SR, Harris JM & Barber DB (2003) Long-term results for Malone antegrade continence enema for adults with neurogenic bowel disease. *Adult Urology*. **61(3)**: 502–6.

Terranova O, Sandei F, Rebuffat C, Maruotti R & Bortolozzi E (1979) Irrigation vs. natural evacuation of left colostomy: a comparative study of 340 patients. *Diseases of the Colon and Rectum*. **22(1)**: 31–3.

Tod AM, Stringer E, Levery C, Dean J & Brown J (2007) Rectal irrigation in the management of functional bowel disorders: a review. *British Journal of Nursing*. **16(14)**: 858–64.

Venturini M, Bertelli G, Forno G, Grandi G & Dini D (1990) Colostomy irrigation in the elderly – effective recovery regardless of age. *Diseases of the Colon and Rectum*. **33(12)**: 1031–3.

Wade B (1989) *A Stoma Is for Life*. Harrow: Scutari Press.

Williams NS & Johnston D (1980) Prospective controlled trial comparing colostomy irrigation with 'spontaneous-action' method. *British Medical Journal*. **12**: 107–9.

Woodhouse F (2005) Colostomy irrigation: are we offering it enough? *British Journal of Nursing*. **14(16)**: S14–S15.

Yerkes EB, Rink RC, King S, Cain MP, Kaefer M *et al*. (2001) Tap water and the Malone antegrade continence enema: a safe combination? *Journal of Urology*. **166**: 1476–8.

Yerkes EB, Cain MP, King S, Brei T, Kaefer M *et al*. (2003) The Malone antegrade continence enema procedure: quality of life and family perspective. *Journal of Urology*. **169**: 320–3.

Chapter 18

Other Stoma Issues

Jennie Burch

Introduction

A number of other topics requiring discussion did not easily fit into the previous chapters. These issues will be discussed here.

Age related issues

The age of the ostomate can have an impact on the care required from the health care professional. The issues related to infants (Nour *et al.* 1996), children, adults (Fitzpatrick *et al.* 2003) and the elderly population are explored. This can include, for the elderly, issues related to poor eyesight (Benjamin 2002) or manual dexterity. Practical advice is provided, such as the use of two-piece appliances for ostomates with dexterity problems.

Babies

The majority of stomas formed on babies are performed as an emergency on neonates, with a temporary colostomy being the most commonly formed stoma (Webster 1985). This is a distressing time for both the baby and their parents (Nour *et al.* 1996). Ideally the parents should be well informed and supported. However the babies are often transferred to a specialist hospital adding further stress.

As babies usually wear a nappy it might be more appropriate to also use this to contain their stomal output rather than an appliance. Barrier cream around the stoma might be required, if using a nappy, particularly if the faeces are loose and corrosive to the peristomal skin.

Children and teenagers

Caring for the child with a stoma can be challenging. Siting is important taking into account any physical disabilities such as callipers. Involving the child can help them to accept their stoma (Webster 1985). It can also be difficult for parents to cope with the concept of their child having a stoma. However, often young children are able to perform their own stoma care so parents need to be encouraged to let children have a degree of independence. School can be problematic due to the concerns of the child, parents and teachers (Rogers 2003). It may be necessary for the parents to meet with the teacher to discuss the situation.

Being a teenager is a difficult time for many without the additional stresses of a stoma. No one wants to be different to their peers, particularly in relation to issues such as their bowels. Often the teenager will have a stoma for ulcerative colitis or a trauma and in many cases this will be temporary. The changes that puberty brings make body image of great importance and may make coping with a stoma more difficult. Each ostomate will need to be individually assessed and involving the parents is vital. Teenagers may have many questions or may prefer to ignore it and avoid talking about their concerns. Careful communication is required by the multidisciplinary team to encourage discussion and some acceptance of their stoma.

Adults

All ostomates are different and need to be considered individually (Fitzpatrick *et al.* 2003). Ideally adult ostomates will become independent with their stoma care needs and be able to return to their roles in society after surgery and recuperation.

Learning disabilities

The degree that a person with learning disabilities will be able to cope with their stoma will depend upon the extent of their disability. If patients are capable of living on their own or with minimal assistance they should be able to become independent with their stoma care needs. However, the training may take longer and other training approaches may be required. People need to be individually assessed to ascertain their potential independence. It may be necessary to include carers in planning and undertaking the care (Black & Hyde 2004).

Older ostomate

The elderly ostomate may encounter additional problems, such as rheumatoid arthritis, that may reduce their manual dexterity. Poor eyesight (Benjamin 2002) or short-term memory loss, for example, may also make the care of the stoma difficult. There are ways in which these issues can be addressed. Those colostomates with arthritis might find that the newer two-piece appliances are simpler to use. In severe cases a community nurse can apply the flange if hand co-ordination is poor, and the colostomate can simply apply the bag when required. The older ileostomate might find a newer type of appliance with an integral clip and a Velcro type fastening easier to use. The older urostomate might find that some taps or openings are easier to use than others. An assessment should also be made to ensure that the appliances are pre-cut as scissors can be difficult to use for those with arthritis.

Poor vision can be addressed in a number of ways. If the ostomate can live independently with their current vision then they should also be able to manage their stoma. Blind ostomates and those with limited vision have successfully learnt how to care independently for their stoma.

For those with memory problems it might be useful to put reminders in the toilet about their stoma. Printed instructions for their stoma care and/or forms to tick to remind the ileostomate to empty the appliance can be useful.

A quality of life study was undertaken on older ostomates by Notter *et al.* (2003) and found that initial dietary problems were overcome by trial and error but this left some with inadequate diets. Diets need to be assessed to ensure a good balance. The study also found a wide variation between levels of activities, with some ostomates reporting doing any type of sport, including white water rafting, while others felt unable to do any exercise at all. Approximately 14% felt that they even needed to give up gardening.

Drugs

There are a number of drugs that are useful for the ostomates, such as laxatives (Peate 2003) and bowel thickening agents. Some nurses are now able to prescribe, however many of the drugs used in stoma care are not on the list for nurse prescribers. The ones that will be discussed are related to:

- laxatives
- bulking agents
- pain management.

Laxatives

Laxatives are suitable for the colostomate and the urostomate. However, other methods such as dietary changes should be tried as the first option. The following will be discussed:

- stimulants
- osmotics
- suppositories
- enemas
- softeners

Stimulants

Stimulant laxatives, such as senna (Peate 2003), increase intestinal motility but often cause abdominal cramps and should be avoided if there is an intestinal obstruction. Stimulant laxatives often take 8–12 hours to be effective and therefore should be taken prior to bed for a morning action. There can be a number of side effects associated with stimulant laxatives such as diarrhoea and hypokalaemia. It is thought that the consistent use of stimulants may lead to a 'lazy' bowel, although there is no conclusive evidence to support this. Dantron should only be used in the terminally ill due to the increased cancer risk. Stimulants in general should not be used for those with inflammatory bowel disease.

Osmotics

Osmotic laxatives increase the amount of water in the colon by retention or drawing water into the bowel. These are used regularly and include medications such as lactulose (10 mg daily) or liquid paraffin. However, there may be some anal seepage if the rectum is in situ. Movicol may be suitable for colostomates who have faecal impaction. The medication is taken orally and several doses are generally required.

Suppositories

Glycerine/glycerol suppositories can be used for acute constipation associated with pain. The glycerol suppository acts as a stimulant as it is a mild irritant. There are, however, no sphincter muscles to hold the suppositories in and thus they are prone to fall out before becoming effective. McClees *et al.* (2004) found that glycerine suppositories were ineffective when not held within the stoma. Therefore it is recommended to insert the suppository as usual using a water-based lubricant and hold the suppository in place with a gloved finger over the opening in the stoma or quickly put an appliance over the colostomy and press gently but firmly over the exit of the stoma through the appliance. Pressure needs to be applied for about 10–15 minutes to allow the suppository to dissolve and become effective.

Enemas

Phosphate enemas work as an osmotic laxative, although they can cause local irritation. A problem occurs trying to retain the enema fluid in the body. Thus enemas are not commonly used.

Softeners

Faecal softeners such as arachis oil enemas can be used with effect for the colostomate but the oil makes subsequent appliance application difficult. As with enemas there can be problems with retaining the oil.

Bulking agents

This group of medications works by increasing the faecal mass and thus promoting peristalsis (Thompson *et al.* 2003) but may take a few days to become fully effective and includes ispaghula husk such as fibrogel. These medications may be beneficial but must be used in conjunction with adequate oral fluids. Side effects can include abdominal discomfort if introduced too rapidly. Bulking agents should never be used for patients with obstruction or recent bowel surgery.

Thickening agents

There are a number of drugs that can thicken the faecal output. These include:

- codeine phosphate
- loperamide
- octreotide
- antidepressants.

Codeine phosphate can be effective in two ways, as a pain relief and also to thicken faeces. However, care should be taken if constipation is an unwanted side effect of this medication and other analgesia may be effective. Loperamide is generally associated with fewer side effects than codeine phosphate. Loperamide can be used alone or in conjunction with codeine phosphate for those with high faecal outputs (see Chapter 16).

Octreotide is used to reduce secretions but is often ineffective in the long-term treatment of high-output stomas. The side effects of antidepressants may be constipation and this needs to be considered if prescribed for the colostomate.

Pain therapy

There can be problems associated with pain for people with fistulae when changing the appliance. This is difficult to resolve with conventional therapies. Medications that have provided some benefit are opioids that are used orally, such as a fentanyl lozenge or morphine. The morphine should be taken 30 minutes prior to the procedure for best effect. Entonox/nitrous oxide has also been used. All of these medications carry a risk and need to be used in accordance with protocols set out by the pain team.

Other options are music therapy or hypnotherapy. These are non-pharmacological strategies that are inexpensive and easily available (Giaquinto *et al.* 2006). Music has helped in a variety of settings and may be useful at dressing changes (Kane *et al.* 2004).

Exercise

When abdominal surgery is performed the abdominal muscles are stitched back together, but will take time to heal and remain weak for several months. While the healing occurs the wound should not be strained as herniation can result at the site of either the incision or the stoma. To strengthen the weakened abdominal muscles it is advantageous to advise the ostomate to perform exercises (Meadows 1997). However, many exercises are not suitable to be performed until several months after the surgery, to ensure that adequate healing has occurred. Each person is different and will need individual assessment prior to beginning any form of exercise. As a general rule the ostomate should continue gentle walking immediately after discharge home and gradually build this up. Four weeks after surgery gentle gym exercises can be performed such as the treadmill or exercise bike but a brisk walk is just as beneficial. It is important for the ostomate to wait three months before swimming with a float (as long as all the wounds are healed) and to wait for six months before powerful swimming strokes and gym work. It should be stressed that it is essential for each individual ostomate to gain advice from their consultant or GP prior to the recommencement of any exercise.

Pre-stoma closure exercises

Prior to stoma closure the anal sphincter muscles may benefit from some exercise. For all ostomates pelvic floor exercises can be a benefit (Wells 1990); for further information, see Chapter 6 on continence.

Lifting

Advice can be given to avoid lifting in the first few weeks after surgery. Lifting should be done by bending the knees and keeping the back straight but not holding your breath. Lifting weights above that of a full kettle should be avoided for three months after surgery. As the abdominal wall is at its weakest immediately after surgery it is useful to give advice to prevent any further stress to the wound/scar. When carrying objects, such as shopping, a smaller load and more trips made to carry these loads may be beneficial, but not for several weeks after surgery.

Simple analogies can be given to patients to help them understand about lifting; for example, carrying full baskets of wet washing or small children is too much in the post-operative period. This can be overcome by carrying washing in small loads and sitting when with children. It is essential that lifting be undertaken correctly to prevent injury. Correct lifting can help to prevent herniation (see Chapter 15 on complications).

Swimming

Swimming is not recommended after surgery for at least three months. To prevent the appliance filter from getting wet and becoming ineffectual when swimming it can be useful to cover the filter. Ideally do not get the appliance wet for an hour after application to ensure a good seal and to be leak free.

Swimwear can be bought from high street stores, the Internet or there is specialist swimwear available. Some ostomates prefer a one-piece suit that covers scars and appliances. However, some find a two-piece swimsuit more appropriate. For men swimming shorts disguise an appliance better than swimming trunks.

Sport

Ostomates have participated in a variety of sporting activities, although some should be undertaken with caution. Ostomates should not undertake sport for many weeks after their stoma is formed, except for walking. Strenuous activities and those involving physical contact should be refrained from until the wounds are well healed. Ostomates have undertaken scuba diving and parachute jumps so it can be seen that a variety of sports are possible. A stoma shield can be worn for protection when undertaking sports that may potentially lead to damage to the stoma itself, such as football. A stoma shield can be ordered through the stoma specialist nurse. It can be useful to consult the stoma specialist nurse or a member of the multidisciplinary team before commencing sports after stoma forming surgery; as each person is individual it can be difficult to give firm guidance about when it is safe to resume sporting activities. It might be useful to wear an abdominal support when undertaking sport. It is also essential for the ostomate to be aware of the risks and signs of dehydration and to drink sensibly when participating in sports.

Psychological issues

Facing stoma-forming surgery can be daunting and worrying. Fear about the surgery and/or the stoma can manifest itself in a variety of psychological responses:

- anger
- depression
- denial
- repression
- low self-esteem
- socio-emotional problems
- psychosexual problems.
  (Kirkwood 2006; Virgin-Elliston & Williams 2003)

Anxiety may be a product of helplessness, accentuated by a hospital admission. Anxiety may be due to misconceptions about stomas, lack of information or worries about body image. It is felt that strengthening patients' self-efficacy can accelerate their adaptation to their stoma (Bekkers *et al.* 1996). However this is made more difficult if there are associated stoma complications. In the short term most ostomates experience negative feelings and each ostomate will react differently. Feelings can change over time (Brown & Randle 2005) and with support from the multidisciplinary team. Some ostomates may require further support in the form of counselling.

The ostomate may experience loss and grief over a variety of actual or potential losses. These can include:

- body parts
- fertility
- relationships.
  (Junkin & Beitz 2005)

The nurse can utilise listening skills and convey a caring attitude to promote trust and collaboration with the ostomate (Sirota 2006b). Interpersonal skills are essential to enable the ostomate to feel comfortable to discuss any areas of concern that they might have.

Body image

Body image can be defined as how we perceive our bodies (White 1998). This perception will alter with age and is related to a variety of factors, such as weight gain (Hunter 2004). The formation of a stoma will alter the body image forever and can have psychological implications for the ostomate, including potential problems with self-concept, self-esteem and self-worth (Williams 2005). Self-concept is related to ideas, values and perceptions that characterise the person and can influence the behaviour, attitude and well-being of the person.

Body image can be broken down into three main components:

- body reality (the physical presentation of the body, which alters following stoma-forming surgery);
- body ideal (the person's desired body image);
- body presentation (the body presented to the world).

(Price 1990)

Altered body image can be associated with a number of feelings that may include degradation, mutilation and restriction (Black 2000a). In relation to the stoma and the lack of bowel control can be feelings of reverting to a 'baby'. In the initial period following stoma formation the perception of body image may be based on the immediate social situation and past experiences (Black 2004).

There are many factors that can affect the ability to adapt to the altered body image including:

- diagnosis
- treatment
- medical and nursing care
- disease process.

It is therefore important for the health care professional to ensure that they assist the patient to cope with these changes. This can be achieved by encouraging the patient to discuss their experiences and fears (Black 2004). This might be in the form of advice on other methods to manage the stoma such as irrigation, which may be beneficial for some colostomates.

Sexual issues

Following stoma formation it is generally possible to have sexual intercourse and even children. However there can be sexual problems after surgery. Sexual issues can be difficult for both the health care professional (Williams 2006) and the ostomate to discuss. However, it is an important topic to address due to the potential risk to sexual function after surgery. Nurses should be able to assist ostomates and their families to cope with the psychological and psychosexual impact of stoma-forming surgery (Borwell 1997a). The sexual problems may not be the result of the surgery, but because of the loss of self-esteem and body image issues (Comb 2003).

There can be male or female sexual dysfunction following stoma formation, which may be temporary or permanent (Baxter & Lloyd 2004). Women may have dyspareunia (Borwell 1997b) and men may have erectile dysfunction (Black 2004). The following will be discussed:

- male sexual problems including impotence;
- female sexual problems;
- homosexuality;
- contraception and fertility issues.

Normal sexual activity can be resumed after stoma-forming surgery in many patients. However, for some it is not of primary importance and others use different ways to express intimacy. Patients should be made aware that the body might respond to illness and surgery with an inability to have sexual intercourse if it is attempted too soon. However, sexuality may also be affected by emotional distress. Even if there are no physical sexual problems associated with the stoma-forming surgery they can often be perceived (White 1998). This can result in a decreased libido for any number of reasons for the ostomate, as with anyone (Baxter & Lloyd 2004). Simple tips to consider prior to commencing lovemaking are to ensure that the appliance is empty and securely attached to the abdomen to prevent the risk of leakage. Some people choose to cover their stoma but this is the personal choice of the ostomate. For males it is possible to make no preparations prior to sexual intercourse; however, some men prefer to wear a cummerbund or similar to cover and support the appliance. For female ostomates if it is felt necessary to disguise the appliance then sexy underwear can be used to conceal the appliance. Male or female ostomates may choose to wear a smaller appliance for times of intimacy.

Sexuality – which can be defined as more than just the sex act – influences self-image, feelings and interpersonal relationships. The ostomate may feel less attractive to their partner (Black 2000a) and may feel rejected by their significant others or worry about the appliance and any potential leakages or noise. There are also biological, psychological and social elements to sexuality:

- biological – reproductive organs and physical appearance;
- psychological – body image and self-esteem;
- social – gender role, cultural expectations and stereotypes.

(Junkin & Beitz 2005)

There are many factors that can affect sexuality and the nurse needs to consider these when assessing and having sexual discussions with the ostomate. Some of the more common factors include their upbringing, environment, culture, religion and personal circumstances (Bond 1997).

Insertion of any foreign body into the stoma can cause damage and should be avoided. This should be discussed if appropriate.

Male sexual dysfunction and impotence

Impotence can be defined as the inability to have sexual intercourse, which may be temporary or permanent. The cause may be nerve damage during surgery, for example, which may cause erectile problems or ejaculatory problems (Black 2004). The reason that the nerves can be damaged during surgery is that they are very close within the pelvis so that it is not always possible to preserve them. Erectile problems commonly affect the middle-aged and older man (Dorey 2002a). There are a number of necessary components for an erection including the pelvis floor strength, thus specific exercises might help to improve muscle strength (Dorey 2002b). Ejaculatory problems may be organic due to nerve damage for example or as a result of psychological problems. If impotence is an issue an erection can be obtained by other methods. Ejaculation is not possible once the bladder and prostate are removed, but many men do achieve orgasm. Figures are improving but impotence may occur in 90% of men after surgery for bladder cancer (Dorey 2000), up to 80% following an abdominoperineal resection of the rectum and 20% following an anterior resection (Davis 1990). Generally there is no increased sexual dysfunction following ileostomy formation.

The urologist will assess the ostomate and treatment can include:

- oral tablets
- vacuum pumps
- penile injections or penile pellets
- penile implants.
        (Rutherford & Duffy 1999)

Viagra can significantly improve sexual function following rectal surgery if there is only partial nerve damage. Vacuum devices are useful to provide an erection if erectile nerves are severed, by drawing blood into the penis, and then a rubber ring is used to keep the erection. Pellets instilled directly into the penis and urethra can also stimulate an erection. Another option is a firm plastic condom that is used in conjunction with a vacuum device. Penile injections and implants can also be useful but are only generally considered if other therapies fail.

Female sexual problems

Less is known about women's sexual dysfunction, but improving surgery is reducing the risk of damage. There may be a number of sexual problems that a female ostomate may incur. These can include a dry vagina which can occur with increased age or following the menopause and can be resolved with increased foreplay or the use of lubrication (Salter 1997). There can also be dyspareunia or pain on intercourse (Borwell 1997b). This may occur for a number of reasons. Anxiety can prevent relaxation and in this situation communication with the partner can help. Pain may also be the result of a change in the position of the vagina if, for example, either the rectum or the bladder is removed. This may be resolved by a change in sexual position (Meadows 1997). There may also be scar tissue from the surgery resulting in a vaginal tightness (Williams 2005) which can be treated with vaginal dilation. Sexual counselling may also be useful for the female ostomate and her partner.

There are a number of sexual aids that can be used to increase arousal that can be beneficial for the ostomate and their partner.

Homosexuality

It cannot be presumed that all gay men choose to have anal sex as there are many other methods that can be used. Some gay men do choose to have anal sex, which may not be possible after certain operations such as the removal of the anal canal and anus.

Contraception

As it is possible for ostomates and people with pouches to become pregnant it may be necessary if children are not desired at that time to use appropriate contraception. Generally the female oral contraceptive pill is effective but ostomates with a high faecal output should seek advice.

Fertility and pregnancy

The risks of surgery to fertility are not yet fully understood. There is thought to be a reduced fertility for females following surgery due to the adhesions. However, there have been many children born to ostomates or those with a pouch. Following the formation of a stoma or pouch it is possible to get pregnant. The method of childbirth can be natural or by caesarean section and the patient's choice and individual assessment needs to be considered. However, there may be problems with conception following abdominal surgery or cancer therapy. Cancer in the younger ostomate may lead to infertility, as a result of radio or chemotherapy, for example.

Prior to planning a pregnancy it is advisable to seek advice from the gastroenterologist or stoma specialist nurse. Once pregnant there may be a number of issues for the pregnant ostomate. Hormonal changes can affect the skin and the appliance adherence. As the abdomen changes shape this can affect the stoma function and size and remeasuring of the stoma appliance aperture may be required. After childbirth the hormones can take a while to settle back down. Practical advice can include making sure that the appliance is emptied prior to feeding the baby, particularly for ileostomates and urostomates.

Specialist clothing

There are abdominal supports and clothing that are designed to disguise the stoma or support the appliance during exercise or sexual activities. This includes a specialised product called ostoshorts that can be worn to hold the appliance to the body. These products are available at a cost to the ostomate and are advertised in the various publications by the support groups or the manufacturers. Specialist clothing for men includes high waisted trousers. For men and women there is specialist swimwear and underwear available. Some of the underwear has a pocket inside to support the weight of the stoma appliance as it fills.

Toilet access

The RADAR key allows access to over 5000 disabled toilets in the UK, see www.radar.org.uk for more information. Some ostomates find this facility useful; although use of a disabled key does not mean that an ostomate is or should be perceived as disabled. There are also credit card sized cards available from various appliance manufacturers or support groups which state that the card holder has a problem and needs to use the toilet urgently.

Cultural issues

Today's multicultural society has implications for ostomates (Pinches 1999). There can be a number of cultural issues that can affect the ostomate. This can include a language barrier, clothing and food (Black 2004). Some issues can be overcome relatively simply, for example the use of a translator to facilitate communication between the nurse and the ostomate. However, a language barrier can lead to isolation or feelings of frustration. It is rarely appropriate to have a family member translate; however, an independent interpreter may also present potential problems (Williams & Da Costa 2006).

Religious issues

It must be remembered that each person is individual and may not follow their religious guidance in the same ways as other people of their faith. Only a few examples of religious considerations that may affect ostomates will be discussed. The Islamic patient may need to seek guidance from the imam at their mosque prior to making decisions about their surgery. Ostomates that follow the Muslim faith traditionally use their left hand for cleansing and their right hand for eating (Black 2004). This may result in problems caring for the stoma. However, there are ways to care for the stoma with only the left hand. Muslims are also expected to pray five times a day and prior to this they need to be clean. This can cause potential problems with skin care and a two-piece appliance might be more appropriate (Black 2000b).

A person's spirituality or religious perspective will affect how the ostomate will cope with their stoma (Sirota 2006a). A strong belief is often associated with a more positive outlook on life. This can assist in coping with a new ostomy.

Diet and religion

Diet choices can vary greatly due to personal or religious reasons. Many people of the Sikh and Hindu religion are vegetarians and this may affect their stomal output. Strict vegetarian/vegan diets may lead to difficulties for a colostomate or ileostomate as the faecal output can increase as can the flatus (Williams & Da Costa 2006). Fasting can also be an issue.

Fasting

Fasting is required for some religions, such as Hindus, Jews, Muslims, Rastafarians and Sikhs (Black 2004) and can cause problems with stoma management and dehydration. It may be possible for the ostomate to speak to their religious leader for advice (Readding 2003), but ostomates can abide by their religious guidelines if carefully planned.

Travel

There are a number of things to consider when planning a holiday. It is possible to obtain a travel certificate from the GP or stoma specialist nurse. If flying the ostomate may find the following suggestions useful.

- Take the appliances as hand luggage (in case of the loss of their hold luggage).
- Take twice as many appliances as are usually needed for the period of time (the heat or swimming may require more frequent appliance change or alterations in diet may increase faecal output).
- Some ostomates find an aisle seat on an aeroplane allows simpler passage to the toilet.
- Some ostomates ask for seats near the toilet – but this is not usually required.
- Some colostomates find more flatus is passed when flying (use a filtered appliance, eat small frequent meals and/or use a two-piece appliance to release the wind).
- Do not take scissors in the hand luggage and if appliances are not pre-cut then cut apertures in any appliances that may be required before the flight.
- Try and use the toilets before the meal as there is often a queue after.

While in a hot climate it is important to avoid dehydration, particularly ostomates with an ileostomy or urostomy. For those with a colostomy it is important to be aware that loose stool may occur due to the different food, water and temperatures as well as from bacteria. It may therefore be useful for the colostomate to request a few drainable appliances to take on holiday. If there are problems obtaining holiday insurance it can be advisable to contact the stoma specialist nurse or an ostomy support group.

Storage of appliances can be problematic as very high or low temperatures can affect the appliance adhesive. This can be resolved by keeping appliances in a room that is comfortable for the ostomate.

Quality of life

There are limited quality of life evaluation tools (Baxter *et al.* 2006). The general consensus is that the quality of life is reduced for ostomates. One study found that the coping strategies for those with a permanent stoma were different from those with a temporary one (Santos *et al.* 2006). Those ostomates with temporary stomas employed the coping technique 'escape avoidance' compared to those ostomates with permanent stomas who coped by planning and problem solving.

Conclusion

There are many issues that have to be considered when caring for the ostomate, whether the stoma is newly formed or after many years. Some people never seem to adjust to their stoma whilst others cope well. Some factors that can help the ostomate are the support of their family and the multidisciplinary team.

Ideally ostomates should be able to undertake a 'normal life' unless they have a poor prognosis. Many ostomates of both sexes have successfully parented after their stoma was formed. They are also able to continue their job, sports and holidays. This should be encouraged.

References

Baxter A & Lloyd PA (2004) Elimination: stoma care. In: Dougherty L & Lister S (eds) *The Royal Marsden Hospital Manual of Clinical Nursing Procedures*. 6th edn. London: The Royal Marsden.

Baxter NN, Novotny PJ, Jacobson T, Maidl LJ, Sloan J et al. (2006) A stoma quality of life scale. *Diseases of the Colon & Rectum*. **49(2)**: 205–12.

Bekkers MJ, Van Knippenberg FC, Van Den Borne HW & Van Berge-Henegouwen GP (1996) Prospective evaluation of psychosocial adaptation to stoma surgery: the role of self-efficacy. *Psychosomatic Medicine*. **58(2)**: 183–91.

Benjamin HC (2002) Teaching the stoma care routine to a patient with low vision. *British Journal of Nursing*. **11(19)**: 1270–7.

Black PK (2000a) *Holistic Stoma Care*. London Baillière Tindall.

Black PK (2000b) Practical stoma care. *Nursing Standard*. **14(41)**: 47–55.

Black PK (2004) Psychological, sexual and cultural issues for patients with a stoma. *British Journal of Nursing*. **13(12)**: 692–7.

Black P & Hyde C (2004) Caring for people with a learning disability, colorectal cancer and stoma. *British Journal of Nursing*. **13(16)**: 970–5.

Bond CF (1997) Men and sexuality in stoma care. *British Journal of Community Nursing*. **2(5)**: 260–3.

Borwell B (1997a) The psychosexual needs of stoma patients. *Professional Nurse*. **12(4)**: 250–5.

Borwell B (1997b) Psychological considerations of stoma care nursing. *Nursing Standard*. **11(48)**: 49–53.

Brown H & Randle J (2005) Living with a stoma: a review of the literature. *Gastroenterology*. **14**: 74–81.

Comb J (2003) Role of the stoma care nurse: patients with cancer and colostomy. *British Journal of Nursing*. **12(14)**: 852–6.

Davis K (1990) Impotence after surgery. *Nursing.* **4(18)**: 23–5.

Dorey G (2000) Conservative treatment of erectile dysfunction 2: clinical trials. *British Journal of Nursing.* **9(12)**: 755–62.

Dorey G (2002a) Outcome measures for erectile dysfunction 1: literature review. *British Journal of Nursing.* **11(1)**: 54–64.

Dorey G (2002b) Outcome measures for erectile dysfunction 2: evaluation. *British Journal of Nursing.* **11(2)**: 120–5.

Fitzpatrick G, Stammers C & Taylor P (2003) The influence of age on patients' problems. In: Elcoat C (ed) *Stoma Care Nursing.* London: Hollister.

Giaquinto S, Cacciato A, Minasi S, Sostero E & Amanda S (2006) Effects of music-based therapy on distress following knee arthroplasty. *British Journal of Nursing.* **15(10)**: 576–9.

Hunter M (2004) A sense of self. *Gastrointestinal Nursing.* **2(8)**: 12–15.

Junkin J & Beitz JM (2005) Sexuality and the person with a stoma. *Journal of Wound Ostomy and Continence.* **32(2)**: 121–8.

Kane FMA, Brodie EE, Coull A, Coyne L, Howd A *et al.* (2004) The analgesic effect of odour and music upon dressing change. *British Journal of Nursing.* **13(19)**: S4–12.

Kirkwood L (2006) An introduction to stomas. *Journal of Community Nursing.* **19(7)**: 12–19.

McClees N, Mikolaj EL, Carlson SL & Pryor-McCann J (2004) A pilot study assessing the effectiveness of a glycerine suppository in controlling colostomy emptying. *Journal of Wound Ostomy and Continence Nursing.* **31(3)**: 123–9.

Meadows C (1997) Stoma and fistula care. In Bruce L & Finlay TMD (eds) *Nursing in Gastroenterology.* London: Churchill Livingstone.

Notter J, Bailey B, Stammers C, Jones D, Lightfoot T *et al.* (2003) *The Quality of Life of Older Ostomates.* Birmingham: The University of Central England and Birmingham.

Nour S, Stringer MD & Beck J (1996) Colostomy complications in infants and children. *Annals of the Royal College of Surgeons of England.* **78(6)**: 526–30.

Peate I (2003) Nursing role in the management of constipation: use of laxatives. *British Journal of Nursing.* **12(19)**: 1130–6.

Pinches F (1999) Cultural issues. In: Taylor P (ed) *Stoma Care in the Community: A Clinical Resource for Practitioner.* London: Nursing Times Books.

Price B (1990) A model for body-image care. (Nurse's role in assisting the patient with an altered body image.) *Journal of Advanced Nursing.* **15(5)**: 585–93.

Readding LA (2003) Stoma siting: what the community nurse needs to know. *British Journal of Community Nursing.* **8(11)**: 502–11.

Rogers J (2003) Successful inclusion of a child with a stoma in mainstream schooling. *British Journal of Nursing.* **12(10)**: 590–9.

Rutherford D & Duffy FJR (1999) Current treatment of impotence: Viagra and other options. *British Journal of Nursing.* **8(4)**: 235–41.

Salter M (1997) *Altered Body Image: The Nurse's Role.* 2nd edn. London: Baillière Tindall.

Santos VLCG, Chaves EC & Kimura M (2006) Quality of life and coping of persons with temporary and permanent stomas. *Journal of Wound, Ostomy and Continence Nursing.* **33(5)**: 503–9.

Sirota T (2006a) Meeting the psychological needs of ostomy patients through therapeutic interaction, part I: the psychosocial needs of ostomy patients and the personal attributes of the nurse who cares for them. *World Council of Enterostomal Therapists Journal.* **26(2)**: 26–32.

Sirota T (2006b) Meeting the psychological needs of ostomy patients through therapeutic interaction, part II: effective use of nurses' professional competencies. *World Council of Enterostomal Therapists Journal.* **26(2)**: 5–15.

Stevens P & James P (2003) Anatomy and physiology associated with stoma care. In: Elcoat C (ed) *Stoma Care Nursing*. London: Hollister.

Thompson M, Boyd-Carson W, Trainor B & Boyd K (2003) Management of constipation. *Nursing Standard*. **18**: 41–2.

Virgin-Elliston T & Williams L (2003) Psychological considerations in stoma care. In: Elcoat C (ed) *Stoma Care Nursing*. London: Hollister.

Webster P (1985) Special babies. *Community Outlook*. July. 19–22.

Wells M (1990) Stress incontinence and pelvic floor exercises. *Professional Nurse*. **6(3)**: 151–6.

White C (1998) Psychological management of stoma-related concerns. *Nursing Standard*. **12(36)**: 35–8.

Williams J (2005) Psychological considerations in gastrointestinal nursing. *British Journal of Nursing*. **14(17)**: 931–5.

Williams J (2006) Sexual health: case study of a patient who has undergone stoma formation. *British Journal of Nursing*. **15(14)**: 760–3.

Williams J & Da Costa M (2006) Cultural aspects of stoma care nursing. *Gastrointestinal Nursing*. **4(1)**: 12–16.

Index